O'Connor Davies's **Ophtha** ~~...~~ **.ugs.**
Diagnostic and Therapeutic Uses

O'Connor Davies's
Ophthalmic Drugs:
Diagnostic and Therapeutic Uses

Fourth Edition

Revised by
Graham Hopkins
BPharm, PhD, MRPharmS
Pharmacist, Cheltenham, Gloucestershire

Optometric Advisor
Richard Pearson
MPhil, FBOA HD, FCOptom, DCLP, DOrth, FAAO
Department of Optometry and Visual Science, The City University, London

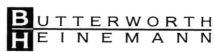

OXFORD   BOSTON   JOHANNESBURG   MELBOURNE   NEW DELHI   SINGAPORE

Butterworth-Heinemann
Linacre House, Jordan Hill, Oxford OX2 8DP
225 Wildwood Avenue, Woburn, MA 01801-2041
A division of Reed Educational and Professional Publishing Ltd

 A member of the Reed Elsevier plc group

First published 1972
Second edition 1981
Third edition 1989
Fourth edition 1998

British Library Cataloguing in Publication Data
A catalogue record for this book is available from the British Library

Library of Congress Cataloguing in Publication Data
A catalogue record for this book is available from the Library of Congress

ISBN 0 7506 2966 5

Typeset by BC Typesetting, Bristol BS31 1NZ
Printed and bound in Great Britain by The Bath Press

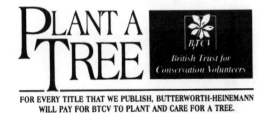

FOR EVERY TITLE THAT WE PUBLISH, BUTTERWORTH-HEINEMANN
WILL PAY FOR BTCV TO PLANT AND CARE FOR A TREE.

Contents

Preface

In carrying out the revision of this text, it was evident that two tasks should be addressed. First, the modern scientific knowledge on the subject of ophthalmic drugs should be reflected, and the more extensive list of references is a measure of the increasing source of information on pharmaceutical products used in the eye. Secondly it was necessary for the revised text to be more relevant to modern ophthalmic practice. Many of the older diagnostic agents have fallen out of use and are no longer commercially available. Their coverage in the text has been drastically reduced, as has reference to obsolete diagnostic techniques. The section on therapeutics has been expanded to give the book a wider appeal. Patients are far more aware of the drugs they receive on prescription and rely on a variety of health professionals for information concerning adverse effects and interactions. In addition, the change in legal status of drugs from POM to P has led to a greater level of self medication, for information and advice on which the optometrist and pharmacist may be the only health professionals they consult.

1 General pharmacological principles

Introduction

In order to use drugs effectively and safely it is necessary, as far as possible, to be able to predict not only a particular agent's clinical effect but also the magnitude and duration of the effect. This is not always straightforward because of a range of variables that can influence the amount of drug that is finally delivered to the site of action and the variation in the sensitivity of the target tissue. Drugs administered in the form of eyedrops have to run a gauntlet of events which will, in the main, reduce the resultant concentration at the effector site.

Like all subjects, the study of drugs is divided into several disciplines which are themselves further subdivided in order to cope with the volume of information that is generated by their study. Below is a list (by no means exhaustive) of the areas that have required study in the use of medicinal agents.

Pharmacognosy – deals with the natural sources of drugs, i.e. from plants and animals.

Pharmaceutics – the science of compounding and formulating drugs into suitable dosage forms for human and veterinary administration.

Pharmacodynamics – the study of the action of drugs on the effector tissues; in brief what the drug does to the body.

Pharmacokinetics – concerned with absorption, modification, detoxification and excretion; what the body does to the drug.

Therapeutics – the application of drugs to produce the desired effect, whether this is therapeutic or prophylactic.

Sources of drugs

Although there are a few inorganic drugs, for example lithium salts, the majority of drugs are organic compounds and can be derived from several sources.

Naturally occurring drugs

These are the oldest type of drugs and are extracted from plants and animals. Depending on the availability of the biological source, they can be expensive and the supply erratic. Utilizing natural drugs first involves making an extract of the crude drug in the form of a tincture or decoction and then formulating the extract into a suitable form for administration to the patient. Because of normal biological variability, such preparations contain varying amounts of the active, beneficial ingredient (if there is one!) and varying amounts of co-extracted harmful agents which just happen to coexist in the same species.

Synthetic drugs

The chemical laboratory has replaced the herbalist's garden and the rainforest as the principal source of pharmacological agents. Not only can such drugs be produced more cheaply and in a purer form than can be extracted from natural sources, but from a knowledge of the chemical structure of the compound and the effect that it produces, a structure–activity relationship can be elucidated, allowing the tailoring of drugs for more specific purposes. This often leads to an increased beneficial effect and a reduced toxic effect as well as an optimization of the time course of the effects.

Semisynthetic drugs

Some natural drugs can be modified in order to enhance their effects. Nature carries out all the hard work in producing the basic compound which, again making use of structure-activity relationships, is tailored to the required use.

Genetic engineering

One of the best examples of an agent produced by this method is human insulin. The genetic makeup of certain bacteria is modified by inserting relevant genes into the chromosome and as a result the required molecules are produced.

Development of new drugs and pharmaceutical compounds

The kind of fortuitous accident that led to the discovery and subsequent development of penicillin is relatively rare, and although the pharmacologist has yet to exhaust nature's storecupboard of physiologically active substances, new drugs and products are most often the result of the screening of a large number of chemical substances through a suitable biological model. The new compounds are sometimes variations on an existing drug, developed either to enhance activity, reduce harmful side effects or to modify the drug's action in a way to make it more suitable for a particular indication. When a substance is found that appears to be active it is subjected to a battery of pharmacological and toxicological tests before humans are exposed, initially as healthy human volunteers. Once these tests have been carried out a Clinical Trials certificate is applied for, which allows for studies of the effectiveness and safety of the drug on patients. After these have been carried out, full product licence may be issued for the production and sale of the product.

Not all new products result from novel chemical entities, especially in the field of ophthalmics where the sales of a product would not justify the large financial investment needed to develop a drug from a novel, untried compound. Many eye preparations are byproducts of developments in other fields, e.g. beta blockers, which were first developed for use in the treatment of cardiovascular conditions and then later found to be of benefit in the treatment of glaucoma. Sometimes substances which are thought to be just of scientific interest find a use in treatment. Botulinum toxin, well known for its potent toxicity, is now used in the treatment of some cases of squint.

Drug nomenclature

A drug can be described by a variety of names:

1. *Its chemical name.* This is a description of the chemical structure of the compound and is usually long and difficult to remember. There would certainly be a lot of problems if prescriptions had to be written by chemical names!
2. *The approved or official name(s).* These are also known as the generic names but unfortunately are sometimes not universal, e.g. adrenaline and epinephrine are used to describe the same catecholamine extracted from the adrenal medulla. Within a country, however, they do allow for one pharmaceutical product to be compared with another.
3. *Proprietary names.* These are almost always trade marks and are given to products to distinguish them from their competitors.

Administration

There are several ports of entry to the body for drugs, and they can be utilized in a variety of ways.

Alimentary tract
The oral cavity

The mouth has a large area of mucous membrane which can be used for direct absorption of drugs. It has the advantage that drugs go straight into the venous system without passing through the liver, which is the fate of drugs absorbed from the lower alimentary tract. This route has several routine applications. Glyceryl trinitrate for the acute relief of angina pectoris is administered under the tongue, as are certain analgesics. Nicotine replacement for people wishing to abstain from smoking is sometimes administered as chewing gum, which is masticated for a while and then left for the nicotine to leach out. Sometimes the oral cavity requires treatment in its own right, e.g. for aphthous ulcers, for which locally acting agents are used.

The oropharynx

Upper respiratory tract infections often cause discomfort in this area, and the pharmacists' shelves are full of remedies such as pastilles, linctuses and sprays for relief in this region.

The stomach and small intestine

This is the most widely used application site for drugs and pharmaceutical products. Sometimes their effects are local, e.g. antacids and other alimentary remedies, but mainly products are swallowed in order that the active ingredient can be absorbed from the gut and gain access to the blood stream. Tablets, capsules, mixtures, draughts, powders, syrups and cachets are just some of the pharmaceutical forms that have been used in this way. This route has the great advantage of convenience and ease of administration, since little or no training is required for the patient to self-medicate. There is no requirement for stability and the dosage forms are relatively cheap to produce. However, the response can be variable as other gut contents can influence the absorption of alimentary-administered drugs. Milk and dairy products, for example, can interfere with the uptake of the tetracyclines. Food in general will reduce the uptake of penicillin which is thus best taken on an empty stomach. Additionally, after absorption from the alimentary tract, the drug must pass through the liver before gaining access to the general blood circulation.

The large intestine

Suppositories and enemas are principally used for local administration of drugs, but sometimes substances for systemic effects are administered by this route. This apparently roundabout route is particularly useful for children and unconscious patients, and for drugs which can cause gastric irritation, e.g. nonsteroidal anti-inflammatory agents.

The respiratory system

The modern treatment of asthma and other respiratory problems relies greatly on the ability of the respiratory mucous membrane to act as an area through which drugs can be absorbed.

The skin

Products for administration to the skin were for a long time just used as a method of local application for either the treatment of skin disorders or as rubefacients (counterirritants which are applied to the skin to promote the blood flow through tissues and impart a feeling of warmth, beneficial in the treatment of soft tissue problems). However, the discovery that the skin is not a complete barrier and that it will absorb certain drugs has brought about the development of the transdermal patch, which is used to deliver hormones as replacement therapy in the relief of postmeno-pausal symptoms, nicotine in the treatment of addiction, hyoscine for travel sickness and drugs for the relief of angina (unlike the sublingual treatment, this route gives a depot effect and is for prevention of attack rather than acute treatment).

Injection

Depending on the site of the injection, a very fast effect (intravenous) or a depot effect (intramuscular) can result. Injections can also be used to circumvent certain absorption barriers that prevent drugs reaching the desired site of action. The terms 'blood/brain barrier' and 'blood/aqueous barrier' are really expressions of the relative impermeability of the blood capillaries in these organs.

Local administration

Many of the routes that are used for systemic administration are also used for local administration. As well as the skin, the gut sometimes requires local treatment with drugs which remain in the lumen of the gut and are not absorbed. Mucous membranes are sites of absorption and can be usefully employed for local actions. The nasal mucosa has long been a target for medicaments for the treatment of the common cold and the relief of hay fever and other allergic problems. The external ear and to a lesser extent the middle ear can be treated with local administration of drops. However, one mucous membrane greatly utilized in the administration of drugs is the conjunctiva.

Drug modifications (pharmacokinetics)

The response of the patient to the drug will to a great extent depend on the concentration of the drug that is available at the site of action. The relationship between the dose or concentration administered and the final concentration at the locus of action is the resultant of normal pharmacokinetic processes which are themselves subject to the effect of other agents.

Absorption

Even if a drug is not going to be absorbed into the systemic blood circulation, it will almost certainly be required to pass across a membrane which has a high lipid content. Thus there is a dual solubility requirement for drugs in that they must be water soluble to dissolve in body fluids such as blood plasma or aqueous humour, and lipid soluble to pass across lipid membranes. There are pores in the membranes which allow small polar water soluble molecules to pass across, but lipid solubility does confer a better ability for absorption.

Many drugs are chemically salts of weak bases and strong acids e.g. cyclopentolate hydrochloride, atropine sulphate, which are highly ionized and water soluble having little lipid solubility. However, the free bases have the opposite properties and are highly lipophilic. In any solution of a drug there will be a mixture of the free base and ionized salts, their relative concentrations being dependent on the concentration of hydrogen ions present, i.e. the pH. Every compound has its own pKa value, which is the pH at which equal concentrations of free base and ionized salt exist. From the pKa, the effect of pH on the concentration of free base and thus the lipid solubility can be determined using this simple equation:

$$pH = pKa + \log_{10} \frac{[base]}{[salt]}.$$

Thus the lower the pKa, the higher will be the proportion of base at a given pH and the greater will be the passage across lipid membranes such as the corneal epithelium. It is not always possible or desirable to change the pH of the medium in which the drug works, e.g. tears, in order to influence the rate of absorption of a drug (Fig. 1.1). However, extremes of pH can be usefully avoided.

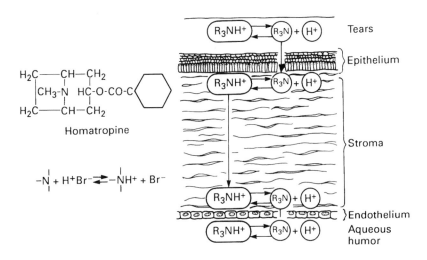

Figure 1.1 Penetration of an alkaloid through the cornea illustrating differential solubility characteristics (reproduced from *Adler's Physiology of the Eye*, 1975, by courtesy of Mosby, St Louis).

Absorption of drugs can be passive or active. Passive transport mechanisms will be enhanced by a greater area for absorption, a high concentration gradient across the membrane and sometimes by hydrostatic and osmotic differences when the absorption process depends on filtration. Additionally, absorption will be enhanced by increased contact time of the drug solution with the absorbing membrane, e.g. drugs will be taken up in greater amounts by the conjunctiva if the solution remains in the conjunctival sac for a longer time.

Specialized active transport processes appear to be responsible for the transfer of certain water-soluble drugs, as well as naturally occurring sugars and amino acids. Carriers (membrane components) form complexes with the selected substance and (with the aid of energy) transport it through the membrane by a diffusion process, releasing it from the complex on the other side, against an electrochemical gradient. These processes rely in part on the Na^+ gradient across the membrane and are affected by drugs that modify Na–K transport. Active transport requires metabolic energy, and exhibits selectivity and saturability.

Distribution

After absorption, the drug will enter or pass through various body fluid compartments depending on the route of absorption. If the drug is absorbed into the blood stream then it passes through the plasma, interstitial fluid and cellular fluids. In the eye it will pass through the intracellular fluid of the corneal epithelium, the matrix of the stroma and then the aqueous humour before being taken up by various ocular tissues. Those drugs that pass through all cell membranes redistribute throughout all fluid compartments, whereas drugs to which these membranes are impermeable will be restricted in their distribution and potential effects.

Many drugs are bound, to varying degrees, to plasma proteins (especially the albumin fraction). Although this binding is reversible, it limits the drug's distribution and therapeutically effective blood concentration, as only the unbound proportion is pharmacologically active. It can also lead to a cumulative effect with successive dosing as the plasma bound proportion acts as a depot. Tissue concentrations of drugs higher than those in plasma result from pH gradients, binding to certain tissues such as fat or pigment, or active transport.

Biotransformation

In order to produce their effects, drugs will have some resemblance to chemicals normally found in the body and thus will be able to act as substrates for a range of enzymes. In fact it is by mimicking the natural substrate that many drugs produce their effects. Other enzymes will have a modifying effect on the drug's activity, either enhancing or, more commonly, reducing its effect. The use of prodrugs takes advantage of the activating mechanisms that exist by administering a substance that is inactive *in vitro* but becomes active *in vivo* due the effect of enzymes (Fig. 1.2). Such enzymatic processes involve oxidation, reduction or hydrolysis. Conjugate reactions can also occur in which the drug is coupled (conjugated) enzymatically with an endogenous chemical entity, e.g. a carbohydrate or amino acid, to render the drug inactive. This is

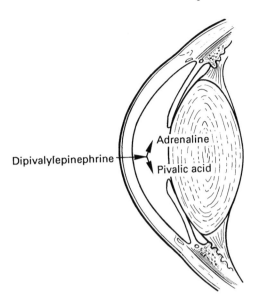

Figure 1.2 Mode of action of a prodrug.

principally a detoxification process and many of these reactions are carried out by the hepatic endoplasmic reticulum.

These enzymic reactions are themselves subject to modification, which accounts partly for the variability of response of the patient not only to the drug's therapeutic effect but also to its unwanted toxic and side effects. Enzymic activity is finite, and although at normal substrate levels increasing substrate levels will increase activity, a saturation level can be reached. In addition, many drug interactions result from the effect of one drug on the deactivating enzyme of another. If the interacting drug enhances the effect of the enzyme, then the drug substrate will be broken down more quickly and will have less effect, and increased doses may be required. However, sometimes deactivation is inhibited and toxic levels can be achieved from doses that would be tolerated in the absence of the interacting drug.

Excretion

The principal route for excretion of both unchanged drugs and metabolites is via the kidneys. The processes by which foreign substances are removed (cleared) from the plasma are exactly the same as for naturally occurring endogenous substances, i.e. glomulerular filtration, active tubular transport and passive tubular reabsorption. Many factors affect the efficiency of this route of excretion. Reduced kidney function is present in neonates, geriatric patients and patients suffering from kidney disease, and for these patients assessment must be made of their normal renal clearance and the dose adjusted appropriately. Plasma proteins do not pass across the glomerular membrane and thus drugs bound to them will not be filtered. Tubular reabsorption will depend on the lipid solubility of the drug or metabolite, and by modifying the pH of urine by administering sodium bicarbonate to raise it or ammonium chloride to reduce it, the reabsorption can be reduced or enhanced depending on the substance's pKa.

Drug responses (pharmacodynamics)
Receptors—concept and variety

Fundamental to the concept of pharmacodynamics is the study of the interaction of the drug with biological tissues at a molecular level. In most cases (but by no means all) the site of action is a specific molecule referred to as a receptor. In the case of drugs acting on effector cells such as muscles and glands, the receptors are localized on the membrane and are either the same as or related to the receptors for endogenous substances. Other drugs produce their effects by reacting with sites on enzymes either in the cytoplasm or in the extracellular space.

The concept of receptors is not a modern one. In 1857 Claude Bernard, in his classical experiments, showed that skeletal muscle poisoned with curare from South American arrows no longer exhibited a contractual response to the electrical stimulation of its nerve, although the nerve still conducted the stimulation and the muscle still contracted to direct electrical stimulation.

Langley (1905) and a number of other scientists including Lewandowsky (1898), Elliot (1905) and Dixon (1907) developed the concept of drug–cell combinations, where the receptors were envisaged as chemically defined areas of large molecules with which foreign molecules such as drugs interacted. How this interaction elicits a biological response has been the subject of much investigation and theorizing. Clark (1933) proposed his occupation theory, in which the drug's action commenced with its occupation of the receptors and terminated when it dissociated, the maximal effect being achieved when 100% of the receptors were occupied. Paton's rate theory (1961), however, maintained that it was not necessary for all the receptors to be occupied to obtain a maximal response. Instead the response would be dependent on the rate of formation of drug–receptor complexes and the rapidity of dissociation, freeing the receptors for further combination with another drug molecule. There are many parallels between the action of drugs on receptors and that of a substrate with the active site of an enzyme and some of our knowledge of drug action is extrapolated from a study of enzyme action.

A further modification of the receptor theory is the concept of spare receptors, which again proposes that the maximum effect may be achieved without all the receptors being occupied.

Agonist/antagonist

The ability of drugs to produce apparently opposite effects by reacting with the same receptors has led to their separation into agonists and antagonists – a division which in itself is too simplistic and requires further subdivision. An agonist, according to the occupation theory, is a drug which combines with the receptor and elicits a physiological response similar to that produced by the natural local transmitter or hormone. It is said to have affinity (the ability to combine with the receptor) and efficacy (produces a response from the membrane). In the rate theory, an agonist is a drug which combines and dissociates rapidly with the receptor.

An antagonist on the other hand still has affinity (if it did not it would not react with the receptor) but has little or no efficacy. Such a drug has, according to the rate theory, an ability to combine with the receptor as rapidly as an agonist, but having formed a complex with the receptor it dissociates very slowly. Again there is a comparison with the inhibition of an enzyme by a false substrate. It would be a very unusual situation in which an antagonist was present at a receptor site in the complete absence of a corresponding agonist. The effectiveness of the antagonist will depend on the relative concentrations of the two agents; i.e. the antagonism is competitive, and the term competitive antagonist is used to describe such drugs. The type of chemical bond formed in the drug–receptor complex will vary from very weak tenuous bonds in the case of agonists, to stronger and, in some cases, permanent bonds. In the latter case the antagonism or blockade will be irreversible and new receptor molecules must be formed.

As our knowledge of pharmacology increases, so does the number of receptor types and subtypes. As well as the well-known receptors for acetylcholine, adrenaline, histamine and serotonin, we now have evidence for specific receptors for opiates, dopamine, adenosine, insulin and glucagon, to mention a few. Many of these receptors are further subdivided into subtypes.

Cholinergic and adrenergic receptors will be further discussed with the autonomic nervous system.

Concentration–response relationships

Many of the concentrations of drugs used in eyedrops have been arrived at empirically and tend to continue to be used, although in many situations a lower concentration would suffice and lead to less opportunity for adverse effects. However, it is important to be aware of the relationships that exist between drug doses and the responses produced. Of course biological variability has an effect and responses of subjects to the same dose will differ.

In this context, the term concentration refers to the amount of the drug which is present at the receptor site and is available to react with the receptor. Drugs do not act at a distance and chemical bonding of a tenuous nature must occur. This concentration will not be the same as the concentration of drug in an eye drop administered to the conjunctival sac, as many pharmacokinetic factors will affect the final concentration. However, the concentration at the receptor is not easy to measure and so the dose or concentration applied is used in calculations.

The term response is a little more difficult to define and will depend on the type of drug and the desired effect. One can choose a continuously measurable response from an individual animal or tissue, e.g. the size of the pupil. With some drugs, for example analgesics, such a convenient measure is not available and populations of subjects must be used choosing a convenient end point such as noticeable relief of pain. Because of biological variability, a proportion of subjects will achieve the end point at a relatively low dose and as the dose increases so will this proportion

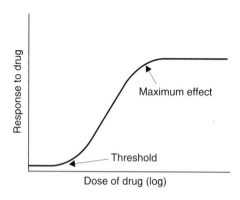

Figure 1.3 Dose–response curve.

until a maximum of 100% is achieved. If a plot were to be made of the proportion of subjects achieving the end point against dose, it would be seen that the relationship is not a linear one. To overcome this a value known as the ED50 is used, which is the dose (or concentration) at which 50% of the subjects achieve the end point. This can be compared with other drugs to gain some idea of relative potency and with the drugs own LD50 (lethal dose 50 – the dose at which 50% of the test animals die) to assess the drug's safety margin.

Returning to graded responses such as our example of the pupil diameter, as opposed to all-or-none responses, it is possible to plot a curve of response (in our example in mm) against the logarithm of the dose applied (see Fig. 1.3). Below a certain level (threshold) no effect will be seen. Between this level and the maximal effect the curve is sigmoid. After the maximum is reached there is no increase in effect with increased dose. The dose–response curve of one drug does not tell us a great deal, but when the curves of several drugs are plotted together, comparisons can be made between them. A drug with a steep slope will quickly pass from threshold level to maximum and will be difficult to use because of the danger of passing quickly to an overdose situation. Different drugs can be compared for their efficacy and potency. These terms are sometimes used interchangeably but mean different things. Efficacy refers to the maximum response that can be achieved, a more efficacious drug producing a greater maximal effect. Potency refers to the dose of a drug required to produce a given effect. Some drugs are more potent than others, i.e. require smaller doses, but have the same efficacy, probably due to better absorption. This may not confer an advantage because the drug with a greater therapeutic potency may also have a greater potency for side effects (Fig. 1.4).

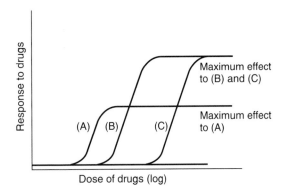

Figure 1.4 Potency and efficacy. (B) is more potent than (C) but both have the same efficacy. (B) and (C) have a greater efficacy than (A).

The peripheral autonomic nervous system (ANS)

Many ophthalmic drugs produce their effect by modifying the actions of the peripheral autonomic nervous system in some way. The study of their mode of action requires a basic knowledge of the anatomy and physiology of ANS.

Divisions and distribution

The autonomic nervous system is responsible for the control of smooth muscle, cardiac muscle and exocrine gland cells which are not normally under voluntary control and is thus sometimes referred to as the involuntary nervous system. The major divisions of the autonomic nervous system are the parasympathetic and sympathetic, and they have many anatomical and functional differences. However, they share one important difference from the somatic nerve fibres that supply skeletal muscle in that they possess a synapse outside the central nervous system. The synapse is a break in the continuity of the nerve pathway and across this gap normal axonal transmission is impossible. Instead, transmission takes place by chemical (humoral) means. These synapses occur in the swellings on nerves called ganglia. The nerve which leaves the central nervous system (CNS) and conducts impulses to the ganglion is referred to as the preganglionic nerve and the nerve which conducts impulses from the ganglion to the effector organ is called the postganglionic nerve.

Parasympathetic preganglionic nerves leave the CNS by two outflows – cranial nerves and sacral nerves (see Plate I). Parasympathetic fibres are found in the IIIrd (oculomotor), VIIth (facial), IXth (glossopharyngeal) and Xth (vagus) cranial nerves and in the pelvic nerves. The parasympathetic nervous system supplies the viscera in the thoracic and abdominal cavities and the autonomic structures in the head (e.g. salivary glands, intraocular muscles and lacrimal glands). The preganglionic nerve fibres are very long, as the ganglia in which they synapse are very close to the organs which the postganglionic fibres innervate (effector organs).

The outflow for the sympathetic nervous system is from the thoracic and lumbar regions of the spinal cord. Most synapses occur in the paravertebral ganglion chain and hence the preganglionic nerve is very short in comparison to that of the parasympathetic system. Some fibres however pass through these ganglia to synapse in the prevertebral ganglia, the coeliac and superior and inferior mesenteric ganglia. One sympathetic nerve does not synapse on its way to its effector organ; this is the supply to the adrenal medulla.

Most involuntary structures (but not all) are innervated by both divisions which normally have antagonistic effects, i.e. if one division stimulates a particular effector organ then the other will inhibit it. The sympathetic prepares the body for situations of stress – the so-called fright, fight and flight response – whereas the parasympathetic dominates during normal sedentary life. However there is normally a balance between the two (see Table 1.1).

Neurohumoral transmission in the autonomic nervous system (Fig. 1.5)

The theory of neurohumoral transmission, which is now generally accepted, proposes that nerve fibres (including those of the ANS) do not act by direct electrical stimulation of a muscle or organ or second (postganglionic) nerve fibre. Instead the impulse is transmitted across most synapses and neuroeffector junctions by means of specific chemical agents known as neurohumoral transmitters, acetylcholine and noradrenaline (usually known as norepinephrine in the USA) in the case of cholinergic and adrenergic nerve fibres respectively.

Most of the so-called 'autonomic' drugs, affecting smooth muscle and gland cells, act in a manner that mimics or modifies the actions of the 'natural' transmitters, released on stimulation of the autonomic nerves at either ganglia or effector cells.

Axonal conduction

Axonal conduction is the passage of an impulse along an axon. The currently most acceptable hypothesis on axonal conduction (Hodgkin and Huxley, 1952) is, briefly, as follows. A stimulus above the threshold level initiates a nerve impulse or nerve action potential (AP) at a local region of the axonal membrane. The internal resting potential of the latter has a negative value and this is reversed through zero, continuing uninterrupted to a positive value. This local reversal is due to a sudden selective increase in the permeability of the membrane to sodium ions, which flow inwards in the direction of their concentration gradient. This occurs because at rest sodium and chloride ions are in much higher concentration in the extracellular fluid than in the axoplasm, the axonal membrane then being relatively impermeable to sodium while allowing comparatively easy traverse for other ions. The reverse operates for potassium ions in the resting potential state, when they are approximately 30–50 times more concentrated in the axoplasm than the extracellular fluid, these concentration gradients being maintained by pump and active transport mechanisms, involving an adenosine triphosphatase (ATPase) at the inner surface of the membrane activated by sodium and at its outer surface by potassium (Thomas, 1972). The rapid inflow of sodium ions is immediately followed by increased membrane permeability for potassium ions which flow in the opposite direction. The local circuit currents produced by these transmembrane ionic currents around the axon activate adjacent regions of the axon, propagating the nerve

Table 1.1 Effector organ responses to autonomic impulses*

Effector organs	Adrenergic impulses		Cholinergic impulses
	Receptor type	Response	Response
Eye**			
Dilator pupillae	mainly α (very few β)	Contraction (mydriasis)	—
Sphincter pupillae	α and β in equal amounts	—	Contraction (miosis)
Ciliary muscle	mainly β (very few α)	Relaxation for far vision (slight effect)	Contraction for near vision (accommodation)
Heart			
S-A node	β†	Increase in heart rate	Decrease in heart rate; vagal arrest
Atria	β†	Increase in contractility and conduction velocity	Decrease in contractility and (usually) increase in conduction velocity
A-V node and conduction system	β†	Increase in conduction velocity	Decrease in conduction velocity; A-V block
Ventricles	β†	Increase in contractility, conduction velocity, automaticity and rate of idiopathic pacemakers	—
Blood vessels			
Coronary	α	Constriction	Dilatation
	β	Dilatation	
Skin and mucosa	α	Constriction	—
Skeletal	α	Constriction	Dilatation
	β	Dilatation	
Cerebral	α	Constriction (slight)	—
Pulmonary	α	Constriction	—
Abdominal viscera	α	Constriction	—
	β	Dilatation	
Renal	α	Constriction	—
Salivary glands	α	Constriction	Dilatation
Lung			
Bronchial muscle	β	Relaxation	Contraction
Bronchial glands		Inhibition (?)	Stimulation
Stomach			
Motility and tone	β	Decrease (usually)	Increase
Sphincters	α	Contraction (usually)	Relaxation (usually)
Secretion		Inhibition (?)	Stimulation
Intestine			
Motility and tone	α, β	Decrease	Increase
Sphincters	α	Contraction (usually)	Relaxation (usually)
Secretion		Inhibition (?)	Stimulation
Gall bladder and ducts		Relaxation	Contraction
Urinary bladder			
Detrusor	β	Relaxation (usually)	Contraction
Trigone and sphincter	α	Contraction	Relaxation

Table 1.1 (*cont.*)

Effector organs	Receptor type	Adrenergic impulses Response	Cholinergic impulses Response
Ureter			
Motility and tone		Increase (usually)	Increase (?)
Uterus	α, β	Variable‡	Variable‡
Male sex organs		Ejaculation	Erection
Skin	α	Contraction	—
Pilomotor muscles			
Sweat glands	α	Slight, localized secretion	Generalized secretion
Spleen capsule	α, β	Contraction Relaxation	—
Adrenal medulla		—	Secretion of adrenaline and noradrenaline
Liver	β	Glycogenolysis	—
Pancreas			
Acini		Decreased secretion	Secretion
Islets	α	Inhibition of insulin and glucagon secretion	Insulin and glucagon secretion
	β	Insulin and glucagon secretion	
Salivary glands	α	Thick, viscous secretion	Profuse, watery secretion
Lacrimal glands	—	Secretion	
Nasopharyngeal glands	—	Secretion	

*Modified from Goodman and Gilman: *The Pharmacological Basis of Therapeutics*, 5th ed., 1975. New York; Macmillan: and Ganong, W. F.: *Review of Medical Physiology*, 9th ed., Lange Medical Publications.
**According to Van Alpen (1976).
β† The receptors of the heart producing excitatory responses have been classified as β_1-receptors, and most of the other β-receptors producing inhibitory responses as β_2-receptors.
‡ Depends on presence or absence of pregnancy, stage of menstrual cycle, amount of circulating oestrogen and progesterone and other factors.

AP along it, the recently activated region remaining momentarily in a refractory state.

Very few drugs in normal therapeutic doses, with the exception of high concentrations of local anaesthetics infiltrated in the immediate vicinity of nerve trunks, modify axonal conduction.

Junctional transmission

Junctional transmission is the passage of an impulse across a synaptic or neuroeffector junction.

The arrival at the axonal terminals of the AP initiates the neurohumoral transmission of an excitatory or inhibitory impulse. The following events occur.

1. *Release of transmitters*. These are largely synthesized in the region of the axonal terminals (some in the cell body) and stored there in synaptic vesicles, either in highly concentrated ionic form, as with acetylcholine (ACh), or as a readily dissociable complex or salt, as with that of nor-adrenaline with adenosine triphosphate (ATP) and a specific protein.

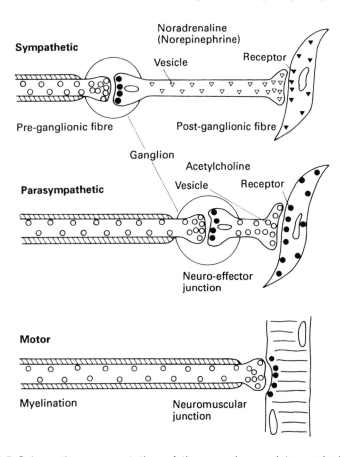

Figure 1.5 Schematic representation of the neurohumoral transmission of autonomic and motor nerves. *Open circles* = acetylcholine storage vesicles; *solid circles* = acetylcholine receptor sites; *open triangles* = noradrenaline (norepinephrine) storage vesicles; *solid triangles* = noradrenaline receptor sites. Only the postganglionic sympathetic fibre has noradrenaline vesicles. Transmission at sympathetic neuroeffector junctions is by noradrenaline in contrast to acetylcholine transmission at all ganglia, at the parasympathetic neuroeffectors, and at neuromuscular junctions. It should be noted that this greatly simplified representation of ganglionic transmission has now been superseded by the concept that such transmission is a far more complex process, involving cholinoceptive and adrenoceptive sites (after Drill: *Pharmacology in Medicine*, 3rd edn, 1965. New York McGraw-Hill).

Slow release of small amounts of these transmitters does take place in the resting state, but these are insufficient to initiate a propagated impulse at the postjunctional site. The AP precipitates simultaneous release of larger amounts of transmitter (several hundred quanta). This process is triggered by the depolarization of the axonal terminal. Although the other intermediate steps are uncertain, one step is the mobilization of the calcium ion, which enters the intra-axonal medium and is thought to promote fusion of the vesicular and axoplasmic membranes. The process by which the vesicles' contents are then discharged to the exterior is termed exocytosis.

2. *Combination of the transmitter with postjunctional receptors and production of postjunctional potential.* Diffusing across synaptic or junctional clefts (a distance of 10–50 nm), the transmitter combines with the specialized macromolecular receptors on the postjunctional membrane (second neurone, muscle fibre or gland cell), generally resulting in a localized non-propagated increase in the permeability of this membrane that can be of two types.

(a) A general increase for all ions (chiefly Na^+ and K^+) in which case a localized depolarization follows, the excitatory postsynaptic potential (EPSP).

(b) A selective permeability increase for smaller ions only (chiefly K^+ or Cl^-) followed by stabilization or actual hyperpolarization of the membrane, the inhibitory postsynaptic potential (IPSP).

3. *Initiation of postjunction activity.* A propagated AP in a neurone, or muscle action potential (AP) in most types of skeletal muscle, or secretion in gland cells, is initiated if an EPSP exceeds a certain threshold value. In smooth muscle and certain types of tonic skeletal muscle, propagated impulses do not occur; instead an EPSP activates a localized contractile response. EPSPs initiated by other neuronal sources at the same time and site as an IPSP will be opposed by the latter, the algebraic sum of these effects deciding whether or not a propagated impulse or other response ensues.

The extraocular muscles are stimulated in the manner described above for most types of skeletal muscle (Koelle, 1975), but some differences in the structure and reaction of these particular muscles should be noted. It is usual in most skeletal muscle for one motor neurone to innervate between 100 and 200 muscle fibres, whereas in the extraocular muscles one neurone may supply one between 5 and 20 fibres. Such small motor units permit a precision of control over extraocular muscles not to be found in other skeletal musculature. This smoothness of ocular movement is further assisted by the exceptionally large amount of elastic connective tissue around the loosely arranged fine extrinsic ocular fibres, not found to the same extent in the dense connective tissue surrounding the bundles of other skeletal muscles.

Vesicles believed to contain acetylcholine are concentrated together with a large number of mitochondria within the axonal terminals of motor nerves. Similar vesicles also occur in the various presynaptic terminals or boutons, but unlike the small discrete motor endplates in skeletal muscle fibres, the presynaptic and postsynaptic neurone processes form complicated patterns of intertwining ramifications amidst the tightly packed cells of the ganglion (for example, approximately 100 000 ganglion cells occur in a cubic millimetre of the superior cervical ganglion). As with the skeletal muscle the transmitter in the autonomic ganglia has proved to be acetylcholine, which has been obtained from the perfusate of isolated ganglia after stimulation of the preganglionic fibres. The superior cervical ganglion of the cat is often used in such experiments.

Eccles (1964, 1973), Katz (1966), McLennan (1970) and Krnjevic (1974) are only a few of the many research scientists who have contributed much to our understanding of synaptic transmission. Koelle (1975), referring to the work of Katz and Miledi (1972), stated that this demonstrated that immediate postjunctional response (of skeletal muscle) to acetylcholine liberated by stimulation of the motor nerve is the development of a localized depolarization at the motor endplate, the EPP (endplate potential), equivalent to EPSP at postsynaptic sites, which on reaching a critical level generates propagated muscle AP leading to a contraction.

Smooth and cardiac muscle, in contrast to cholinergically innervated skeletal muscle exhibits an inherent activity that is independent of a nerve supply, although this property probably does not apply to all smooth muscles equally.

This activity may be modified but is not initiated by nerve impulses, and though it is less sensitive to electrical stimuli than striped, smooth muscle is more sensitive to chemical stimulation. It has been suggested that the inherent activity of smooth muscle may be regulated by acetylcholine synthesized and released by the muscle fibres. Spikes or waves of reversed membrane polarization travel from cell to cell at rates considerably slower than the action potentials of axons or of skeletal muscle. Rhythmic fluctuations in the membrane resting potential in smooth muscle seem to initiate spikes which, as in skeletal muscle, in turn initiate contractions, which in some tissues pass as a wave along the muscle sheet: for example, peristalsis in the small intestine.

Experiments have demonstrated that depolarization of the smooth muscle fibres of the rabbit's colon, occurring after a delay of 400 ms after stimulation of the cholinergic postganglionic fibres to this tissue, produces a spike which persists for approximately 600 ms. As the response occurred simultaneously in all the muscle fibres and the rate of depolarization is proportional to the stimulus, Gillespie (1962) concluded that each muscle fibre is probably innervated by more than one nerve fibre.

Membrane potential changes of single smooth muscle cells of the guinea pig vas deferens, where the excitatory fibres from the hypogastric nerve are adrenergic, show a somewhat similar state of affairs, although on stimulation of the nerve the delay in depolarization is much briefer. The actions of acetylcholine and adrenaline at membrane level have been described by Bulbring (1958). Burnstock and Holman (1961) also found in the vas deferens of the guinea pig miniature potentials similar to those at motor endplates of skeletal muscles in the absence of nerve stimulation, probably due to spontaneous release of small amounts of noradrenaline. Burnstock and Holman (1961) include among their conclusions the remark:

> Our results have shown that the mechanism of transmission of excitation from sympathetic nerve to smooth muscle is essentially similar to that of transmission at other neuro-effector junctions,

stimulation of the effector nerve producing depolarization of the postjunctional membrane.

As in skeletal muscle, the spike initiates a contraction.

4. *Destruction or dissipation of the transmitter.* As Koelle (1975) remarks, when impulses can be transmitted across junctions at frequencies ranging from a few to several hundred a second an efficient means of disposing of the transmitter subsequent to each impulse is essential. Acetylcholinesterase (AChE) is the highly specialized enzyme available at most cholinergic junctions for disposing of ACh released there as the transmitter. It is abundantly present in skeletal muscle tissue and is concentrated in the region of the motor endplates. Diffusion may account for the termination of action of acetylcholine at some synapses. It seems likely that this contributes to the method, which is mainly uptake by the axon terminals themselves and by other cells, of ending the activity of the adrenergic transmitter noradrenaline. There are two enzymes capable of metabolizing noradrenaline and adrenaline, catechol-O-methyltransferase (COMT) found in practically all tissues, and monoamine oxidase (MAO), which is present in nervous tissue and the liver. These enzymes have not the importance or speed of action of acetylcholinesterase in cholinergic transmission.

Neuroeffector junctions are those junctions where two cells are in more or less close physical relationship, the term being confined to nerve and effector cells (which respond characteristically to a stimulus) of cardiac muscle, smooth muscle and gland. A synapse is the area of proximity between two neurones where impulses are transmitted from one nerve cell to another across an ultramicroscopic gap (20 nm) called the synaptic cleft. Ganglia contain many such synapses.

Ganglionic transmission is a highly complex process, incorporating many of the elements of transmission at the myoneural junctions of both skeletal and smooth muscles. It is now considered that interneurones and additional transmitters may also be involved. In addition to the primary pathway involving ACh depolarization of postsynaptic sites (described above), secondary pathways for the transmission of excitatory and inhibitory impulses have also been described. Specific nondepolarizing ganglion blocking drugs effect the primary pathway but the secondary pathways are insensitive to these agents (Volle and Koelle, 1975). There is some evidence indicating the participation of a catecholamine (dopamine or noradrenaline, from a catecholamine containing cell or interneurone within the ganglion) acting on the ganglion to cause hyperpolarization (IPSP) (Eccles and Libet, 1961). It has been suggested that multiple cholinoceptive and adrenoceptive sites exist in the mammalian superior cervical ganglion (Greengard and Kebabian, 1974).

Neuromuscular junctions are the spaces that occur between motor nerve fibre endings and skeletal muscle motor endplates, and are comparable to synaptic clefts at synapses.

Myoneural junction is a term that embraces neuroeffector junctions with smooth muscle and neuromuscular junctions, i.e. it includes all types of motor nerve endings.

Evidence for neurohumoral transmission

Evidence for neurohumoral transmission may be deduced from the following experimental data.

1. The demonstration at appropriate sites of the presence of a physiologically active compound and of the enzymes involved in its metabolism.
2. Recovery of the compound from the perfusate during stimulation of an innervated organ, the substance not being present (or only in vastly reduced amounts) in the absence of such stimulation.
3. Appropriate administration of the compound produces the same responses as nerve stimulation.
4. The demonstration that these responses to nerve stimulation and administration of the compound are modified in the same way by various drugs.

This evidence is further supported by that important feature of junctional transmission, the irreducible latent period, that is, the time lag between the arrival of an impulse at the axonal terminal and the manifestation of the postjunctional potential. The evidence for the existence of neurohumoral transmitters is well substantiated by Otto Loewi's classical experiment in 1921 to demonstrate the release of a vagus substance ('vagustoff') on stimulation of the parasympathetic fibres of the cardiac nerve to the frog's heart.

Further substantiation has been produced by identification by various pharmacological, chemical and physiological tests of the substance present in perfusate from an innervated structure during the period of nerve stimulation, that is not present in the absence of stimulation. In addition, it has been demonstrated that the substance so obtained is capable of producing responses identical to those of nerve stimulation and that both responses are modified in the same manner by various drugs.

Most of the general principles concerning the physiology and pharmacology of the autonomic nervous system and its effector organs are applicable, with some reservations, to the neuromuscular junctions (for example, those of extraocular voluntary muscles) and in some respects to the central nervous system, although here knowledge of the transmitters involved is far from complete.

The autonomic nervous system (involuntary, visceral or vegetative nervous system) consists of nerves, ganglia and plexuses that innervate the heart, blood vessels, glands, viscera and smooth muscles throughout the body. The motor nerves of this system supply all structures of the body except skeletal muscle. Somatic nerves with their synapses occurring entirely in the central nervous system supply the latter, whereas the most distal synaptic junctions in the autonomic system are in ganglia occurring outside the spinal cord, for example, the superior cervical ganglion (SCG) and ciliary ganglion (CG) (see Fig.1.4) which are the final relay stations for the sympathetic and parasympathetic autonomic innervation respectively of the eye. The motor nerves to skeletal muscle, including the extraocular muscles, are medullated (myelinated), where the postganglionic autonomic nerves are nonmyelinated, with the exception of the short ciliary nerves.

Acetylcholine

Acetylcholine is the neurohumoral transmitter of all preganglionic autonomic nerve fibres, all parasympathetic postganglionic fibres, and a few postganglionic sympathetic fibres (as previously mentioned, those which innervate the sweat glands, vasodilator fibres to skeletal muscle arteries, and postganglionic fibres to the adrenal medulla) (Fig. 1.6).

The complex sequence of enzymatic reactions in the formation of acetylcholine (ACh) may be outlined as follows (Moses, 1975).

Choline present in the extracellular fluid is taken up by active transport into the axoplasm. Choline acetylase (choline-acetyltransferase) which occurs in all cholinergic nerves, is synthesized within the perikaryon and then transported, by unknown means, along the axon to its terminal. The axonal terminals, in addition to their vesicles, contain the large number of mitochondria in which the acetyl coenzyme A is synthesized. The final step in the synthesis of ACh probably takes place within the cytoplasm, and subsequently most of this transmitter is stored within synaptic vesicles. These are mostly concentrated at the synaptic and neuroeffector junctions and are spherical structures approximately 40–50 nm in diameter.

It has been estimated that each synaptic vesicle contains from 1000 to over 50 000 molecules of ACh, and a single motor nerve terminal contains 300 000 or more vesicles (Koelle, 1975). The simultaneous discharge of 100 or more quanta (vesicles), following a latent period of 0.75 ms, occurs when an AP arrives at the motor nerve terminal (Katz and Miledi, 1965). The action potential appears to depolarize the terminal, increasing the permeability of the terminal axoplasmic membrane and permitting the inflow of calcium ions. This causes the liberation of ACh into the synaptic cleft by the process of exocytosis, that is, the membranes of the vesicles (ACh is found in clear and noradrenaline in granulated vesicles) fuse to the nerve cell membrane and the area of fusion breaks down, extruding the contents on the outside of the cell, the membrane of the latter remaining intact (Ganong, 1979).

Combination of the transmitter with postjunctional receptors and the subsequent effects of this have already been discussed, the effects of this mediator being rapidly terminated by (a) diffusion and/or (b) the antagonistic enzyme AChE. The storage, release and disposal of ACh at synaptic and other cholinergic neuroeffector sites is considered to be essentially the same at neuromuscular junctions.

Acetylcholinesterase

Acetylcholinesterase (AChE) is an enzyme present at neuromuscular junctions and in the neurones of cholinergic nerves throughout their entire lengths. It is also found in large amounts in erythrocytes. Also called specific or true cholinesterase (ChE), this enzyme is capable of rapidly hydrolysing acetylcholine liberated in the process of cholinergic transmission to choline and acetic acid (the latter has no action, and the choline very little, on cholinergic receptors) in time periods as little as a millisecond. The transmitter acetylcholine is its preferred or only substrate. Butyro–cholinesterase is another type of enzyme found in the body tissues and fluids (nerves, plasma, liver and other organs), and is also capable of hydrolysing acetylcholine, but at a slower rate. It is known as nonspecific or pseudocholinesterase, but its physiological function is unknown as its experimental inhibition with certain drugs produces no apparent functional derangement at most sites.

Some drugs known as anticholinesterases (for example, physostigmine) neutralize acetylcholinesterase, and then the liberated acetylcholine continues to act until it diffuses away; for example, after physostigmine has been instilled in the eye, the constriction of the ciliary and pupil sphincter muscles continues long after parasympathetic stimulation of these muscles has ceased.

Noradrenaline

Noradrenaline is the neurohumoral transmitter for the great majority of postganglionic sympathetic fibres, and these latter are termed adrenergic. Sir Henry Dale (1934) was the original proposer of the terms 'cholinergic' and 'adrenergic' to describe neurones that liberated acetylcholine and noradrenaline respectively.

Elliott (1905) suggested that postganglionic sympathetic fibres might transmit their impulses to autonomic effector cells by liberation of an adrenaline-like substance, later called sympathin. Euler in the 1940s conclusively identified sympathin as noradrenaline. This transmitter is

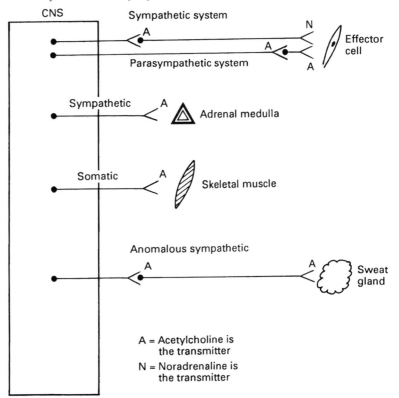

Figure 1.6 Autonomic nervous system.

released from all stimulated postganglionic sympathetic fibres except those to certain sweat glands and vasodilator fibres in man, which were discovered to be cholinergic (Dale and Feldberg, 1934).

The steps in the enzymatic synthesis of noradrenaline and adrenaline (known in the USA as norepinephrine and epinephrine, respectively) proposed by Blaschko (1939) and confirmed by demonstration (using radioactive labelled phenylalanine in rats) by Gurin and Delluva (1947) are as follows.

        Phenylalanine to
(1) (enzyme hydroxylase)
        Tyrosine to
(2) (enzyme hydroxylase)
        Dopa to
(3) (enzyme L-aromatic amino acid decarboxylase)
        Dopamine to
(4) (enzyme dopamine β-hydroxylase)
        Noradrenaline to
(5) (enzyme phenylethanolamine n-methyltransferase)
        Adrenaline

Tyrosine is taken up into the neurone from the extracellular fluid, the other steps of the enzymatic synthesis occurring within the neurone, steps (2) and (3) taking place in the cytoplasm. Dopamine then enters the granules to be converted into noradrenaline (step 4).

Most of the noradrenaline in the adrenal medulla leaves the granules and is converted in the cytoplasm to adrenaline (step 5), re-entering another group of granules for storage until released. Adrenaline accounts for approximately 80% of the catecholamines in the adult human adrenal medulla, noradrenaline contributing most of the remainder.

Under very high magnification (electron micrographs) varicosities can be seen on adrenergic nerve fibres which contain noradrenaline stored in granular vesicles (Ruskell, 1967, 1969).

The Falk–Hillarp fluorescein technique for the demonstration of catecholamines may be used to show these. Briefly, this involves treating the neurones with formaldehyde vapour and examining the resultant histochemical stain under ultraviolet light. The noradrenaline can be seen within the vesicles as fluorescent material.

Adrenergic fibres can sustain the output of noradrenaline for long periods of stimulation, but the maintenance of adequate reserves to allow this is dependent on an unimpaired synthesis and re-uptake of the transmitter, by active transport, into the adrenergic neurone terminals. Cocaine inhibits the re-uptake of catecholamines by adrenergic nerve endings, which temporarily prolongs the activity of noradrenaline, and instillation of cocaine in the eye results in mydriasis as an additional effect to its local anaesthetic property.

It is considered that some of the noradrenaline within the granules is in a smaller mobile pool in equilibrium with some held in reserve as a salt of ATP (four molecules of the catecholamine to one of ATP) along with a specific protein. A much larger mobile pool of noradrenaline exists in

the cytoplasm within the nerve terminal. The cytoplasmic and intragranu-
lar mobile pools are kept in equilibria by active transport mechanisms,
passive diffusion, enzymatic synthesis, and destruction (by mitochondrial
monoamine oxidase (MAO)).

The noradrenaline is discharged rapidly from the neurone terminal by
the nerve action potential, the latter requiring the presence of calcium
ions. The possible involvement of acetylcholine, contained in the sympathetic neurone, as an essential or facilitatory step in the release of noradrenaline, the Burn and Rand hypothesis (1965), is still controversial.
In the adrenal medulla, according to Koelle (1975), ACh liberated by
the preganglionic fibres combines with the receptors on the chromaffin
cells to produce a localized depolarization, which is followed by the
entrance of calcium ions into these cells. This results in their granular content (adrenaline, ATP, chromogranin, dopamine β-hydroxylase) being
extruded by exocytosis into the extracellular fluid and thus into the
circulation.

In the release of noradrenaline at adrenergic terminals calcium ions
again appear to play an essential role in conjunction with the nerve
impulse, but the sequence of steps in this case is not fully understood.

The termination of the effects of noradrenaline, released at adrenergic
terminals, at the adrenoceptive sites of effector cells, other than those in
blood vessels, is mostly by active reabsorption into the adrenergic nerve
terminal, and partly by diffusion and subsequent enzymatic inactivation
by extraneuronal catechol-O-methyl-transferase.

Although much slower acting than AChE, catechol-O-methyltransferase (COMT) and monoamine oxidase, are of major importance in the
initial metabolic transformation of noradrenaline, adrenaline and other
catecholamines in humans. Both enzymes are widely distributed in
tissues, including the brain, throughout the body, their highest concentrations being found in the liver and the kidney.

MAO is associated chiefly with the mitochondria, including those
within the adrenergic fibre terminals and is concerned with the metabolism of intraneuronal catecholamines, by such processes as oxidative
deamination. COMT, on the other hand, is mainly concerned with
extra-neural degradation of catecholamines by way of 3-O-methylation
to 3-methyoxy compounds (Penn, 1980).

Cholinergic receptors

Based on their ability to be stimulated by either nicotine (the well known
alkaloid from tobacco) or muscarine (an alkaloid found in the poisonous
toadstool *Amanita muscaria*), cholinergic receptors are divided into two
groups – muscarinic receptors which are found on the effector cells of
autonomic structures, and nicotinic receptors on which acetylcholine
acts at autonomic synapses and skeletal muscle. Further subdivisions
are necessary for both receptors. There is a difference in susceptibility to
the effects of blocking agents between the nicotinic receptors at the
synapses and those at the motor endplates of skeletal muscle. The neuromuscular blocking drugs such as tubocurarine are less effective on autonomic ganglia, while the reverse is true for ganglion blocking agents
such as hexamethonium. There is also more than one type of muscarinic

receptor – M1 receptors are found in autonomic ganglia while M2 predominate at autonomic effector sites. Additionally, different organs are affected to different degrees by antimuscarinic agents.

Drugs producing their effects by acting on cholinergic receptors

In clinical usage, there are three main types of drugs which produce their effects by acting on cholinergic receptors:

1. Stimulant or mimicking drugs
2. Anticholinesterases
3. Antagonist or blocking drugs.

Cholinomimetics

While it is known that chemicals exist that will produce the same effect as endogenous acetylcholine at nicotinic receptors, these have little clinical significance other than possibly as side effects. However, drugs acting on muscarinic receptors have been used for many decades to produce effects similar to that of stimulating the parasympathetic nervous system – such drugs are known as the parasympathomimetics. They are divided into two types depending on their structure and origin.

The oldest group is that of naturally occurring cholinomimetic alkaloids which have a plant source. They are muscarine (of course), pilocarpine and arecoline. Of these, the most widely and probably the only one regularly used is pilocarpine, whose employment in ophthalmic medicine extends back into the nineteenth century.

Traditionally, the supply of plants from exotic locations from which drugs can be extracted has been erratic and expensive, so a search for synthetic alternatives was made. Derivatives of acetylcholine, choline esters, were made and were found to mimic acetylcholine to varying degrees. Methacholine is still broken down by true cholinesterase at a slow rate while carbachol and bethanechol are resistant. Methacholine has only muscarinic effects while carbachol will affect nicotinic receptors.

Anticholinesterases

There is a natural background release of acetylcholine from cholinergic terminals which is broken down by cholinesterase before it can accumulate in physiologically active quantities. Anticholinesterases are compounds which bind to cholinesterase in a similar manner to acetylcholine. The difference between the two is that acetylcholine can be broken down very quickly whereas anticholinesterases are only slowly metabolized. While anticholinesterases are occupying the cholinesterase site they are not available to hydrolyse acetylcholine, and the transmitter can build up to pharmacologically active levels.

Anticholinesterases very greatly in duration of action and can be divided into two types:

1. Reversible anticholinesterases.
2. Irreversible anticholinesterases.

Reversible anticholinesterases. The best known example of these compounds is physostigmine from the calabar bean, while neostigmine is a more modern synthetic copy which has the advantage of greater stability.

Irreversible anticholinesterases. Originally developed as nerve gases and insecticides, the organophosphorus compounds produce an inhibition of cholinesterase which is so prolonged that it is thought that the body produces a new enzyme before the original has been regenerated. One of the original compounds was di-isopropylfluorophosphate (DFP) which has been superseded by more stable compounds.

The effects of anticholinesterases are similar to those of parasympathomimetics, with additional effects (due to the nicotinic actions) of causing enhanced transmission which is sometimes evident as muscle fasciculation or twitching. Anticholinesterases, in addition to their ophthalmic application, are used in the treatment of myasthenia gravis.

Antagonistic or blocking drugs

The ability of drugs to combine with receptors without producing the same effect as the natural transmitter has been discussed above. To some extent the classification of receptors has been based on the differential effects of blocking drugs.

Different cholinergic receptors are susceptible to the effects of different agents and as in the classification of cholinergic receptors, there are drugs which block muscarinic receptors (the antimuscarinic agents) and nicotinic blocking drugs which are divided into ganglionic blocking agents and neuromuscular blocking drugs.

The archetypal antimuscarinic agent is atropine but this has been to a great extent supplanted by newer agents designed for the treatment for stomach ulcers and other conditions in which a reduction in parasympathetic tone is desirable. The action of antimuscarinic agents is widespread and is due to an inhibition of those structures which are normally parasympathetically stimulated. Exocrine gland secretions are inhibited (particularly the salivary glands, and the glands in the gut). Although they are sympathetically innervated, the sweat glands are also affected resulting in a marked reduction in the production of sweat and a rise in temperature. Gut motility is reduced, a property which leads to the use of antimuscarinic agents as travel sickness remedies.

Ganglion blocking drugs were extensively used thirty years ago in the treatment of systemic hypertension. These drugs prevent the transmission of impulses across autonomic synapses without an apparent effect on skeletal muscle. Both divisions of the autonomic nervous system are equally affected, but the blood vessels are only innervated by the sympathetic nervous system and blockage of transmission of impulses results in a lowering of blood pressure from the widespread dilation of blood vessels. The effects were not restricted to blood vessels and the side effects were most unpleasant. They have to a large extent been replaced by more modern drugs which are kinder to the patient.

Neuromuscular blocking agents are used as adjuvants in surgery and relax skeletal muscle by preventing the normal transmission of impulses across the neural muscular junction. They produce their effect by one of two methods – (a) by competitive blockade or (b) by depolarizing blockade. In the former the motor endplate is maintained in its polarized unstimulated resting state by the blocking drug, which occupies the receptor without producing the action potential necessary for muscle contraction. Drugs like tubocurarine work in this manner and as they are competitive agents will be reversed by increasing the amount of normal transmitter at the motor endplate. Thus their effects can be reversed to some extent by the use of an anticholinesterase.

Depolarizing blocking drugs on the other hand maintain the motor endplate in a depolarized state and prevent repolarization which is necessary for a new action potential to be initiated. For normal skeletal muscle this results in a relaxation, but certain muscle fibres such as those found in the oculorotatory muscle respond by going into a sustained contraction – contracture. The administration of an anticholinesterase will result in a deepening of the blockade.

Adrenergic receptors

Noradrenaline, adrenaline and other members (for example, dopamine) of the catecholamines acting as neurohumoral transmitters can cause either excitation or inhibition of smooth muscles, depending on the site and amount of catecholamine present. Catecholamines are a group of chemical compounds (catechol is dihydroxybenzene) distributed throughout the tissue of the body in cells called chromaffin cells, due to the brown colour of the latter produced when they are treated with dichromate. The actual percentage of these catecholamines in various tissues depends on the site in the body, for example the adrenal medulla secretes 80% adrenaline, the remainder of its secretion being noradrenaline, very little dopamine being present. On the other hand, the transmitter liberated from adrenergic nerve fibres is noradrenaline with perhaps a little adrenaline.

The most potent excitatory catecholamine is noradrenaline, which has a correspondingly low activity as an inhibitor, whereas adrenaline is relatively potent in both excitatory and inhibitory activities.

Ahlquist (1948) studied the excitatory and inhibitory actions of various catecholamines (including *l*-adrenaline, *dl*-adrenaline, noradrenaline, methyl-noradrenaline, methyl-adrenaline, and isopropyl noradrenaline [isoprenaline]), using vascular, bronchial, stomach and intestinal, uterine and ureter smooth muscle, cardiac muscle and the smooth muscle in the nictitating membrane of the cat. He proposed the terms alpha and beta receptors for adrenoreceptive sites on smooth muscles where catecholamines produce excitation or inhibition respectively. Both types may be present in the same tissue. This occurs in blood vessels where, with the usual amounts of physiologically circulating adrenaline, beta receptor response (vasodilation) predominates in the blood vessels of the skeletal muscle and the liver; alpha receptor response (vasoconstriction) occurs in blood vessels of the abdominal viscera, skin and mucosa (including the conjunctival vessels).

Exceptions to the general proposal associating alpha receptors with excitation and beta receptors with inhibition are recognized. An inhibitory response is mediated by both alpha and beta receptors in the intestine, the latter being generally relaxed by catecholamines. Developments in the study of adrenergic receptors have led to the division of alpha receptors into alpha$_1$ and alpha$_2$, based on their molecular mode of action.

Lands *et al.* (1967) have shown on the basis of relative selectivity of effects of both excitatory and antagonist agents that there are at least two different types of beta receptors.

As excitatory responses, positive chronotropic and inotropic effects (increased rate and force respectively) are the response of cardiac nodes and muscle which have beta receptors, these latter in the heart have been classified as beta$_1$. Most of the other beta receptors, where inhibition is produced, are termed beta$_2$. There is now a beta$_3$ receptor which is found in fat cells and brings about lipolysis in the intestine.

Whichever beta receptor is involved, the basis of its action is the activation of a membrane enzyme which leads to the conversion of adenosine triphosphate into cyclic adenosine monophosphate, cAMP, which leads to a series of complex events culminating in the pharmacological response.

Drugs producing their effects by acting on adrenergic receptors

Drugs acting on the sympathetic nervous system can produce their effects by a variety of mechanisms.

1. Direct acting sympathomimetics.
2. Indirect acting sympathomimetics.
3. Drugs which interfere with the neuronal re-uptake of noradrenaline.
4. Adrenergic receptor blocking drugs.
5. Adrenergic neurone blocking drugs.

Directly acting sympathomimetics

These drugs are directly comparable with parasympathomimetics in that they mimic the effect of a natural transmitter on the adrenergic receptor which is normally (but not exclusively) found opposite nerve terminals. Because their action is direct they do not need the presence of the nerve terminal. Since the basis of the classification of the adrenergic receptors is the differential effects of the various sympathomimetics, then it follows logically that some drugs will predominantly effect alpha stimulators e.g. noradrenaline, while others like isoprenaline will predominately affect beta receptors. The two groups are not mutually exclusive and noradrenaline will stimulate the heart and produce bronchial dilation while isoprenaline will constrict blood vessels and cause a rise in blood pressure. Their effect is enhanced by sympathetic denervation.

Indirectly acting sympathomimetics

These drugs have little direct effect on the receptors but serve to enhance the release of natural catecholamine from the sympathetic nerve terminals. They will only produce an effect in the presence of functional adrenergic nerve terminals and their effect will be abolished by denervation. Such drugs are amphetamine, phenylpropanolamine and pseudoephedrine.

Drugs which interfere with neuronal reuptake of noradenaline

When catecholamine is released from nerve terminals not all of it is destroyed as is the case with acetylcholine. Instead, its action is limited by the reuptake of the chemical. Some drugs inhibit the reuptake of the transmitter and thus increase its duration of action, producing an enhanced effect. Cocaine produces its effect in this manner.

*Adrenergic receptor
blocking drugs*

Adrenergic receptor blocking drugs may be of the alpha adrenergic blocking type (for example, thymoxamine; this is used in eyedrops for reversing
pupillary blockage caused by sympathomimetic mydriatics), or beta
adrenergic blocking agents (for example, atenolol and timolol).

The development of alpha blocking drugs preceded beta blockers by
many years but it is now the latter which predominate in clinical medicine
for the treatment of hypertension and other cardiovascular problems.
They have also been used in the treatment of open angle glaucoma,
inhibiting the production of aqueous humour.

One of the first beta blockers was propranolol which affected both beta$_1$
and beta$_2$ receptors equally and was termed nonselective. Thus it would
have an effect on the heart reducing the rate and force and also on the
respiratory system causing a narrowing of the airways. The latter effect
would not be a problem except for patients with pre-existing obstructive
airway disease such as asthma. To overcome this problem beta blockers
with a more specific effect on beta$_1$ were developed, such as betaxolol.
However they still have some beta$_2$ effect and are not ideal drugs for
asthmatic patients. Some beta blockers are partial agonists and the term
intrinsic sympathomimetic activity is used to describe this property.

Labetalol is unusual in that it has both alpha and beta blocking activity.
Clinically it has the benefits of both type of drugs as well as, unfortunately,
their adverse effects. It is used in the treatment of hypertension.

Adrenergic blocking drugs

These drugs do not interfere with the adrenergic receptor, but interfere
with the natural release of noradrenaline by preventing synthesis, storage
or neurogenic release. Reserpine depletes the store of noradrenaline
from the nerve terminals by preventing the synaptic vesicles storing the
chemical, resulting in pharmacological denervation. Bretylium and guanethidine work in a similar manner. They are little used today.

Denervation supersensitivity

When the nerve to an effector cell is cut or destroyed, the cell becomes
supersensitive to the transmitter normally supplied by the nerve or to
any drug capable of mimicking its effects. This supersensitivity is brought
about by the lack of a neurotropic factor which is present when the nerve
is functioning.

The mechanism of supersensitivity is due to an increased number of
receptors and an absence of the reuptake mechanism in the case of sympathetic nerves. It can be produced chemically using 6-hydroxydopamine
or pharmacologically with guanethidine, as well as surgically. It also, of
course, occurs spontaneously in Horner's and Adie's syndromes, in
which the sympathetic and parasympathetic systems are affected, respectively. When the nerve returns to normal (regenerates), the effector cell
loses its supersensitivity.

References

Ahlquist, R. P. (1948) A study of the adrenotropic receptors. *Am. J. Physiol.*, **153**, 586–600

Blashko, H. (1939) The specific action of L-dopa decarboxylase. *J. Physiol. (Lond.)*, **96**, 50–51

Bulbring, E. (1958) Physiology and pharmacology of intestinal smooth muscle. *Lect. Sci. Basis Med.*, **7**, 374–397

Burn, J. H. and Rand, M. J. (1965) Acetylcholine in adrenergic transmission. *A Rev. Pharmac.*, **5**, 163–182

Burnstock, G. and Holman, M. E. (1961) The transmission of excitation from autonomic nerve to smooth muscle. *J. Physiol. (Lond.)*, **155**, 115–133

Clark, A. J. (1933) *The Mode of Action of Drugs on Cells*. London: Edward Arnold

Dale, H. H. (1934) Chemical transmission of the effects of nerve impulses. *Br. Med. J.*, **I**, 835–841

Dale, H. H. and Feldberg, W. (1934) Chemical transmitter of vagus effects to stomach. *J. Physiol. (Lond.)*, **81**, 32–334

Dixon, W. D. (1907) On the mode of action of drugs. *Med. Mag.*, **16**, 454–457

Eccles, J. C. (1964) *The Physiology of Synapses*. Berlin: Springer-Verlag, New York: Academic Press

Eccles, J. C. (1973) *The Understanding of the Brain*. New York: McGraw-Hill

Eccles, R. M. and Libet, B. (1961) Origin and blockade of the synaptic responses of curarised sympathetic ganglia. *J. Physiol. (Lond.)*, **157**, 484–503

Elliot, T. R. (1905) The action of adrenaline. *J. Physiol. (Lond.)*, **32**, 401–467

Ganong, W. F. (1979) *Review of Medical Physiology*, 9th edn., p. 57. Los Altos: Lange Medical Publications

Gillespie, J. S. (1962) The electrical and mechanical responses of intestinal smooth muscle cells to stimulation of their extrinsic parasympathetic nerves. *J. Physiol. (Lond.)*, **162**, 76–92

Greengard, P. and Kebabian, J. W. (1974) Role of cyclic AMP in synaptic transmission in mammalian peripheral nervous system. *Fedn. Proc. Fedn. Am. Socs. Exp. Biol.*, **33**, 1059–1067

Gurin, S. and Delluva, A. (1947) The biological synthesis of radioactive adrenaline from phenylalanine. *J. Biol. Chem.*, **170**, 545–550

Hodgkin, A. L. and Huxley, A. F. (1952) A quantitative description of membrane current and its application to conduction and excitation in nerves. *J. Physiol. (Lond.)*, **117**, 500–544

Katz, B. (1966) *Nerve, Muscle and Synapse*. New York: McGraw-Hill

Katz, B. and Miledi, R. (1965) The measurement of synaptic delay, and the time course of acetylcholine release at the neuromuscular junction. *Proc. R. Soc. B.*, **161**, 483–495

Katz, B. and Miledi, R. (1972) The statistical nature of acetylcholine potential and its molecular components. *J. Physiol. (Lond.)*, **224**, 665–699

Koelle, G. B. (1975) In *Goodman and Gilman's The Pharmacological Basis of Therapeutics*, 5th edn., pp. 404–444. New York: Macmillan

Krnjevic, K. (1974) Chemical nature of synaptic transmission in vertebrates. *Physiol. Rev.*, **54**, 418–540

Lands, A. M., Arnold, A., McAnliff, J. P., Luduena, F. P. and Brown, R. G., Jr. (1967) Differentiation of receptor system activated by sympathomimetic amines. *Nature (Lond.)*, **214**, 597–598

Langley, J. N. (1905) On the reactions of cells and nerve-endings to certain poisons, chiefly as regards the reactions of striated muscles to nicotine and curare. *J. Physiol.*, **33**, 374–413

Lewandowsky, M. (1898) Ueber eine Wirkung des Nebennierenextractes auf das Auge. *Zent Bl. Physiol.*, **12**, 599–600

McLennan, H. (1970) *Synaptic Transmission*, 2nd edn., Philadelphia: Saunders

Moses, R. A. (1975) *Adler's Physiology of the Eye–Clinical application*, 6th edn., p. 326. St Louis: Mosby

Paton, W. D. M. (1961) A theory of drug action based on the rate of drug-receptor combination. *Proc. R. Soc. B.*, **154**, 21–69

Penn, R. G. (1980) *Pharmacology*, 3rd edn., London: Ballière Tindall

Ruskell, G. L. (1967) Vasomotor axons of the lacrimal gland of monkeys and the ultrastructural identification of sympathetic terminals. *Z. Zellforsch. microsk. Anat.*, **83**, 321–33

Ruskell, G. L. (1969) Changes in nerve terminals and action of the lacrimal gland and changes in secretion induced by autonomic denervation. *Z. Zellforsch. Microsk. Anat.*, **94**, 261–281

Thomas, R. C. (1972) Electrogenic sodium pump in nerve and muscle cells. *Physiol. Rev.*, **52**, 563–594

Volle, R. L. and Koelle, G. B. (1975) In *Goodman and Gilman's The Pharmacological Basic of Therapeutics*, 5th edn., pp. 565–566. New York: Macmillan

2

Ocular autonomic innervation

Effector structures in the eye and orbit

Many of the diagnostic drugs used in ophthalmic practice, in particular cycloplegics, mydriatics and miotics, directly or indirectly produce their effects by stimulating or inhibiting a part of the autonomic nervous system (ANS) supplying the intraocular muscles. They may also have an effect on other smooth muscles or glands in the orbit. Therefore, it is essential before proceeding to a more detailed discussion on the actions and uses of ophthalmic autonomic drugs to have a basic understanding of the structure and function of this involuntary nervous system in the orbital region.

Intraocular muscles
Ciliary muscle

This muscle consists of flat bundles of unstriped fibres which may be classified as follows:

1. Meridional fibres (Brücke's muscle)
2. Radial fibres
3. Circular fibres (Müller's muscle) (Fig. 2.1).

Pupil sphincter muscle

This is a circular band of smooth muscle fibres 1 mm wide just inside the pupillary border of the iris. In order to produce the tremendous variation in pupil diameter these muscle fibres have a prodigious ability to shorten. They are not arranged as a simple 'drawstring', and pupil constriction is still achieved after sector iridectomy. The pupil sphincter and pupil dilator muscles do not originate embryonically from mesoderm as do the great majority of muscles, but from neural ectoderm; a fact that makes them unique.

Pupil dilator muscle

This consists of radially arranged smooth muscle fibres, processes of the cells of the anterior layer of the pigment epithelium of the iris; it is innervated by the sympathetic nervous system.

Palpebral smooth muscle

This also known as Müller's muscle and arises from the global surface of the levator palpebrae superioris muscle (striped muscle). It is dependent on the tone of the levator to provide a firm base for the effect of the contraction of the smooth muscle.

Lacrimal gland

As an exocrine gland the lacrimal is subject to autonomic control, and the quantity and quality of secretions will be affected by changes in ANS tone and the administration of drugs with an autonomic mode of action.

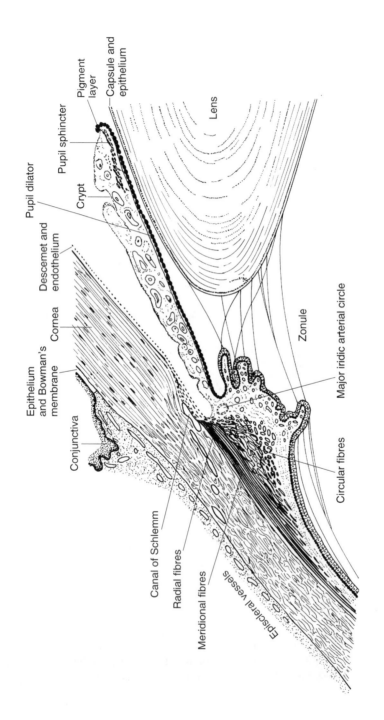

Figure 2.1 Antero-posterior section through the anterior portion of the eye.

Epithelium and Bowman's membrane

Conjunctiva

Cornea

Descemet and endothelium

Canal of Schlemm

Radial fibres

Meridional fibres

Episcleral vessels

Circular fibres

Major iridic arterial circle

Zonule

Pupil dilator

Pupil sphincter

Pigment layer

Capsule and epithelium

Crypt

Lens

Parasympathetic innervation of the eye (Colour Plate I)

The ciliary muscle is innervated by cholinergic fibres of the parasympathetic running in the third cranial nerve (the oculomotor), and their origin is in the Edinger–Westphal nucleus near the third nucleus in the floor of the aqueduct of Sylvius. From there they pass out of the midbrain in the main trunk of the third nerve which, just before entering the orbit, divides into superior and inferior divisions. The parasympathetic fibres continue in the inferior division and pass into its inferior oblique branch, which they leave to form the motor root of the ciliary ganglion. In this ganglion the parasympathetic fibres synapse, their postganglionic components (which are atypical in being medullated) entering the globe via the short ciliary nerves (six to ten), which pierce the sclera around the optic nerve. The parasympathetic fibres then pass forward in the perichoroidal space to supply the ciliary and pupil sphincter muscles.

The Edinger–Westphal nucleus, according to Miller (1978), receives excitatory connections from the frontal and occipital (psycho-optical) cortex.

The parasympathetic (secretomotor) fibres to the lacrimal gland have their origin in cells forming a discrete subnucleus located very close to the superior salivatory nucleus, which lies lateral to the nucleus of the seventh cranial nerve beneath the floor of the pontine part of the fourth ventricle. Leaving the brain stem in the nervus intermedius, between the pons and inferior cerebellar peduncle, they run with the seventh nerve, fusing with the latter at the geniculate ganglion.

From this ganglion arises the great (superficial) petrosal in which the parasympathetic fibres run to join the deep petrosal (sympathetic) to form the nerve of the pterygoid canal (the Vidian). This nerve joins the pterygopalatine (sphenopalatine; Meckel's) ganglion, where only the parasympathetic component relays, the postganglionic parasympathetic fibres then travel via the maxillary nerve to enter its zygomatic branch and reach the lacrimal gland via a connecting branch of this nerve.

Sympathetic innervation of the eye and orbit (Colour Plate I)

The preganglionic sympathetic nerve fibres of the dilatator tract supplying the pupil dilatator muscle probably have their origin in the hypothalamus not far from the constrictor centre (Edinger–Westphal) to which they are connected, Miller (1978) considers, by an inhibitory pathway, in addition to having connections with the cerebral cortex. The dilatator nerve fibres pass downwards, with partial decussation in the midbrain, through the medulla oblongata into the lateral columns of the cord. They leave the latter by the anterior roots of the first three thoracic nerves and perhaps the last cervical nerve, passing to the corresponding lateral ganglion chain on each side via the white rami communicantes. These sympathetic nerve fibres then run to the first thoracic or the stellate ganglion (as the frequently fused first thoracic and inferior cervical ganglion is termed), and from there into the cervical sympathetic chain in the neck, synapsing in the superior cervical ganglion which is the peripheral ganglion in their path from the central nervous system to the orbit. The nonmedullated postganglionic fibres enter the cranial cavity in company with the internal carotid artery around which they form networks, the carotid plexus, and a little further on (where this artery lies within the cavernous sinus) the cavernous plexus. It is mainly from the latter that most of the sympathetic nerves to the eye and orbit are derived. The dilatator fibres pass from the cavernous plexus to run over the anterior part of the trigeminal (Gasserian) ganglion before entering the ophthalmic division of the fifth cranial nerve, the sympathetic fibres continuing in its nasociliary branch. They leave this nerve to join the long ciliary nerves which enter the eye on either side of the optic nerve. Running forward in the perichoroidal space, the sympathetic fibres then pass through the ciliary body to reach the pupil dilator in the iris.

Other postganglionic sympathetic fibres from the cavernous plexus form the sympathetic root of the ciliary ganglion, passing through it without further synapse to enter the eye via the short ciliary nerves to supply the intraocular blood vessels of the uvea. Also, from the cavernous plexus, further vasomotor sympathetic fibres supply the ophthalmic artery and its branches to the extraocular muscles.

It has been suggested in the past that some sympathetic fibres may supply the ciliary muscle itself (not just its blood vessels), adrenergic impulses affecting receptors on the muscle fibres: the resultant 'negative' accommodation might assist for distance vision.

Work by Van Alpen (1976) using material obtained from eye banks, showed that the ciliary muscle has mostly beta receptors, the pupil dilator muscle mostly alpha receptors, and the pupil sphincter muscle both alpha and beta receptors. Adrenergic impulses to the intraocular muscles should therefore simultaneously induce relaxation of the ciliary muscle and contraction of the pupil dilator, and cause an uncertain response in the pupil sphincter.

According to Wolff (1976), postganglionic (vasomotor) sympathetic fibres to the lacrimal gland may reach the gland coming from the superior cervical ganglion via: (1) sympathetic nerves along the lacrimal artery from the internal carotid plexus; (2) the deep petrosal nerve; and (3) those sympathetic fibres that run in the lacrimal nerve with the latter's sensory fibres.

It is now thought that the sympathetic lacrimal innervation is to its blood vessels, while the parasympathetic probably controls normal tear secretion. This supposition is supported by the fact that drugs inhibiting the parasympathetic reduce the secretion of the gland, for example, atropine. Electron microscopic investigations by Ruskell (1969) would appear to confirm this view.

Sensory innervation of the eye and orbit
(Colour Plate I)

It may not be out of place here, although it is not a part of the ocular autonomic innervation, to mention that the third root (the sensory) of the ciliary ganglion (the other two being the sympathetic and parasympathetic) is a branch of the ophthalmic division of the fifth cranial nerve (the trigeminal), which is the sensory nerve for the whole of the eye and orbit. The short ciliary nerves carry the sensory fibres from the intraocular structures of the globe, particularly the cornea. These fibres leave the ciliary ganglion as its sensory root to join the nasociliary nerve, which has already received the two long ciliary nerves from the eye, carrying sensory fibres from the ciliary muscle, the iris and the cornea; in addition these two nerves carry sympathetic fibres running in the naso-ciliary forwards to the pupil dilator. Proceeding back towards the trigeminal (Gasserian) ganglion, the nasociliary is joined by the (sensory) frontal and lacrimal nerves (the latter also carries sympathetic fibres), the three branches uniting to form the ophthalmic nerve, the first (or ophthal-mic) division of the trigeminal ganglion of the fifth cranial nerve. Drugs known as local anaesthetics are used to block the conduction of impulses back along these sensory nerves from the eye and orbit.

Ocular effects of drugs acting on autonomic receptors

Because of the extensive autonomic innervation of the eye and orbit, drugs acting on autonomic receptors as detailed in Chapter 1 will produce a variety of effects when administered to the eye in a form which allows the drugs to act on the ocular tissues. These effects will be manifested as modifications of the following:

1. Pupil diameter
2. Pupillary light reflex
3. Accommodation
4. Intraocular pressure
5. Ocular vasculature
6. Lacrimal secretion
7. Palpebral fissure.

Pupil diameter

The diameter of the pupil is a result of the balance of the parasympathetic and sympathetic nervous system, with the former normally predominant. However, even in bright light the iris still has the ability to be stimulated to bring about further miosis by the application of drugs which stimulate the cholinergic receptor such as pilocarpine and other parasympatho-mimetics, and the anticholinesterases. These drugs will be fully discussed in Chapter 8 – Miotics. Equally, drugs which block cholinergic receptors will bring about the opposite effect of mydriasis, the mechanism of which will depend on the type of receptor that is blocked. Drugs blocking muscarinic receptors (antimuscarinics such as atropine) will paralyse the pupil sphincter directly and reduce the miotic action of parasympathomi-metic miotics. Ganglionic blocking agents whose action is on nicotinic receptors will block both the ciliary and superior cervical ganglia. Although both dilator and sphincter muscles will be paralysed, the normal dominance of the latter will result in a pupil dilation. Both muscles will be amenable to stimulation by agents that act on effector cell receptors.

Due to the sympathetic innervation of the iris muscles, drugs and agents acting on adrenergic receptors will also affect the diameter of the pupil. Sympathomimetic drugs will cause a mydriasis by stimulating the pupil dilator muscle to contract. Because of reciprocal innervation, there is a corresponding relaxation of the pupil sphincter. Adrenaline blocking drugs, in particular the alpha blocking drugs, will antagonize the effect of locally released noradrenaline and exogeneous sympathomimetics and cause a degree of miosis which is probably not as great as that produced by most parasympathomimetics. Adrenergic neurone blocking drugs such as guanethidine will deplete the catecholamine stores in the sympathetic nerves to the iris dilator leading to miosis. However, unlike the alpha blocker, the iris will become supersensitive to sympathomimetics and the pupil will dilate when low concentrations of such drugs are administered.

Pupillary light reflex

Stimulation of the pupil sphincter by parasympathomimetics and anticholinesterase will only result in a loss of light reflex if a supramaximal dose of drug is used, such that the muscle is in spasm, and normal mechanisms are swamped by a miotic drug such as a long acting irreversible anticholinesterase. Potent antimuscarinics such as atropine and cyclopentolate will prevent the pupil from reacting to light because the sphincter is unable to contract. This is also true for the ganglion blocking agents, but not for the sympathomimetics which leave the pupil sphincter still sensitive to stimulation and able to contract the pupil.

Accommodation

In spite of the suggestion of adrenergic innervation, it is the drugs that act on cholinergic receptors that have the most profound effects on the amplitude of accommodation.

Parasympathomimetics and anticholinesterases will cause a spasm of the ciliary muscle and of accommodation, the amplitude and duration of which will depend on several factors such as the type and concentration of drug and the age and pigmentation of the patient. A pseudomyopia will result.

Antimuscarinic drugs will act directly on the ciliary muscle to cause a paralysis and a cycloplegia. As for drugs causing a cyclospasm, the depth and duration of the cycloplegia will be dependent on the drug, its concentration and the pigmentation of the patient. Antinicotinic drugs, in particular ganglionic blocking agents, paralyse accommodation by interfering with the transmission of impulses across the ciliary ganglion. The latter effect is of little clinical use, and was one of the many side effects of ganglionic blocking drugs that led to their discontinuation in the treatment of systemic hypertension.

The effects of adrenergic drugs on ciliary muscle are of little importance.

Intraocular pressure

Intraocular pressure is a result of the balance between aqueous humour secretion and aqueous humour drainage, and as some drugs can affect both mechanisms in different ways it will be beneficial to separate the two for the purposes of considering the actions of various drugs.

Aqueous secretion

Aqueous production comprises a passive component (ultrafiltration) and an active component (secretion). Ultrafiltration will be subject to many factors, but an important one will be the blood pressure in the ciliary body vasculature and any mechanism which impedes flow into the ciliary capillaries will result in a reduction in aqueous secretion. To some extent ciliary blood vessels are sensitive to adrenergic agents. Active secretion is dependent on energy using enzymes such as the ATPases. Since the stimulation of beta receptors leads to a conversion of adenosine triphosphate into cyclic AMP, adrenergic drugs will have an effect on secretion which is a resultant between their vascular and biochemical effects. The end result is normally a reduction in secretion. It is somewhat confusing to find that beta blockers also have the effect of reducing secretion.

Aqueous drainage

Irrespective of their miotic effects in unblocking the filtration angle in angle closure glaucoma, cholinergic stimulant drugs increase the outflow of aqueous humour. This effect is probably secondary to their stimulant effect on the longitudinal ciliary muscle, which has its origin opposite the uveal trabecular meshwork which is opened up by the spasm of the smooth muscle. Antimuscarinic drugs can cause a reduction in drainage by two mechanisms; first, by causing a mydriasis which causes the iris to bunch up in the angle and embarrass the flow when the angle is narrow, and more commonly by relaxing the ciliary muscle.

Sympathomimetics will, conversely, increase the drainage of aqueous humour, probably acting via a metabolic route increasing active transport of aqueous across the trabecular meshwork.

Sympathetic blocking drugs have little effect on the outflow of aqueous humour.

Ocular vasculature

Most blood vessels are controlled by the sympathetic system and it is the drugs which act on the adrenergic receptors that have the most effect on the blood vessels of the eye. However, even if blood vessels are not innervated they will contain muscarinic receptors which can be acted upon by cholinergic drugs. Not all blood vessels are equally affected, and as a general rule the farther back in the eye the blood vessels are located the less they will be affected. The most sensitive blood vessels are those found in the conjunctiva, and administration of parasympathomimetics will cause a vasodilation and a conjunctival hyperemia. Dilation of deeper vessels can sometimes lead to a rise in intraocular pressure followed by a more persistent fall. The permeability of the blood/aqueous barrier may be increased, allowing larger molecules to pass into the aqueous humour. The blood vessels of the retina are little affected by autonomic drugs.

Antimuscarinic drugs have little direct effect on the blood vessels because the cholinergic receptors are normally not innervated.

Sympathomimetics produce a marked constriction of the conjunctival blood vessels causing blanching of the conjunctiva, and this leads to their use as conjunctival decongestants. They will also constrict uveal blood vessels leading to an increase in uveal vascular resistance. They have little effect on retinal blood vessels.

Lacrimal secretion

There are two parameters which can be affected when drugs act on the lacrimal gland; the quantity and the quality of secretion. Drugs acting on cholinergic receptors, in particular parasympathomimetics, will stimulate the gland to produce an increased secretion of both mucous and serous components. Antimuscarinics will produce the opposite effect and bring about a reduction in secretion.

Stimulation of the sympathetic receptors will cause a vasoconstriction in the gland and lead to the production of a more viscous secretion.

Palpebral fissure

There are two types of muscle in the upper lid, the striped skeletal muscle fibres of the levator palpebrae superioris and the smooth muscles cells of Müller's muscle. Cholinergic drugs with nicotinic effects, in particular anticholinesterase drugs, will affect the former and administration of these drugs will sometimes cause the lid to twitch due to fasciculation of the muscle fibres.

Müller's muscle is principally affected by adrenergic drugs and these will cause an increase in the palpebral fissure if they are absorbed across the bulbar conjunctiva. Adrenergic blocking drugs, particularly the neurone blocking drugs such as guanethidine, will paralyse the muscle and lead to ptosis.

References

Miller, J. H. S. (1978) *Parsons' Diseases of the Eye*, 16th edn., pp. 34–36. London: Churchill Livingstone

Ruskell, G. L. (1969) Changes in nerve terminals and action of the lacrimal gland and changes in secretion induced by autonomic denervation. *Z. Zellforsch. Microsk. Anat.*, **94**, 261–281

Van Alpen, G. W. H. M. (1976) The adrenergic receptors of the intraocular muscles of the human eye. *Invest. Ophthal.*, **15**, 502

Wolff, E. (1976) *Anatomy of the Eye and Orbit*, 7th edn., p. 226. London: Lewis

3

Basic microbiology

An understanding of the basic science of microbiology is essential for the optometrist. It will help him deal with matters such as:

1. patients with 'red eye'
2. contact lens solutions and the claims made for them by manufacturers
3. preventive measures following contact tonometry and foreign body removal
4. the constituents of eye drops and the maintenance of sterility.

The science of microbiology covers organisms invisible to the naked eye. Micro-organisms include protozoa, fungi, bacteria, rickettsia, chlamydia and viruses.

Protozoa and fungi are the only micro-organisms which have eucaryotic cells similar in structure to those of higher organisms. Such cells have inclusions like nuclei and an endoplasmic reticulum. Fungi and protozoa can be either parasitic or free-living. Bacteria are simpler cells (procaryotic cells) but some species are capable of an independent existence in simple environments. However, many bacteria are parasitic or saprophytic and live off the tissues of living or dead organisms. Rickettsia and chlamydiae lack many of the structures found in more complicated cells and are thus obligate intracellular parasites.

Viruses are the simplest micro-organisms and can only multiply by utilizing the host cell's biochemical systems. Of the above, it is the bacteria that have received most attention.

Bacteria

Bacteria are important because of their ubiquity, i.e. their ability to infect and multiply in varied environments, and the ability of many types to cause disease – their pathogenicity. In order to reduce problems caused by bacteria, it is important to understand something of their structure, growth, environmental and metabolic requirements, classification, relationship with disease and the particular problems they can cause to the eye.

Structure (Figs 3.1 and 3.2)

The cytoplasm of bacterial (procaryotic) cells is notable because of the absence of discrete structures normally found in eucaryotic cells. There are no mitochondria; the respiratory enzymes are instead located on the cell membrane. There is no endoplasmic reticulum or Golgi apparatus and the ribosomes are found free in the cytoplasm. There is also no nucleus and no nuclear membrane, and when the cell divides there is no mitosis. Genetic material is carried on a single strand of DNA, unlike that of eucaryotic cells which is organized into chromosomes.

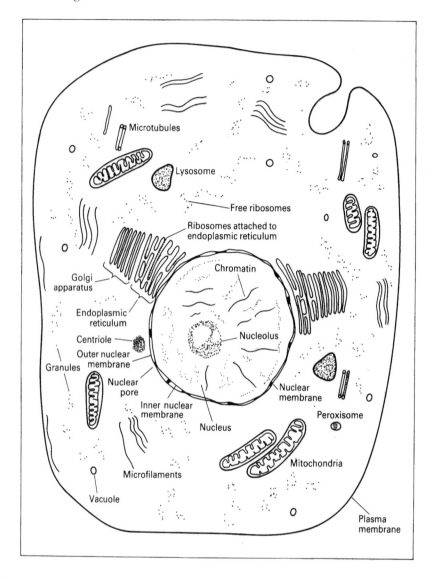

Figure 3.1 Eucaryotic cell.

Some bacteria contain additional DNA molecules called plasmids which are not essential for the organism's life but can confer on it very special properties such as resistance to antibiotics. Plasmids are most commonly found in Gram negative bacteria and can spread from one cell to another.

Surrounding the cytoplasm is a thin, selectively permeable lipoprotein elastic membrane – the plasma membrane. It is the site of action of many of the bacterial enzymes and controls entry of substances into the cell. Being elastic, the cell membrane does not determine the shape of the bacterial cell. This is the function of the cell wall, a rigid permeable structure principally composed of a substance called murein. Because of the osmotic pressure of the cytoplasm, the cell membrane is usually

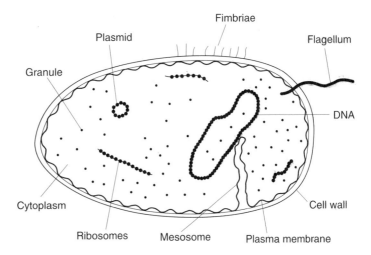

Figure 3.2 Procaryotic cell.

pushed hard against the inside of the cell wall by a pressure of up to 20 atmospheres. The cell wall is relatively thick, especially in Gram positive bacteria, and is chemically unrelated to the cell walls of higher plants.

In some bacteria the cell wall is surrounded by a layer of extracellular material referred to as the capsule (if it is closely associated with the cell wall) or slime layer (if the relationship is looser). This is a poorly organized layer of large molecules such as polysaccharides or polypeptides. The effect of this layer is to impede the ingress of substances (useful and harmful) into the cell wall. The result is that the cells tend to grow and divide at a slower rate but are more resistant to antibacterial chemicals, viruses (bacteriophages), phagocytes and other adverse agents. It may also inhibit antibody formation against the bacteria, thereby rendering the bacteria more harmful to the body. Additionally, it can act to form an adhesion between the bacterial cell and a host cell which also increases its virulence. One of the best known bacteria which forms a capsule is *Mycobacterium tuberculosum*, the causative organism of tuberculosis.

On the outside of some types of bacteria are found flagella. The number of flagella per cell is constant for each species. Flagella are long filamentous structures containing a contractile protein, flagellin, which is similar to muscle myosin. The presence of flagella normally confers the ability of motion which it is assumed allows the bacterium to migrate to better environments. Other bacteria have the ability to move without possessing flagella. These are the spiral forms which move by twisting the whole body.

Projecting from the surface of some bacteria are fimbriae, also formed of protein, which instead of facilitating motion act to hold the bacterial cell to a host cell or another bacterial cell. The fimbriae are very specific to the molecule to which they attach and fimbriated bacteria are found to be more virulent than those which lack these appendages.

Environmental and metabolic requirements

Bacteria are ubiquitous and can exist in many environments that are far too hostile for the cells of higher organisms. More fastidious bacteria have requirements closer to those of the internal environment of animals and hence are more likely to be parasitic and pathogenic.

Nutritional requirements

All organisms have a requirement for carbon, hydrogen, oxygen and nitrogen. Since hydrogen and oxygen can be obtained from water, it is the requirement for the other elements that is most critical. Some bacterial species can obtain their nutrient requirements from inorganic sources. They obtain energy from other sources, e.g. bacterial chlorophyll allows some bacteria to use sunlight as a source of energy and synthesize simple organic compounds. Others have the ability to utilize inorganic nitrogen providing they are supplied with an organic source of carbon. Such organisms are found in soil and are responsible for maintaining its fertility.

Others require both organic carbon and nitrogen to survive. Pathogenic bacteria need other complicated growth factors and minerals.

Oxygen requirement

Although oxygen can be obtained from water, some types of bacteria need atmospheric oxygen and cannot exist without it. These bacteria are termed obligate aerobes. Others are the exact opposite and cannot exist in the presence of oxygen, requiring anaerobic situations (obligate anaerobes). The majority, however, are facultative anaerobes, which means they can exist in either the absence or presence of oxygen.

Physical conditions

Different bacteria can exist at both high and low extremes of pH and temperature. Pathogens prefer the medium state of pH7 and 37°C. Acidophilic bacteria prefer a low pH, while basophiles like a high one. Thermophilic bacteria grow best at between 55 and 80°C, while the spores of *Bacillus stearothermophilus* can withstand boiling. Some organisms can exist at very low temperatures.

Growth

Reproduction of bacteria is by binary fission. The cell divides and two equal daughter cells are formed. As there is no nucleus there is no mitosis. The time between a daughter cell being formed and itself dividing to form two new cells is called the generation time and varies greatly between species. It also varies with environmental conditions and the supply of nutrients. Some bacteria multiply very quickly and divide every 20 minutes. Others, like *M. tuberculosus*, take hours or even days.

When a new sterile environment with finite limits is colonized the bacterial cell population goes through four phases (see Fig. 3.3).

1. Lag phase, when the original inoculum remains dormant and no increase in numbers is seen.
2. Log phase, during which there is an exponential growth in the number of organisms and the logarithm of the number of cells is directly proportional to time. It is during the early stages of this phase that the bacterial population is most susceptible to antibacterial agents.

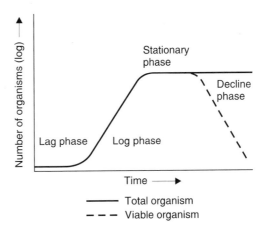

Figure 3.3 Bacterial growth.

3. Stationary phase, which represents a time when the number of viable organisms remains constant because the number of new organisms is equal to the number dying. This phase can be brought about by a depletion of essential nutrients, a change in the oxygen level or an accumulation of metabolites which regulate the growth.
4. Decline phase, in which the number of viable organisms declines.

Sporulation

It is the property of certain bacteria to produce endospores. They are produced inside the vegetative cell as compact masses with a very resistant coat. Once formed, the rest of the cell disintegrates releasing the spore.

Spores have the ability to withstand adverse environments which would be lethal to the vegetative cell. When the conditions are right the spore germinates into one vegetative cell (sporulation is not a form of multiplication).

Classification

Once a pure colony of an organism has been isolated by successive culturing, it is often necessary to find out which organism is present. Not only genus and species require elucidation but also the particular strain. To elicit this information the following techniques can be used:

1. Microscopy and staining
2. Differential media and biochemical tests
3. Serological testing
4. Bacteriophage typing.

Microscopy and differential staining

Gram's stain divides bacteria into Gram positive and Gram negative bacteria. Bacteria are fixed onto a microscopy slide and stained with a dark purple stain. The slide is then covered with an iodine solution to act as a mordant, i.e. to fix the stain onto the organisms. The next step is the decolorizing process in which the slide is treated with a solvent. A counterstain completes the process and the slide is viewed under the microscope. If the organism has resisted decolorization it is termed Gram positive and will appear purple under the microscope. If the original stain has been lost the colour of the counterstain will show through and the organism will be deemed Gram negative. This is a fundamental method of classifying bacteria.

Other differential stains have been used, e.g. acid fast staining, in which the organisms are subjected to a decolorizing process using acid. Specific stains can be used to show the presence of spore-forming bacteria.

Examination under the microscope not only gives information about the organisms' staining characteristics but, of course, about the shape. Basically, bacteria can be spherical (cocci), rod-shaped (bacilli) or spiral. Cocci can be divided according to their form of aggregation. Some bacteria appear in just one direction and form chains (Streptococci) while others give the appearance of a bunch of grapes (Staphylococci). However, the appearance of aggregations under the microscope can sometimes be deceptive and other tests are necessary to differentiate between Streptococci and Staphylococci.

Differential media and biochemical tests

Special media which can be designed to support the growth of some types of bacteria and not others can be useful in bacterial typing. Other tests examine the organism's ability to break down hydrogen peroxide, to liquefy protein and to ferment certain sugars. Media containing blood are useful in differentiating Streptococci.

Serological testing

Bacteria possess many potentially antigenic substances and one of the body's defences against bacterial invasion is to produce antibodies to these antigens. These antibodies are specific to the antigens and this specificity can assist in the determination not only of the genus and species but also the strain of bacteria present.

Bacteriophage typing

Bacteriophages are viruses that attack bacteria. They invade the bacterial cell just like any other host cell, and once inside they combine with the bacterial DNA and change the genetic material. This effect can be destructive and the whole cell is taken over, producing new phage particles. Bacteriophages are species specific to the bacterium they invade.

Viruses (see Fig. 3.4)

Viruses are much smaller than bacteria (18–300 nm). All known bacteria will be trapped by a 0.22 μm filter (sterilizing filter). Many viruses will pass through, hence the term filtrable viruses. Viruses can infect any form of higher organism and are usually divided into animal viruses, plant viruses and bacteriophages.

Viruses consist of either RNA or DNA (never both), surrounded by a layer of protein (capsid) or a membrane (referred to as the envelope). The outer covering of the virus particle plays a vital role in the initial infection of the cell and the spread of a virus within the host. The components of the covering layer are very antigenic and are involved in the host's immune response. Capsids are rigid structures and tend to be very protective against adverse environments such as desiccation and detergents. Such viruses tend to retain their infectivity on fomites and will withstand the adverse conditions in the gut, i.e. low pH and the presence of

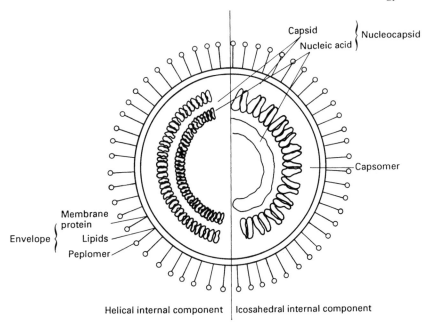

Figure 3.4 Diagram of a virus.

proteases. Envelopes are less protective and can be disrupted by acids, detergents and drying out. Thus the virus particles must remain in aqueous solution in order to survive and these viruses are transmitted by droplet infection or blood or other body fluids; they will not survive in the gut.

The nucleic acid may be single strand or double strand. Viruses contain few if any enzymes and are entirely reliant on the host cell to bring about replication; they are obligate intracellular parasites. They vary greatly in size and in the number of genes they carry (from three to several hundred).

Virus reproduction

Virus reproduction does not take place by binary fission. It generally takes the following pattern:

1. The virus particle (virion) becomes attached to the surface of the cell. There are usually specific receptors involved and this leads to the viral preference for certain cells within the host. For example, the HIV (AIDS) virus binds to CD4 receptors which are found on T cells.
2. The virus particle passes into the cell.
3. The virus particle loses its coat, releasing the viral genetic material into the host cytoplasm if it is RNA. For DNA viruses the genetic material must be delivered into the nucleus.
4. The viral genetic material induces the cell to produce different macro-molecules essential for the production of new viral particles.
5. Assembly of new virus particles takes place within the host cell and these are then released. The release may bring about disruption of the host cell. The new virus particles are available to infect new cells.

Classification of viruses

The classification of viruses is more difficult than that of bacteria. Many criteria are used in classifying viruses.

1. Morphology
2. Nucleic acid type
3. Immunological properties
4. Transmission methods
5. Host and cell tropisms
6. Symptomatology and pathology.

The following are the main groups of animal viruses:

Single strand DNA viruses

Parvo viruses e.g. Parvovirus B19

Double strand DNA viruses

Papova viruses, e.g. papilloma (wart virus)
Adeno viruses, e.g. adeno virus 8 – epidemic keratoconjunctivitis
Herpes viruses, e.g. Herpes simplex, varicella-zoster, cytomegalovirus
Pox viruses, e.g. smallpox, molluscum contagiosum
Hepatic viruses, e.g. Hepatitis B virus

Single strand RNA viruses

Picorna, e.g. poliomyelitis, Hepatitis A virus
Toga viruses, e.g. human respiratory disease, Rubella
Arena viruses, e.g. Lassa fever
Corona viruses, e.g. human respiratory disease
Retro viruses, e.g. HIV (AIDS)
Bunya viruses, e.g. insect borne diseases – California encephalitis
Orthomyxo viruses, e.g. influenza
Paramyxo viruses, e.g. measles, mumps
Rhabdo viruses, e.g. rabies

Double strand RNA viruses

Reoviruses, e.g. California tick fever

Chlamydiae

These organisms are more complex than viruses but less complex than bacteria. They can only multiply in susceptible cells but unlike viruses contain both DNA and RNA. They multiply by binary fission and are susceptible to certain antibiotics.

They exist in two forms: (a) as an elementary body (300 nm) which can exist outside the body and is the infectious unit, and (b) as a reticulate body (1000 nm) which only exists inside the cell and is not infectious.

Chlamydiae attack mucous membranes and inhibit host cell protein synthesis. They rely on the host to provide ATP, which they cannot generate. They synthesize their own nucleic acids and proteins. There are two species, *C. trachomatis* (trachoma, inclusion conjunctivitis) and *C. psittaci* (psittacosis).

Fungi

As causative organisms of disease, fungi are less important than bacteria and viruses. Out of the tens of thousands of species probably only about 100 are pathogenic. Some of these, however, are capable of producing very severe infections (filamentous keratitis) as well as the more trivial, such as athlete's foot. Fungi have the ability to colonize nonliving structures and lead to spoilation, e.g. hydrogel contact lenses.

Fungi are composed of eucaryotic cells with the normal inclusions, e.g. a nucleus and mitochondria. They can be divided into four groups according to their structure.

Moulds

These grow as a mycelium, which is composed of filamentous multicellular structures called hyphae. The mycelium is divided into the vegetative mycelium, which grows into the substrate and assimilates nutrients, and the aerial mycelium, which produces the spores either asexually by budding or sexually by the fusion of two cells.

Yeasts

These fungi occur as single cells and reproduce by budding.

Yeast-like fungi

Both hyphae and yeast cells exist together.

Dimorphic fungi

Dimorphic fungi exist either as yeasts or filaments. If they are grown on artificial media they appear as hyphae. When they inhabit a living host they occur as yeast cells.

Protozoal parasites

Protozoal parasites are best known for their ability to colonize and in some cases parasitize the alimentary tract, particularly in tropical countries. However, they are capable of living in other parts of the body and causing serious pathological conditions. The most important of these are the various forms of amoebae, which are primitive acellular organisms with a simple life cycle. They exist in two forms, the active trophozite which moves around its environment by the use of pseuodpodia (extensions of the cytoplasm in one direction and the drawing up of the rest of the organism), and the dormant cyst which lives in the spores of bacteria and is more resistant to unfavourable environments. Reproduction is either by simple binary fission of the active trophozite or the formation of multi-nucleated cysts.

Some amoebae are free living while others such as *Entamoeba coli* and *Entamoeba gingivalis* inhabit parts of the alimentary tract as commensals. Others are potent pathogens such as *Entamoeba hystolytica*, the causative organism of ameobic dysentery. *Naegleria fowleri* causes a rapidly fatal (4 to 5 days) meningoencephalitis.

Micro-organisms and disease

The human plays host to a large number of bacteria which normally do no harm and to varying degrees contribute to the body's wellbeing. For example, bacteria live on the dead surface of the skin and prevent other more potentially dangerous organisms from occupying the site. Bacteria which inhabit the gut provide the body with vitamin K, essential for the production of prothrombin, in exchange for nutrients. These commensal organisms only maintain this mutually advantageous relationship providing they remain in their proper place. One tissue's commensal is another's pathogen.

It is not always the micro-organism itself that causes the harm, but substances that the organism produces. Some bacteria live and multiply in food, producing toxins as they do so. When the food is ingested the toxins produce adverse effects. *Clostridium botulinum* is such an organism and the toxin it produces, botulinum toxin, is fatal in minute quantities. *Staphylococcus aureus* is also capable of bringing about food intoxication.

Most micro-organisms, however, cause disease by acting as parasites on the body, gaining access by a variety of routes.

Direct contact. This normally means sexual contact and the disease is classed as a venereal one. This method of transmission favours the very fastidious bacteria which exist only with difficulty outside the human body. *Treponema pallidum* (syphilis) is so fastidious that it has never been grown on lifeless media.

Indirect transmission. Infection is passed from one person to another by an inanimate object (called a fomite), e.g. bedclothes, used dressings, etc.

Dust-borne infection. Dust contains discarded human cells and dried water droplets. These are likely to carry bacteria, especially spores.

Droplet infection. Bacteria are present in the fine spray that is exhaled with forced expirations such as coughing and sneezing.

Water borne infection. Water is an excellent medium for transmitting infection. Public health and sanitation prevent this until some disaster interrupts the supply of clean drinking water.

Insect borne infection. Biting and sucking insects have the ability to take organisms from an infected host and transfer them to a new one.

Maternal transmission. In addition to the routes mentioned above, infections can also be passed from mother to child either while the child is still in the womb or during birth (e.g. ophthalmia neonatorum).

Microbiology of the eye

The eye is at risk from infection by opportunistic and invasive organisms via a variety of routes. In addition to congenital ocular infections, micro-organisms can gain access as a result of:

1. Direct contact e.g. Herpes simplex
2. Airborne infections
3. Insect-borne infections, e.g. trachoma
4. Migration of bacteria from the nasopharynx
5. Metastatic infection from other loci in the body
6. Trauma, especially penetrating injuries
7. Infected contact lenses
8. Infected eyedrops and lotions
9. Infected instruments.

Obviously the lids, cornea and conjunctiva are the most exposed and hence the most at risk from infection. Infections of these tissues are far more common than those of deeper tissues, but they are also less serious.

The eye is covered with tears which contain a number of antimicrobial agents in order to reduce the incidence of infections. The result is a fairly low level of microbial contamination in the fornices. Tears contain immunoglobulins A, G and M (IgA, IgG and IgM) (Reim, 1983) in different proportions to those found in plasma, suggesting that their origin is secretory rather than just the result of filtration.

There are also two agents with marked antibacterial properties, lysozyme and betalysin. Lysozyme is an enzyme capable of dissolving the cell wall of bacteria, especially Gram positive bacteria. The level of lysozyme decreases with age and is reduced in patients with dry eye syndrome (Mackle and Seal, 1976). Betalysin, on the other hand, acts principally on the cell membrane (Ford *et al.*, 1976) and works in concert with lysozyme. Since the cell membrane is the site of action of the bacterial enzymes, the effect is quite marked. Betalysin is also present in aqueous humour.

Some common ocular pathogens
Gram positive cocci
Staphylococcus aureus

Some Staphylococci are normal inhabitants of the skin and mucous membranes, whilst other species are capable of producing conditions such as boils, abscesses and even a fatal septicaemia. They are capable of bringing about a form of food poisoning by the liberation of an enterotoxin. Resistance to certain antibiotics develops easily and the term 'hospital Staph' is applied to some resistant forms, while the modern term is now MRSA (methicillin resistant *Staphylococcus aureus*).

Staphylococci are differentiated from Streptococci by the presence of an enzyme capable of breaking down hydrogen peroxide (catalase). Pathogenic Staphylococci possess coagulase, which clots blood plasma.

In the eye Staphylococci can cause infections of the lids, lacrimal apparatus, conjunctiva and cornea (Davis *et al.*, 1978). Infections of the lash follicle lead to the formation of a stye (hordeolum). Staphylococci can also produce acute or chronic blepharitis. This is sometimes associated with acute conjunctivitis (Brook, 1980; Brook *et al.*, 1979; Brown, 1978). This organism has also been found to be present in a large number of cases of ophthalmia neonatorum in one study (Jarvis *et al.*, 1987). The routine use of prophylactic eye ointments to prevent ophthalmia neonatorum can lead to the emergence of resistant strains. Hedberg *et al.* (1990) reported an outbreak of erythromycin resistant staphylococcal conjunctivitis in a newborn nursery in which erythromycin eye ointment was used as a prophylactic agent. Following septicaemia, Staphylococci have caused endophthalmitis (Bloomfield *et al.*, 1978).

Because *Staphylococcus aureus* is so common, it is often employed in the efficiency testing of preservative systems. *Staphylococcus epidermidis* is normally considered to be a commensal and is a normal inhabitant of the skin. Unlike *Staph. aureus* it produces white colonies. Maske *et al.* (1986) found a higher than normal incidence in a group of patients with bacterial corneal ulcers. It has been suggested that *Staph. epidermidis* releases a toxin to cause some of the signs of blepharitis and keratopathy (McGill *et al.*, 1982).

Streptococci

Streptococci lack the enzyme catalase and are characterized by their ability to cause haemolysis. Complete haemolysis is brought about by beta haemolytic Streptococci while the haemolysis produced by alpha haemolytic species is incomplete and leads to the formation of a green pigment. There are also non haemolytic Streptococci.

Streptococci are capable of producing local and general infections. One of the most common local infections of beta haemolytic Streptococci is the Streptococcal sore throat which in young children can extend into the middle ear to cause otitis media. On the skin they can cause impetigo.

Beta haemolytic Strep. infections give rise to puerperal fever, wound sepsis and endocarditis. It is fortunate that penicillin continues to be effective against many strains of Streptococci.

In the eye, infections may cause conjunctivitis, dacryoadenitis, dacryocystitis and blepharitis (Brook, 1980). Jones et al. (1988) reported corneal ulcers, endophthalmitis, conjunctivitis and dacryocystitis resulting from streptococcal infections. The ability of Streptococci to cause sight-threatening infections is of concern because many strains are not susceptible to gentamicin, an antibiotic often chosen to treat such infections.

Gram negative cocci

The Neisseriae are a group of Gram negative bacteria which include the normal flora of the respiratory system and the pathogens which cause meningitis (N. meningitidis) and gonorrhoea (N. gonorrhoeae).

In the eye Neisseriae can infect the lids, lacrimal apparatus and conjunctiva but N. gonorrhoeae is best known as the one-time principal cause of ophthalmia neonatorum, an infection which occurs as the infant passes down the birth canal. The disease becomes manifest between the second and fifth day after birth when the lids become swollen and there is a bilateral purulent discharge. The lids are tightly closed and difficult to open and the acute phase lasts for four to six weeks. The condition is treated with topical and systemic antibacterials. If treatment is not carried out, the cornea may become involved and the eye lost. However, other organisms such as Chlamydia and other causes (paradoxically the overenthusiastic use of silver nitrate) are more important today (Jarvis et al.,1987).

Gram positive rods
Corynebacterium diphtheriae

Corynebacteria are nonmotile Gram positive rods which do not form spores. Species are found normally resident in the human respiratory tract. C. diphtheriae when infected with the appropriate bacteriophage produces a powerful exotoxin which causes the pathology of diphtheria. The disease results in the growth of a membrane across the throat, leading to suffocation. It can similarly affect the eyelids, with the appearance of such membranes on the inner surface of the lids. The conjunctiva may become involved in the same way. Diphtheroids have been isolated in a proportion of infected conjunctivae (Brook et al., 1979; Brown, 1978).

Clostridia spp.

The Clostridia are a group of obligate anaerobes notorious for their pathogenicity. In particular, they include Cl. botulinum, which when it infects food produces botulinum toxin. Although botulinum toxin ingestion is potentially fatal, this substance has been used to paralyse the antagonist muscles in cases of paralytic strabismus (Elston and Lee, 1985) and other ocular disorders (Alpar, 1987). Cl. tetani is a possible infectant of deep wounds and prophylaxis against the effects of its toxin is routine. Other Clostridia such as Cl. perfringens, Cl. welchii and Cl. oedematiens cause gangrene. Gas gangrene of the lids has been reported (Crock et al., 1985).

Gram negative rods

This is by far the biggest group of pathogens, most of which are facultative anaerobes.

Pseudomonas aeruginosa

Pseudomonas aeruginosa is perhaps the most notorious of bacteria for causing ocular problems and is normally found in small numbers in the gut and on the skin. It is a common contaminant of water and has been cultured from jacuzzis (Brett, 1985). Its numbers are kept in check by the presence of other organisms, but since it is resistant to many antibiotics it can gain dominance if the surrounding organisms are suppressed. *Pseudomonas aeruginosa* produces a bluish green colour when grown on media, has a characteristic odour and is pyogenic, the presence of green pus suggesting the presence of a *Pseudomonas* infection.

Pseudomonas aeruginosa is an opportunistic organism and is normally kept at bay by the body's defence mechanisms. Once these are breached a serious infection often results. It can infect burns, especially those of large area, and can also gain a hold in patients who are immune-compromised. *Ps. aeruginosa* is an extremely versatile organism in that it can metabolize fluorescein and hydroxybenzoates as carbon sources for energy, which means that it can survive in conditions which are alien to most other organisms. This organism is only susceptible to antibiotics such as gentamicin and polymixin.

In the eye, *Ps. aeruginosa* can produce meibomitis, conjunctivitis and corneal ulcers and is one of the causes of ophthalmia neonatorum (Cole *et al.*, 1980). Should access be gained to the sterile interior of the eye, then panophthalmitis may result and indeed has been responsible for causing more than one serious case of hospital acquired disease leading to the loss of an eye (Crompton, 1978). It is an important test organism for contact lens solutions and eyedrop preservative systems, not only for its virulence when an infection is established but also because of its biochemical versatility which sometimes makes it difficult to eradicate.

Haemophilus spp.

These are small aerobic organisms which get their name from their requirement for enriched media containing blood for culturing *in vitro*. They include certain important human pathogenic organisms. *H. influenzae* is a secondary invader which helps to produce some of the symptoms of influenza and can produce inflammation in most parts of the respiratory tract. *Bordetella pertussis* is another of this group to affect the respiratory system, causing whooping cough which is transmitted by airborne infections from one person to another. It cannot exist for long periods outside the body. Similarly, *H. ducreyi* is so fastidious in its requirements that it can only be transmitted sexually and is the causative organism of chancroid, a form of venereal disease.

H. influenzae and *H. ducreyi* are capable of infecting ocular tissues. There are two members of this group which are particularly noted for their ability to cause conjunctivitis. *H. aegyptius* (*H. conjunctivitidis*, Koch–Weeks bacillus) is often the cause of acute epidemic conjunctivitis, especially in schoolchildren. *Moraxella lacunata* (Morax–Axenfeld bacillus) is another well-known causative organism of conjunctivitis.

Viruses
Herpes viruses

The most important members of the Herpes group as far as the eye is concerned are H. zoster, H. simplex and Cytomegalovirus.

H. zoster (varicella) virus leads to chickenpox in children. This is a mild, highly contagious disease characterized by a vesicular rash. The disease leaves the patient with a continuing immunity to the disease. In the adult, a reactivation of the virus leads to shingles, in which an area of the body becomes covered with a painful rash. Evidently the virus becomes stored in a sensory ganglion, the attack being caused by a migration of the virus along the nerve root. When the nerve affected is the ophthalmic division of the trigeminal nerve, the area served by it exhibits signs, i.e. the eye, the orbit and surrounding areas. This is known as Herpes zoster ophthalmicus, in which the cornea becomes inflamed and oedematous, and sensitivity may be impaired permanently. Secondary infection can occur, leading to ulceration and scarring.

Herpes simplex can be differentiated into Types I and II. Type II is associated with genital herpes and neonatal herpes. Transplacental infection with Type II virus has led to the development of neonatal cataract (Cibis and Burge, 1971). Type I causes cold sores, inflammation of the oral cavity, encephalitis and dendritic ulcers.

Dendritic ulcers are so called because of their branching pattern. As the ulcer extends it may lose this appearance and become amoeboid or geographic. The patient complains of pain, photophobia, blurring of vision and a watery discharge (unlike that from bacterial conjunctivitis). In the early stages, infection only affects the epithelium, later progressing to the superficial stroma. The cornea becomes oedematous and there is further loss of stroma and possible vascularization. The condition is treated with intense local antiviral therapy. Herpes simplex can also produce a keratoconjunctivitis similar to that caused by adenovirus 8 (Darougar et al., 1978) (see below).

The third virus in this group is Cytomegalovirus, which normally inhabits the female reproductive tract giving rise to congenital infections. Congenital infections can give rise to chorioretinitis, optic atrophy and cataract.

Adenovirus 8

Adenovirus 8 gives rise to epidemic keratoconjunctivitis, sometimes called 'eye hospital eye' because of its possible transmission by contaminated instruments. The infection produces severe acute conjunctivitis which can spread, leading to keratitis. Marked discomfort can last for months. Adenovirus was the cause of 8% of cases of acute conjunctivitis in one study (Wishart et al., 1984).

Pox viruses

This group of viruses includes smallpox and cowpox. There is a relatively uncommon skin condition affecting young adults and children, Molluscum contagiosum, which is caused by a pox virus. Transparent nodules (2–3 mm in diameter) appear on the skin of the arm, legs, back and face, with possible involvement of the lid margins and conjunctiva. This condition is sometimes seen in patients with AIDS and AIDS related complex (ARC).

Toga viruses

The best known member of this group is rubella (German measles), which can be passed from mother to baby in the uterus, leading to congenital defects in 30% of the children of mothers suffering rubella in the first trimester of pregnancy. Particularly affected are the heart, ears and eyes. Ophthalmic defects lead to microphthalmia, cataracts and congenital glaucoma.

Retroviruses

The Human Immunodeficiency Virus (HIV) is present in many of the body fluids of affected individuals, including tears. Although there has been no recorded case of transmission via infected contact lenses, it has become a point of concern for contact lens practitioners. The virus has also been recovered from contact lenses worn by patients with AIDS and ARC (AIDS related complex) (Tervo *et al.*, 1986). AIDS can have certain ocular manifestations, partially because the patients are from the very nature of the disease more likely to develop opportunistic infections such as Cytomegalovirus retinitis. Conjunctival Kaposi's sarcoma is another ocular complication (Kanski, 1987).

Fungi
Candida albicans

This is a dimorphic opportunistic fungus which is normally found in the mucous membranes of the mouth, vagina, gut and eye (Liotet *et al.*, 1980). It causes oral thrush in newborn infants and terminally ill patients. In the eye it can cause corneal ulcers, conjunctivitis and severe uveitis.

Aspergillus niger

This fungus, which is not dimorphic, grows in the form of mycelia. Often found in vegetable matter, it can cause bronchial problems. It is also capable of producing severe local infection in the eye, especially following the injudicious use of local corticosteroids which tend to mask the clinical signs of the infection, allowing it to get a stronger foothold. A case of Aspergillus panophthalmitis has been reported in a patient after excision of a pterygium, who received beta radiation treatment (Margo *et al.*, 1988). *A. niger*, which also can be found in the healthy eye (Liotet *et al.*, 1980), has the ability to infect hydrogel contact lenses and destroy them. Other species of *Aspergillus* have been implicated in contact lens contamination. For example, Yamaguchi (1984) reported growth on a contact lens of *A. flavus* and Filppi *et al.* (1973) found that *A. fumagatus* penetrated soft contact lenses. Aspergillus species are not the only ones to infect contact lenses. Yamamoto *et al.* (1979) found *Cephalosporium acremonium* growing on a contact lens worn for the treatment of metaherpetic keratitis.

Chlamydia
Trachoma
(C. trachomatis)

Trachoma affects a large proportion of the world's population, being endemic in many areas where it affects over 90% of the population. Associated with poor living conditions, this organism is passed on by insects and contaminated objects such as bedclothes (fomites). It is sometimes a resident of the female genital tract (Barton *et al.*, 1985) and can produce a form of ophthalmia neonatorum (Markham, 1979). The incidence of Chlamydial ophthalmia neonatorum varies. In one study in America, 1.4% of all newborn babies acquired chlamydial conjunctivitis (Schacter *et al.*, 1979) and similar findings were reported in Sweden (Persson *et al.*,

1983) and Wolverhampton (Preece *et al.*, 1989). In the latter report it was concluded that screening for chlamydial antigen was not justified as the condition could easily be treated with oral erythromycin. This condition starts as a mild inflammation of the conjunctiva with the development of small follicles which become larger. The cornea is invaded and vascularized, resulting in pannus which can lead to severe scarring and contraction which causes deformity of eyelids. Symblepharon and trichiasis are also seen. In temperate climates, the organism results in inclusion conjunctivitis.

Amoebae

Acanthamoebae like *Naegleria* can infect the brain, but they produce a different amoebic encephalitis (Ma *et al.*, 1990). Amoebic keratitis has been reported as a result of infection with *Acanthamoebae* (Moore *et al.*, 1986). The patients in the report were myopes corrected with soft contact lenses who had used salt tablets dissolved in distilled water during disinfection procedures. This infection has so far proved to be difficult to treat.

Antimicrobial agents

There are many 'agents' which have the ability to kill or inactivate microorganisms. Within this broad term we encompass the body's defence mechanisms, i.e. the white blood cells and circulating antibodies of the blood, the gastric hydrochloric acid and the lyzosyme and betalysin of tears, whilst other micro-organisms such as bacteriophages must also be considered as antimicrobial agents.

Here we are concerned with three basic groups:

1. Physical agents capable of rendering objects and chemicals free of contamination
2. Antimicrobial preservatives which are incorporated into solutions to maintain sterility
3. Chemotherapeutic agents used either to treat or prevent an infection in the body.

It is important to define certain terms which are relevant to this subject and are sometimes used incorrectly.

Sterilization means the killing or removal of all viable organisms (including bacterial spores) from an object or pharmaceutical product by the use of chemical or physical agents.

Disinfection is a lesser process by which the capacity of an object to cause infection is removed. A disinfected product may not be 'sterile'. Antisepsis is a similar degree of decontamination, but refers to solutions and chemicals that are safe to apply to surfaces of the body.

Chemotherapeutic agents are described as bactericidal or bacteriostatic; the former are actually capable of killing the bacteria (although not necessarily bacterial spores) while bacteriostatic agents prevent bacteria from growing and rely on the body's own defence mechanism to get rid of the organisms.

Physical agents

All physical agents are forms of energy and the antimicrobial action is dependent on supplying sufficient energy to cause disruption to the cell.

Bacteria and other micro-organisms are far more resistant to adverse situations than animal cells and can withstand environments which would quickly be lethal to us. The effect of antimicrobial agents follows a first order reaction in which the log number of survivors is inversely proportional to the time. The time for one log cycle reduction, i.e. the time taken for 90% of the bacteria to be killed, is called the D value or decimal death time, this value reducing as the antimicrobial effect increases.

Heat

Heat is one of the best known disinfecting and sterilizing agents. It is used for sterilizing solutions (providing that the substances are thermostable), dressings and some instruments. The effectiveness of heat is increased by the presence of water, especially if the pH is raised, the use of moist heat bringing hydrolysis to bear on the organisms as well as pyrolysis. Temperatures of around 60°C will kill most viruses as well as the vegetative cells of pathogenic bacteria and fungi, whereas boiling brings about the demise of spores of pathogenic bacteria.

However, there are organisms whose spores will withstand boiling for lengthy periods. Therefore, to obtain sterility without compromising the product, autoclaves are used. These work on the 'pressure cooker' principle by heating the product in steam (not air) to a defined temperature for a specified time, which is usually 121°C for 15 minutes.

The use of dry heat is far less efficient and temperatures of up to 160°C for one hour are needed to kill spores.

Disinfection, as opposed to sterilization, can be brought about by boiling for 10–15 minutes.

Temperatures below boiling can reduce the number of micro-organisms present and are used for materials which cannot withstand heating at high temperatures. Milk is pasteurized at 60–70°C, for example. The temperature inside a soft lens storage case subjected to heating by steam will not reach boiling point, but the temperature attained (95°C) is very bactericidal. Thermal disinfection of contact lenses is discussed in Chapter 14.

Freezing

Freezing the cultures of bacteria will markedly reduce the number of bacteria as a proportion may be damaged by the formation of ice crystals, but the rest will survive in a dormant state even at temperatures as low as that of liquid nitrogen. Indeed this process is used to store cultures of bacteria.

Ionizing radiation

This technique is used for disposable plastic items and for paper products such as fluorescein impregnated strips. All types of rays are lethal to micro-organisms (alpha, beta and gamma rays). Usually gamma rays are used, at a dosage of 2.5–3.5 MRad.

Ultraviolet radiation

Light is only bactericidal at low wavelengths (240–280 nm – the UVC region) and at this level does not penetrate well, making it suitable only for surface and aerial disinfection.

Filtration

Solutions of thermolabile drugs can be sterilized by passing the solution through a 0.22 μm filter which retains all bacteria (the smallest bacterium is about 0.5 μm). The filters, which are sterilized before use, will not remove viral contamination.

Ultrasonics

Sound will kill bacteria, but high power inputs are required. Ultrasonic cleaners with antibacterial agents have been used on contact lenses.

Antimicrobial preservatives

There are a whole range of substances incorporated into products to prevent the growth of micro-organisms. These are used in foods, drinks and cosmetics, but are most important in multidose sterile pharmaceutical solutions to ensure that the product is protected from microbial attack while it is in use.

These compounds are selected for their ability to kill or inhibit the growth of micro-organisms, particularly bacteria and fungi. The rate of kill represented by the D value is dependent upon the concentration of the preservative, but is not always a simple inverse relationship, i.e. with the D value inversely proportional to the concentration of the preservative compound. With some compounds the effect is exponential, with a reduction of concentration to half of the original leading to an increase in D value of a factor of 2^8, or 256. Such compounds are thus quickly inactivated by dilution.

These agents are capable of producing damage to human cells, and it is necessary to use them in as low a concentration as possible to reduce toxicity, the final concentration therefore representing a compromise between safety and efficacy. In order to achieve greater efficacy without increasing the toxic effects, mixtures of preservatives are often used. Many such agents have been used in the past; the following are those in common use.

Benzalkonium chloride (BAK)

Benzalkonium chloride has a detergent action which causes disruption of the cell membrane, and it is by far the most commonly used preservative for eye drops. Benzalkonium chloride has a disruptive effect on the tear film when used in concentrations of 0.01% and greater (Wilson *et al.*, 1975). This preservative is often found combined with EDTA (ethylene diamine tetra acetic acid, sodium edetate). EDTA is a chelating agent which combines with divalent ions (normally calcium) to form a nonionizable complex. This agent has a slight antibacterial action of its own but is principally used to enhance the bactericidal action of benzalkonium chloride.

Mercury compounds

Mercurial compounds include thiomersal and phenylmercuric nitrate. They produce mercury ions which react with sulphydryl groups of essential enzymes and are slower in action against certain organisms but are less quickly inactivated by dilution than other compounds. Unlike benzalkonium chloride, mercury compounds are not potentiated by the addition of EDTA (Richards and Reary, 1972). In fact, Morton (1985) found that EDTA actually reduces the antimicrobial efficacy of thiomersal. Significant penetration of mercury-containing compounds into the aqueous humour following their use has been recorded by Winder *et al.* (1980). These compounds have been demonstrated to have cytotoxic effects which are time and concentration dependent (Takahashi, 1982), but which are less than those of benzalkonium chloride (Gasset *et al.*, 1974), and their use in many contact lens solutions has led to the increasing incidence of allergic reactions (Gold, 1983).

Chlorhexidine gluconate

Chlorhexidine is a useful alternative to benzalkonium chloride and is used when the latter is incompatible with the active ingredient. It is very toxic to the corneal endothelium in concentrations of 20 µg/ml and if the epithelium is perfused the result is a sloughing of the cells without corneal swelling (Green *et al.*, 1980).

Oxidizing agents

Strong oxidizing agents are very bactericidal. Probably the best known is hydrogen peroxide, which kills most vegetative forms at a concentration of 3 to 6% while stronger concentrations (>10%) will dispose of spores. The halogens are also strong oxidizing agents and part of the action of iodine and chlorine based disinfectant systems is the oxidation of essential enzymes. Although iodine in simple solution is still occasionally used it is most often complexed with another compound to form an iodophor. Iodine can be complexed with poly-vinylpyrrolidine to form povidone iodine.

Other compounds

Other compounds that have been used include chlorbutol, cetrimide, phenylethanol, hydroxybenzoates and chlorocresol.

Chemotherapeutic agents

The treatment of infections has evolved somewhat since the treatment of syphilis with mercurial compounds. Developments have led to the introduction of agents which are more effective against the infecting organism and less toxic to the host.

Anti-infectives tend to be specific against groups of organisms, e.g. antibacterials, antifungals, although there is some overlap. Certain antibacterials are effective against chlamydiae.

The mode of action of antibacterial agents varies greatly. In order to produce the desired effect without causing a toxic reaction from the patient they must interfere with some specific function important to the parasitizing cells. Modes of action include the following.

Inhibition of the formation of the cell wall

Many of the common antibiotics produce their activity by interfering with the formation of cell walls. Penicillin and the other beta-lactam antibiotics such as cephalosporins work in this manner, as well as vancomycin and bacitracin. The antibiotic molecules combine with enzymes responsible for cell wall synthesis preventing new wall being laid down and causing the destruction of existing material. In the normal bacterial cell the membrane is pushed against the cell wall by osmotic pressure. Without this constraint water balance is not maintained and cell death occurs. These antibiotics are most effective against populations which are actively growing as this is the stage of maximum cell wall production. Such agents are normally bactericidal.

Inhibition or damage to the cell membrane

The cell membrane of the procaryotic cell is even more important than that of the eucaryotic cell because the former lacks mitochondria and respiratory membranes are located on the membrane. Any disruption of the membrane, as well as interfering with the transport of substances into and out of the cell, will have an effect on cell respiration.

Inhibition of protein synthesis

Many of the more modern antibiotic groups can be found under this heading – the tetracyclines, aminoglycosides, macrolides chloramphenicol and clindamycin. Their site of action is the ribosomes where they either bind directly or prevent the binding of tRNA. Many of these antibiotics are bacteriostatic.

Inhibition of nucleic acid synthesis

The most important group in this section are the quinolones, of which new members are constantly introduced. Also included are rifampicin, used in the modern treatment of tuberculosis, and metronidazole, often used in the treatment of dental anaerobic infections. Rifampicin inhibits the formation of RNA while the quinolones interfere with the development of DNA.

Antimetabolites

The best known antimetabolites are the sulphonamides which interfere with the uptake of para-amino-benzoic acid (PABA), which prevents the synthesis of folic acid. Trimethoprim is taken up by an enzyme necessary for the ultilization of folic acid. Interference with the metabolism of folic acid inhibits the production of new genetic material.

The administration of antimicrobial agents for the treatment of infection requires the achievement of adequate levels of the antimicrobial agent as quickly as possible. For many antibiotics, this level is referred to as the Minimum Inhibitory Concentration (MIC), which is the concentration which prevents visible growth after a 24 hour incubation period. Unless the route of administration can achieve a level substantially higher than the MIC for the invading organism, it is unlikely that successful treatment of the infection will be achieved. For bactericidal agents the figure quoted is Minimum Bactericidal Concentration (MBC), which is the concentration that kills 99.99% of the bacterial cells.

The higher the concentration of the agent the greater will be the effect on the organism. Failure to achieve high levels may lead to the development of resistant strains. In any population there will be a proportion of organisms which are resistant to the agent, and in the presence of the agent these will be selected and will form the majority of the population.

Some bacteria develop resistance by altering their metabolic pathways to avoid those with which the antimicrobial interacts. Other bacteria produce enzymes capable of destroying the chemical, e.g. penicillinase, which is an enzyme produced by certain strains of Staphylococci and is capable of breaking down penicillin.

Hygiene in practice

Whilst there has been no recorded case of a patient contracting AIDS from a contaminated contact lens, this condition has highlighted the necessity for good practice hygiene. The AIDS virus is not the only organism (opportunist or invasive) that could be transmitted in an optometrist's practice and simple disinfection procedures should be employed in order to protect both practitioner and patient.

The first consideration is one of cleanliness, since clean objects and surfaces are easier to disinfect and will remain uncontaminated for longer. Normal contaminants will harbour bacteria, protect them from antibacterial agents, provide them with nutrients and inactivate disinfectants.

Jacobs (1986) has laid down simple infection control guidelines for optometrists and contact lens practitioners. Basically, anything that can be boiled without adversely affecting its performance should be, e.g. bowls, soft contact lenses. Items of equipment that will touch the eye should be swabbed with 70% alcohol, e.g. tonometer heads, chin rests, trial frames. Working surfaces should be treated with 1% sodium hypochlorite solution, which is effective against bacteria and viruses. At levels as low as 500 ppm (0.05%) it destroys Herpes simplex, Adenovirus 8 and Enterovirus 70 within ten minutes (Naginton *et al.*, 1983). Such procedures will protect the patient more than will a prophylactic eye drop.

In the interests of self protection the practitioner should have no open cuts uncovered, but the added precaution of wearing gloves is only necessary for high risk patients, e.g. patients who are HIV positive.

References

Alpar, A. I. (1987) Botulinum toxin and its uses in the treatment of ocular disorders. *Am. J. Optom. Physiol. Optics*, **64**, 79–82

Barton, S. E., Thomas, B. J., Taylor Robinson, D. and Goldmeier, D. (1985) Detection of *Chlamydia trachomatis* in the vaginal vault of women who have had hysterectomies. *Br. Med. J.*, **27**, 250

Bloomfield, S. E., David, D. S., Cheigh, J. S., Kim, Y., White, R. P., Stengel, K. H. and Rubin, A. L. (1978) Endophthalmitis following staphylococcal sepsis in renal failure patients. *Arch. Int. Med.*, **138**, 706–708

Brett, J. (1985) *Pseudomonas aeruginosa* and whirlpools. *Br. Med. J.*, April 6, 1024–1025

Brook, I. (1980) Anaerobic and aerobic bacterial flora of acute conjunctivitis in children. *Arch. Ophthalmol.*, **98**, 833–835

Brook, I., Pettit, T. H., Martin, W. J. and Finegold, S. M. (1979) Anaerobic and aerobic bacteriology of acute conjunctivitis. *Ann. Ophthalmol.*, **11**, 389–393

Brown D. H. (1978) The conjunctival flora of nursing home patients and staff. *Ann. Ophthalmol.*, **10**, 333–334

Cibis, A. and Burge, R. M. (1971) Herpes simplex virus induced cataracts. *Arch. Ophthalmol.*, **85**, 220–223

Cole, G. F., Davies, D. P. and Austin D. J. (1980) Pseudomonas ophthalmia neonatorum: a cause of blindness. *Br. Med. J.*, August 9, 440–441

Crock, G. W., Heriot, W. J., Janakiraman, P. and Weiner, J. M. (1985) Gas gangrene infection of the eye and orbit. *Br. J. Ophthalmol.*, **69**, 143–148

Crompton, D. O. (1978) Medical ethics and hospital-acquired disease. *Lancet*, July 15, 146

Darougar, S., Hunter, P. A., Viswalingam, M., Gibson, J. A. and Jones, B. R. (1978) Acute follicular conjunctivitis and keratoconjunctivitis due to Herpes simplex virus in London. *Br. J. Ophthalmol.*, **62**, 843–849

Davis, S. D., Sarff, L. D. and Hyndiuk, R. A. (1978) Staphylococcal keratitis. *Arch. Ophthalmol.*, **96**, 2114–2116

Elston, J. S. and Lee, J. P. (1985) Paralytic strabismus: the role of botulinum toxin. *Br. J. Ophthalmol.*, **69**, 891–896

Filppi, J. A., Pfister, R. M. and Hill, R. M. (1973) Penetration of hydrophilic contact lenses by *Aspergillus Fumagatus*. *Am. J. Optom. Physiol. Optics*, **50**, 553–557

Ford, L. C., DeLange, R. J. and Petty, R. W. (1976) Identification of a nonlysozymal bacteriocidal factor (betalysin) in human tears and aqueous humour. *Am. J. Ophthalmol.*, **81**, 30–33

Gasset, A. R., Ishn, Y., Kaufman, H. E. and Miller, I. (1974) Cytotoxicity of ophthalmic preservatives. *Am. J. Ophthalmol.*, **78**, 98–105

Gold, R. M. (1983) The war on thiomersal. *Contemporary Optometry*, **2**, 7–10

Green, K., Livingston, V., Bowman, K. and Hull, D. S. (1980) Chlorhexidine effects on corneal epithelium and endothelium. *Arch. Ophthalmol.*, **98**, 1273–1278

Hedberg, K. *et al.* (1990) Outbreak of erythromycin resistant staphylococcal conjunctivitis in a new born nursery. *Paediatr. Infect. Dis. J.*, **9**, 268–273

Jacobs, R. J. (1986) Infection control guidelines for optometrists and contact lens practitioners. *Clin. Exp. Optom.*, **69**, 40–45

Jarvis, V. N., Levine, R. and Asbell, P. A. (1987) Ophthalmia neonatorum. Study of a decade of experience at the Mount Sinai Hospital. *Br. J. Ophthalmol.*, **71**, 295–300

Jones, S. *et al.* (1988) Ocular streptococcal infections. *Cornea*, **7**, 295–299

Kanski, J. J. (1987) Ocular manifestation of AIDS. *The Optician*, 2 March, 24–25

Liotet, S., Krzywkowski, J. C., Warret, V. N. and Jacqui, C. (1980) Conjunctival flora of healthy people. *J. Fr. Ophthalmol.*, **103**, 557–560

Ma, P. *et al.* (1990) Naegleria and Acanthamoeba infections. *Rev. Infect. Dis.*, **12**, 490–513

Mackie, I. A. and Seal, D. V. (1976) Quantitative tear lysozyme essay in units of activity per microlitre. *Br. J. Ophthalmol.*, **60**, 70–74

Margo, C. E., Polack, F. M. and Mood, C. I. (1988) *Aspergillus panophthalmitis* complicating treatment of pterygium. *Cornea*, **7**, 285–289

Markham, J. G. (1979) Genital tract to eye infection – tissue culture of *Chlamydia trachomatis*. *N.Z. Med. J.*, **90**, 186–188

Maske, R., Hill, J. C. and Oliver, S. P. (1986) Management of bacterial corneal ulcers. *Br. J. Ophthalmol.*, **70**, 199–201

Moore, M. B., McCulley, J. P., Kaufman, H. E. and Robin, J. B. (1986) Radial keratoneuritis as a presenting sign in acanthamoeba keratitis. *Ophthalmology*, **93**, 1310–1315

Morton, D. J. (1985) EDTA reduces the antimicrobial efficacy of thiomersal. *Int. J. Pharm.*, **23**, 357–358

McGill, J., Goulding, N. J., Liakos, G., Jacobs, P. and Seal, D. V. (1982) Pathophysiology of bacterial infection in the external eye. *Trans. Ophthalmol. Soc. UK*, **102**, 7–10

Naginton, J., Sutehall, G. M. and Whipp, A. (1983) Tonometer disinfection and viruses. *Br. J. Ophthalmol.*, **67**, 674–676

Persson, K., Ronnerstam, R., Svanberg, L. and Pohla, M.-A. (1983) Neonatal chlamydial eye infection: an epidemiological and clinical study. *Br. J. Ophthalmol.*, **67**, 700–704

Preece, P. M., Anderson, J. M. and Thompson, R. G. (1989) Chlamydia trachomatis infection in infants. A prospective study. *Arch. Dis. Child.*, **64**, 525–529

Reim, M. (1983) Normal and pathological components of tears and conjunctival secretion. *The Ophthalmic Optician*, May 21, 346–350

Richards, R. M. E. and Reary, J. M. E. (1972) Changes in antibacterial activity of thiomersal and PMN on autoclaving with certain adjuvants. *J. Pharm. Pharmacol.*, **24**, 84P–85P

Schacter, J., Holt, J., Goodmer, E., Grossman, M., Sweet, R. and Mills, J. (1979) Prospective study of chlamydial infection in neonates. *Lancet*, August 25, 377–379

Takahashi, N. (1982) Cytotoxicity of mercurial preservatives in cell culture. *Ophthalmic Research*, **14**, 63–69

Tervo, T., Lahdevirto, J., Vaheria, A., Valle, S. L. and Suni, J. (1986) Recovery of HTLV-III from contact lenses. *Lancet*, February 15, 379–380

Wilson, W. S., Duncan, A. J. and Jay, J. (1975) Effect of benzalkonium chloride on the stability of the precorneal tear film in rabbit and man. *Br. J. Ophthalmol.*, **59**, 667–669

Winder, A. F., Astbury, N. J., Sheraidah, G. A. K. and Ruben, M. (1980) Penetration of mercury from ophthalmic preservatives into the human eye. *Lancet*, **2**, 237–239

Wishart, P. K., James, C., Wishart, M. S. and Darougar, S. (1984) Prevalence of acute conjunctivitis caused by chlamydia adenovirus, and Herpes simplex virus in an ophthalmic casualty department. *Br. J. Ophthalmol.*, **68**, 653–655

Yamaguchi, T. (1984) Fungus growth on soft contact lenses with different water contents. *Contact Lens J.*, **10**, 166–171

Yamamoto, G. K., Pavan-Langston, D., Stowe, G. C and Albert, D. M. (1979) Fungal invasion of a therapeutic soft contact lens and cornea. *Ann. Ophthalmol.*, **11**, 1731–1735

Further reading

Coster, D. J. (1979) Treacher Collins Prize Essay. Inflammatory diseases of the outer eye. *Trans. Ophthalmol. Socs UK*, **99**, 463–480

Coster, D. J. (1978) Herpetic keratitis and corneal destruction. *Trans. Ophthalmol. Socs UK*, **98**, 372–376

4

Ophthalmic dosage forms

Routes of administration

Drugs will only produce their desired action if they are present at the site of action in sufficient quantities, and the design and choice of the route of administration must take this into account. Certain parts of the eye are more accessible to drugs given by one route than they would be by another. Drugs also vary in their ability to cross capillary and mucous membrane barriers.

Basically, there are three routes by which drugs can be administered to the eye.

Direct injection

This can be either periocular (subconjunctival or retrobulbar) or intra-vitreal. These routes are used when relatively large doses of drug are required at a site very quickly. Antibiotics such as gentamicin are poorly absorbed and for deep infections intravitreal injection may be the only possible route. In the treatment of serious corneal and anterior segment infections, subconjunctival injections of 500 000 units or more of crystal-line penicillin with adrenaline may be repeated every three hours. In desperate cases of intraocular suppuration an absolutely pure penicillin solution injection may be given directly into the anterior chamber or the vitreous (Miller, 1978). A Tenon's capsule injection should result in more effective penetration of the drug than a subconjunctival one, in Havener's opinion (1978).

Local anaesthesia of the eye may be produced by retrobulbar injection of local anaesthetics.

Systemic administration

This route makes use of the ocular blood supply to carry drugs to the eye. While some parts of the eye are richly supplied with blood vessels, others are not. The systemic route, of course, means that the rest of the body receives a dose of the drug which may not be desirable. Drugs may gain access to the systemic blood supply by a variety of routes, but for ophthalmic treatment they are given either orally or parenterally. Acetazolamide (a diuretic for the treatment of glaucoma) is not effective topically and is administered as tablets for the emergency treatment of chronic open angle glaucoma or by injection for the emergency treatment of closed angle glaucoma. Antibiotics are sometimes given orally to supplement their topical use. In fluorescein angiography the dye is normally injected.

Topical application

This is by far the most common route of administration of drugs for the eye. Topically applied agents produce effective levels mainly in the anterior segment. However, if the lens capsule is removed during intra-capsular cataract extraction drugs can gain access to deeper layers. As far as the optometrist is concerned, the topical route is the only one that is applicable.

Dosage forms for topical ophthalmic use

The following is a list of dosage forms that have been developed as a means of delivering ophthalmic drugs. Some are in common use, some are merely experimental while others are no longer used.

1. Aqueous eye drops
2. Oily eye drops
3. Eye ointments
4. Eye lotions
5. Paper strips
6. Lamellae
7. Ocuserts
8. Iontophoresis
9. Contact lenses
10. Collagen shields
11. Ophthalmic rods.

Aqueous eye drops

Aqueous eye drops have the advantage of quick absorption and effect and there is little or no interference with viewing the media, the fundus or its reflex in such examination procedures as ophthalmoscopy, slit lamp microscopy and retinoscopy. The effects of eye drops are briefer than those of eye ointments, which constitutes an advantage in their diagnostic application but a disadvantage in their therapeutic or prophylactic use. Aqueous eye drops carry the risk of systemic toxicity due to their absorption by the alimentary tract following drainage through the nasolacrimal duct.

Viscous or oily eye drops reduce this possibility, while eye ointments allow for even less drainage. Retention of the medicament in the conjunctival sac will give better therapeutic results and fewer systemic toxic effects.

Although eye drops may appear to be an efficient method of drug application, their effects are subject to many variables. In spite of these, reproducible results may nevertheless be obtained from their use. For example, it is calculated that only 1.5% of topically applied pilocarpine is absorbed (Patton and Francoeur, 1978). The volume of the drop varies and so does that of the conjunctival sac into which it is instilled, a problem which is exacerbated by multiple instillations of eye drops. At least 10 minutes should be allowed between drops to allow absorption. Normally the volume of the drop exceeds the volume of the conjunctival sac, leading to an immediate loss of some of the drug. There is some controversy about the volume of a drop delivered by a dropper bottle, Brown *et al.* (1985) finding volumes of between 50 and 70 µl, whereas Akers (1983) reported a normal drop size of 25–50 µl. Both investigators agreed that the conjunctival sac volume is between 7 and 10 µl. Certainly there would be an advantage in reducing the size of the drop administered. Wheatcroft *et al.* (1993) studied the mydriatic response to solutions of phenylephrine 2.5% and cyclopentolate 0.5% in premature infants when the drop size was reduced from the standard 26 µl to 5 µl. They found no difference in response between the two drop sizes. When drops the size of which exceed that of the conjunctival sac are administered, the excess is mostly lost into the nasolacrimal system, where it poses the risk of possible systemic toxicity. Virtually all eye drops sting on instillation and thus will cause reflex tearing, resulting in further loss of drug. Some of the compound will be absorbed by the conjunctival blood vessels and be unavailable for absorption by the cornea.

The state of the corneal epithelium will have a great influence on the rate at which drugs will be absorbed, especially water soluble (polar) drugs (Akers, 1983). Furthermore, the level of pigmentation of the eye, the state of health of the eye and concomitant systemic medication will also influence the response. If the eye is inflamed then the increased blood flow will serve to carry drugs away from the eye.

Aqueous eye drops are solutions of the drug in water, often with other ingredients.

Preservatives. All multidose containers contain a preservative (see Chapter 3) to prevent bacterial growth during use. As an additional safeguard against infection, multidose drop bottles should be discarded after 28 days if used on one patient or seven days if used on several patients. The level of preservative in eye drops is important and is often higher than that in those contact lens solutions that come in contact with the eye. Adverse reactions to preservatives may develop after chronic use of drops, e.g. in glaucoma (Hiratsuka *et al.*, 1994) or dry eye patients who require continuing therapy. In many eye drops, benzalkonium chloride is the chosen preservative, and these should not be administered to patients wearing soft contact lenses because it binds to hydrogel materials. When soft lens patients require such an eye drop, the lens should be removed and not reinserted for at least an hour after instillation.

With some drugs the choice of preservative is determined by the limited compatibility of some drugs and preservatives.

Preservatives will only cope with small inocula of micro-organisms. Good hygiene is still necessary to prevent contaminated eye drops. Harte *et al.* (1978) found contamination in 44% of the residues of eye drops returned to the pharmacy after use in hospitals. This figure is very high and should not be encountered routinely. Aslund *et al.* (1978), however, found a much lower level of contamination in eye drops. In their study only 10 out of 436 containers produced positive cultures. In a laboratory test they found that contamination was likely to be much higher when untrained personnel used eye drops.

pH adjusters. Some drops are buffered while others contain small amounts of acid or alkali to adjust the pH. The correct pH is necessary to avoid adverse effects, to produce adequate therapeutic effect, to stabilize the preparation and to allow the preservative the correct conditions for action.

Unfortunately, some of these desirable effects have conflicting demands on pH and the value chosen for any particular eye drop may be a compromise. Adrenaline, for example, is most active at a high pH but stable at a lower one. A pH of around neutral is normally chosen. However, for pilocarpine there was no difference in ocular hypotensive effect and stability between solutions of pH 4.1 and pH 5.8 (David *et al.*, 1978) and it was concluded that because of enhanced comfort, near neutral solutions should be used. Buffers are used when the pH is critical and cannot be allowed to vary widely.

Viscosity agents. The dwell time of a drop in the conjunctival sac is very short and the reduction in the tear concentration reduces the amount available for absorption. Any modification of the drop which will increase the dwell time will therefore increase the therapeutic effect and reduce the potential for adverse effect. Hardberger *et al.* (1975) found the following halflives for radioactive sodium pertechnate when instilled into human eyes in different vehicles. (The halflife is the time taken for half of the concentration to disappear. Thus one halflife after instillation, half of the original concentration will remain, after two halflives a quarter, after three an eighth, and so on.)

Ointment   – 9.7 minutes
Polyvinyl alcohol   – 7.2 minutes
Methylcellulose   – 4.2 minutes
Saline   – 4.6 minutes

Haas and Merrill (1962) demonstrated a much greater effect from pilocarpine in reducing intraocular pressure and causing miosis when the solution was made viscous with methylcellulose compared with an aqueous solution, and Davies *et al.* (1977) found a similar effect from polyvinyl alcohol.

Similar dramatic increases in activity were seen when pilocarpine was made viscous with carbomer gel (Schoenwald *et al.*, 1978), but there is a level at which a viscous eye drop stops being an eye drop and becomes a gel. Mattila *et al.* (1968) found varying modifications of response to drugs made viscous with methylcellulose, which modified the cycloplegic effect of tropicamide but not the mydriatic effect. Conversely, it quickened the onset of miosis from physostigmine but had less effect on the resulting cyclospasm. The results would seem to demonstrate the variability of drug response rather than the lack of effect from methylcellulose. More modern viscolizing agents are now available. Camber and Edman (1989) studied the effect of sodium hyaluronate of differing molecular weights and at different concentrations on the bioavailabity of pilocarpine in rabbits. A greater miotic effect was found with solutions viscolized with sodium hyaluronate at concentrations around 0.1%. Snibson *et al.* (1992) compared the contact times of three viscolized solutions in patients with keratoconjunctivitis sicca. They found that sodium hyaluronate was significantly superior to both hypromellose and polyvinyl alcohol. Sodium hyaluronate is presently very expensive to produce, being a natural product, and this precludes its wider use as a viscolizer or artificial tears.

Viscosity agents such as polyvinyl alcohol, methylcellulose or hydroxy ethyl cellulose are added to drops, particularly therapeutic drops, to retard the loss of drugs down the nasolacrimal duct. Viscous drops may also be more comfortable than simple aqueous ones.

Antioxidants. Antioxidants such as sodium metabisulphite or N-acetyl cysteine are incorporated into eye drops containing oxygen sensitive chemicals such adrenaline. Antioxidants are reducing agents which are preferentially attacked by the oxygen, leaving the active ingredient unaffected.

Tonicity agents. At one time, tonicity was thought to be all important and hypotonic drops were made isotonic by the addition of solutes such as sodium chloride. In practice problems are only really encountered with hypertonic drops which, of course, cannot be adjusted. Hypotonic drops are well tolerated and only for products such as artificial tears is isotonicity important.

Oily eye drops

Oily eye drops can be used for three reasons: to produce an emollient effect, to protect a compound liable to hydrolysis and to obtain an enhanced effect. Liquid paraffin and castor oil eye drops are used to form a protective film over the eye following trauma or for an unconscious patient. They can also be used prior to making an eye impression for scleral contact lens fitting. Some drugs such as DFP are broken down in an aqueous solution and are supplied in arachis oil to prevent this.

Since lipophilic substances cross the epithelial barrier more easily than hydrophilic ones, it would appear logical to provide drugs in the former state rather than the latter. Smith *et al.* (1978) found that pilocarpine in oil had a greater and longer miosis than a similar amount given in aqueous solution.

Containers for eye drops

The containers for eye drops are very important because not only do they hold the solution and protect them from the potentially destructive effects of air, light and micro-organisms but they also act as a method of application. For many of the drops the optometrist may wish to use in practice, there is the choice of using a multidose or single dose container.

Multidose containers. The old-fashioned amber ribbed dropper bottle made of neutral glass is now becoming less frequently used, but has the advantage that the eye drops can be autoclaved in the final container. In modern pharmaceutical manufacturing methods, the plastic container into which the dropper is incorporated is favoured. Sterilization of the container is by means of gamma irradiation and the solution is sterilized by filtration, with the two being brought together under aseptic conditions. This type of container usually has an inbuilt tamper evident seal while the glass dropper bottle has a plastic sleeve around the cap. Tamper evidence is now very important for all pharmaceutical preparations and in the case of eye drops constitutes a guarantee of sterility. The integral plastic dropper is much easier to use for both patient and optometrist than the separate pipette found in the glass bottle.

Single use containers. Unit dosing of eye drops has been available for a long time and has been recommended since the mid 1960s as the most appropriate container for use where patients are likely to be treated, e.g. hospital outpatient departments, operating theatres, accident and emergency departments.

Single use containers have the following advantages:

1. The drop is always sterile – there is no possibility of cross-contamination. Claoue (1986) subjected single use containers to extreme challenges of contamination and found that under conditions likely to be encountered in practice the contents remained sterile.
2. The units contain no preservative so that patients with preservative allergies may be safely treated. Marquardt and Schubert (1991) found a significant increase in tear break up time when patients previously treated with preserved solutions of timolol were switched to unpreserved single dose units of the same drug. Hiratsuka *et al.* (1994) found a relief from keratitis in a patient who had developed a reaction to preservatives when they used nonpreserved timolol.
3. There are cost savings because there is no need to discard a partly used container at the end of the week.

Single use containers are ideal for use in optometric practice and should be selected whenever possible.

Instillation of eyedrops

Eyedrops are normally instilled into the lower conjunctival sac. The patient's head should be tilted backwards, almost horizontal and slightly to the temporal side of the eye concerned, with the eyes looking back over his head and the lower lid pulled gently away by the examiner. The end of the eyedropper must be held just clear of the sweep of the lashes, being less than an inch or so above the sac, before releasing the drop. The sterile glass tube of the eyedropper must not be allowed to touch the lashes, eye or cheek of the patient or the examiner's hand in order to avoid, as far as possible, contamination of the eyedrops. The dropper must be firmly screwed back in place immediately after use.

The patient is instructed previously that as soon as the drop has fallen (below the cornea, to minimize the force of the blink reflex, and directly into the sac) he must close his eyes gently, with no lid squeezing. A small pad of cotton wool or fresh paper tissue (held ready between the fingers of the same hand that holds the bottle, or the other hand when employing a sterile single dose eyedrops unit) is used to control any tearing. Only one or two drops are instilled at a time as any in excess of this amount will only be expelled on closure of the lids (Fig. 4.1).

Following the instillation of an ophthalmic drug, it has long been common practice to occlude the puncta by applying pressure across the bridge of the nose using thumb and forefinger for about a minute or so, in order to reduce drainage into the nasolacrimal duct and increase the amount of drug available for absorption by ocular tissues. Whether the duct is amenable to closure in this manner is open to doubt, and the possibility exists that such a procedure enhances drainage by expressing the contents of the lacrimal sac on application of pressure, allowing it to fill up

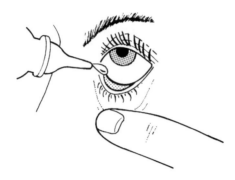

Figure 4.1 Drop installation and punctal occlusion: adults.

with the contents of the conjunctival sac on its removal. There is no doubt, however, if drainage is properly impeded then enhanced absorption by ocular tissues will take place and less drug will be available for systemic absorption through the alimentary tract. The latter can lead to possible toxic effects and interaction with other drugs. Linden and Alm (1990) blocked the nasolacrimal ducts with punctal plugs which are normally used in the treatment of dry eye conditions and applied solutions of fluorescein. Measurements of fluorescein in the cornea and aqueous humour showed a significant increase in the blocked eye compared with the unblocked eye. Attempts to produce similar effects by applying pressure to the lacrimal sac were unsuccessful.

The intraocular penetration of a drug via the cornea does not contribute appreciably to any rapid systemic concentration following instillation of eyedrops because of the relatively slow diffusion of any unchanged drug from the eye via its blood or aqueous drainage. Occlusion of the canaliculi, therefore, only leaves that fraction of the drug not absorbed via the cornea to enter the systemic system via the conjunctival membrane. Normally this amount is not sufficient to produce undesirable systemic effects as long as due observance is given to the contraindications for certain drugs where particular medical conditions exist, or the patient is receiving specific systemic medication: for example, pilocarpine, carbachol and bethanechol are contraindicated in asthmatics; sympathomimetic drugs are contraindicated in patients receiving MAO inhibitors, tricyclic anti-depressives and antihypertensive drugs.

Eye ointments

Eye ointments have the advantage that they may be instilled by an adult in the home, and they are far safer when poisonous alkaloids are involved. For example, eye ointment is the preparation of choice for home use when an atropine cycloplegic refraction of a child is considered necessary. It is a standard dosage recommendation that this ointment should not be used on the day of refraction because the greasy film can interfere with the retinoscopic reflex. Cable *et al.* (1978) employed ointments of cyclopento-late and tropicamide for cycloplegia and mydriasis and found that if small volumes of ointment were applied, there was minimal irritation and inter-ference with the subsequent ocular examination.

Eye ointments are also useful as protective agents following trauma. They do not adversely affect corneal wound healing (Hanna *et al.*, 1973). As well as being fairly safe and well tolerated, eye ointments have the advantage of prolonged contact with the ocular conjunctival membrane with slow but continued absorption of the medicament (Robin and Ellis, 1978). This continuous absorption necessitates less frequent application and can give comfort to inflamed tissues. Hanna *et al.* (1985) found that administration of sulphacetamide eye ointment four times daily was sufficient to maintain a minimum inhibitory concentration in tear flow. Of course, this advantage of prolonged action becomes a disadvantage when ointments are used diagnostically as opposed to therapeutically or prophylactically.

Eye ointments drain from the lacrimal sac by the same route as eye drops, namely through the nasolacrimal duct into the oral cavity (Scruggs *et al.*, 1978).

Eye ointments, like eye drops are susceptible to contamination (Harte *et al.*, 1978), and are also subject to variations in formulation leading to differences in consistency and drug release patterns (Ford *et al.*, 1982).

The traditional greasy eye ointment has a base of soft paraffin. Hydrophilic hydrogel bases have been developed which give the benefit of longer duration in the conjunctival sac without the disadvantage of greasiness. The drug is also released better into aqueous environments from a hydrogel base than from a greasy one (Kecik *et al.*, 1993).

Instillation of eye ointments

Eye ointments are again instilled into the lower conjunctival sac, a grape pip size amount being applied on the end of a clean glass eye rod. The patient is instructed to hold his head more upright than for the instillation of eyedrops, and the examiner again pulls the lower lid gently away, placing the ointment on the end of the rod into the lower conjunctival sac. On instruction the patient closes his eyes, the examiner (or parent in domiciliary cases) holds the upper lid gently but firmly closed, and the glass rod is given a gentle twirl and smoothly withdrawn horizontally via the outer canthus, leaving the eye ointment behind (Fig. 4.2). Gentle

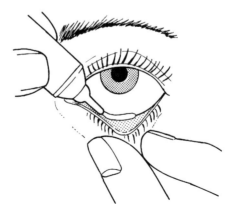

Figure 4.2 Instillation of eye ointment.

massage by the examiner or parent for a few moments, with the lids remaining closed, is followed by removal of any excess ointment from their outer edges with cotton wool. Alternatively, the eye ointment can be applied directly from a tube without the aid of a glass ointment rod, and this is the recommended practice in the consulting room or clinic when using sterile single dose application packs. The practitioner applying an eye ointment in his own consulting rooms, if using a glass rod, should disinfect immediately beforehand. This can be done by wiping the rod with a cotton wool pad soaked in a solution of one in six Savlon Liquid Antiseptic (ICI) in Surgical Spirit (*BPC*), then rinsing the rod in sterile saline solution (a suitable preserved proprietary 'rinsing' solution) and drying with a fresh paper tissue. For domiciliary use where a glass rod is being used, the patient (or parent when a child is involved) should be cautioned to avoid contaminating the medicament and observe good hygiene; a clean glass rod should be used and hands and rod washed and dried on a clean towel. In hospital outpatient clinics and ophthalmic wards either single dose containers should be used (whenever available), or a separate multiple dose tube of eye ointment should be reserved for each patient. The ointment should be applied with a sterile applicator used for one application only (recommendation of *Codex* 1979), a small portion of ointment being discarded on each occasion, before squeezing the material on to the applicator (H.M. (69) 86). The *BPC* (1973) recommended that eye ointment for domiciliary use, after the 'sterile' seal or plastic envelope has been broken, should be discarded after one month, but the *Pharmaceutical Codex* (1979) does not stipulate a time factor. When eye ointments are used in the practice by an optometrist, a small amount of ointment should be squeezed out and discarded each time before applying any to a freshly disinfected eye ointment rod when administering to each new patient. Opened tubes should be discarded after one week.

Eye lotions

Although these are ophthalmic pharmaceutical products they are not strictly speaking a method for administering drugs to the eye. They are large volume isotonic solutions normally containing sodium chloride or sodium bicarbonate. Commercial products may additionally contain substances such as astringents. Apart from first aid, they have little application in modern ophthalmic treatment.

Paper strips

Filter paper is very absorbent and has the ability to become impregnated by solutions with which it comes in contact. If the paper is allowed to dry the solute is retained in the paper even though the solvent has disappeared, and immersion in a suitable solvent will allow the solute to dissolve again. Although this ability could theoretically be used for any substance, it has its principal application in the administration of dyes to the eye e.g. fluorescein and rose bengal. Because the dyes are coloured, it is easy to control the amount released onto the surface of the eye and achieve the desired effect.

Lamellae

These are only included for historic completeness and examples of this method of drug administration probably now only exist in museums. The solution of drug was mixed with a solution of gelatin which was allowed to solidify and dry out, giving a sheet in which the drug was incorporated. Small discs (about 5 mm in diameter) were punched out and stored for use. They were applied to the conjunctival sac where they took up fluid from the tear film and dissolved, releasing the drug.

Ocuserts

The Ocusert (May & Baker) is in some regards a modern, more sophisticated prolonged (depot) version of the older lamellae, and is a method of continuous release of pilocarpine to control the intraocular pressure of glaucomatous patients responsive to this therapy. It is an elliptically shaped unit approximately 0.5 mm (vertical axis) by 13.5 mm (horizontal axis) by 0.3–0.6 mm thick, depending on the dosage of pilocarpine enclosed in the permeable outer membrane. The former thickness represents 5 mg and the latter 11 mg of the drug, the 5 mg reservoir possibly being suitable for patients previously on pilocarpine 1 or 2% eyedrops, and the 11 mg for those previously on higher concentrations of the eyedrops. The slow release of the pilocarpine in both strength Ocuserts is by diffusion into the tears fluid over a period of one week after the Ocusert has been placed in the lower conjunctival sac. The strength of the Ocusert system chosen by the ophthalmologist will be that which achieves adequate reduction of the intraocular pressure. Each individual sterile unit is replaced by the patient every seven days, and the inconvenience of three or four daily instillations of pilocarpine eyedrops is obviated.

Iontophoresis

Iontophoresis is a technique for overcoming the impermeability of the cornea to many molecules, particularly the water soluble polar compounds such as the salts of weak bases and strong acids. A solution of the drug to be administered is held against the cornea by a special rigid contact lens containing an electrode and another electrode is attached somewhere else. A direct current is applied across the two electrodes with the contact lens electrode becoming the positively charged anode. This repels the positively charged anions which are the drug molecules and these are driven across the cornea. It is mainly used as a research tool to investigate the effects of new molecules on intraocular tissues before engaging in expensive formulation work. Hobden *et al.* (1990) used iontophoresis to administer ciprofloxacin to eyes infected with *Pseudomonas aeruginosa*, which was resistant to the aminoglycoside antibiotics, and found it superior to frequent topical administrations. Similar results were found by Grossman and Lee (1989) who used iontophoresis to deliver high concentrations of ketoconazole (an antifungal agent) into the rabbit eye and found it superior to subconjunctival injection.

Hydrogel contact lenses

By their very nature hydrogel lenses can take up solutions into the matrix of the lens, which can be released when the lens is placed in fresh solvent. It was assumed that this property would provide a means of applying a depot of drug to the eye so that it could be released over a period of time, giving a longer duration of action than a simple drop. For a variety of reasons the soft contact lens has not become a routine method of drug delivery.

Collagen shields

Collagen shields were originally prepared as a protective layer to place over damaged corneae to reduce abrasion and promote healing, (Spraul et al., 1994; Simsek and Kozer-Bilgin, 1994). Like soft lenses they will take up drugs from solutions and release them when applied to the eye. Friedberg et al. (1991) found them more clinically acceptable than iontophoresis or constant delivery pumps. Reidy et al. (1990) demonstrated their superiority over aqueous eye drops using fluorescein in human volunteers and assessing the concentration in the aqueous humour. Willey et al. (1991) used collagen shields to test the uptake of antiviral agents in mice as a model for screening these drugs. Being similar to contact lenses some difficulty has been experienced in their administration. This led Kaufman et al. (1994) to use pieces of collagen shield to deliver drugs and agents for the relief of dry eye. Application was simpler and there was no blurring of vision.

Ophthalmic rods

The Alani rod (Alani, 1990; Alani and Hammerstein, 1990) is a novel concept in ophthalmic drug delivery and consists of a rod made from nontoxic plastic which is dipped into an unpreserved solution of the drug to be administered. As the solution dries it forms a thin homogeneous coat on the rod which can then be packed and sterilized by gamma irradiation. For administration, the tip of the rod is rubbed against the palpebral conjunctiva releasing the drug. The system has not received a lot of commercial interest.

Drug classification

Ophthalmic drugs may be conveniently if somewhat arbitrarily classified into two main groups: (1) therapeutic and (2) diagnostic.

Many ophthalmic drugs are used for both therapeutic and diagnostic purposes (for example atropine, homatropine, physostigmine, pilocarpine, etc.), but if their main interest for the optometrist is as a diagnostic agent, they will be discussed in the second grouping with appropriate references to their therapeutic applications.

Diagnostic and prophylactic drugs

Diagnostic ophthalmic drugs may be subdivided as follows.

1. Cycloplegics: used to inhibit or paralyse the accommodation.
2. Mydriatics: used to produce dilation of the pupil.
3. Miotics: used to constrict the pupil.
4. Topical local anaesthetics: drugs applied to the surface of the mucous membrane of the eye to produce local insensitivity in this area.
5. Staining agents: used to stain corneal or conjunctival abrasions, in applanation tonometry and contact lens fitting procedures.
6. Decongestants: used as vasoconstrictors of congested conjunctival blood vessels.
7. Prophylactic anti-infective preparations: these are therapeutic anti-infective drugs used to prevent pathological conditions developing after the minor abrasions of the ocular epithelial tissues that may

occur in many situations, including certain diagnostic procedures and contact lens practice.

Therapeutic drugs

The principal groups of therapeutic drugs are:

1. Drugs for the treatment of infections and inflammations.
2. Drugs for the treatment of glaucoma.
3. Artificial tears.

References

Akers, M. J. (1983) Ocular bioavailability of topically applied drugs. *Am. Pharm.*, **NS23**, 33–36

Alani, S. D. (1990) The ophthalmic rod: A new ophthalmic drug delivery system I. *Graefes. Arch. Clin. Exp. Ophthalmol.*, **228**, 297–301

Alani, S. D. and Hammerstein, W. (1990) The ophthalmic rod – A new drug-delivery system II. *Graefes Arch. Clin. Exp. Ophthalmol.*, **228**, 302–304

Aslund, B., Oslund, O. T. and Sandell, E. (1978) Studies on the in use microbial contamination of eyedrops. *Acta. Pharm. Suec.*, **45**, 389–394

Brown, R. H., Hotchkiss, M. L. and Davis, E. B. (1985) Creating smaller eye drops by reducing the eyedropper tip dimension. *Am. J. Ophthalmol.*, **99**, 460–464

Cable, M. K., Hendrickson, R. D. and Hanna, C. (1978) Evaluation of drugs in ointment for mydriasis and cycloplegia. *Arch. Ophthalmol.*, **96**, 84–86

Camber, O. and Edman, P. (1989) Sodium hyaluronate as an ophthalmic vehicle: Some factors governing its effect on the ocular absorption of pilocarpine. *Curr. Eye Res.*, **8**, 563–567

Claoue, C. (1986) Experimental contamination of Minims of fluorescein by *Pseudomonas aeruginosa*. *Br. J. Ophthalmol.*, **70**, 507–509

David, R., Goldberg, L. and Luntx, M. H. (1978) Influence of pH on the efficacy of pilocarpine. *Br. J. Ophthalmol.*, **62**, 318–339

Davies, D. J. G., Jones, D. E. P., Meakin, B. J. and Norton, D. A. (1977) The effect of polyvinyl alcohol on the degree of miosis and intraocular pressure reduction induced by pilocarpine. *Ophthalmol. Dig.*, **39**, 13–26

Ford, J. L., Rubinstein, M.H., Duffy, T. D. and Ireland, D. S. (1982) A comparison of the physical properties of some sulphacetamide eye ointments commercially available in the U.K. *Int. J. Pharm.*, **12**, 11–18

Friedberg, M. L., Pleyer, U. and Mondino, B. J. (1991) Device drug delivery to the eye: Collagen shields iontophoresis and pumps. *Ophthalmology*, **98**, 725–732

Grossman, R. and Lee, D. A. (1989) Transcleral and transcorneal iontophoresis of ketoconazole in the rabbit eye. *Ophthalmology*, **96**, 724–729

Haas, J. S. and Merrill, D. L. (1962) The effect of methylcellulose on response to solutions of pilocarpine. *Am. Ophthalmol.*, **54**, 21–27

Hanna, C., Fraunfelder, F. T., Cable, M. and Hardberger, R. E (1973) The effect of ophthalmic ointments on corneal wound healing. *Am. J. Ophthalmol.*, **76**, 193–200

Hanna, C., Hof, W. C. and Smith, W. G. (1985) Influence of drug vehicle on ocular contact time of sulphacetamide sodium. *Ann. Ophthalmol.*, **17**, 560–564

Hardberger, R., Hanna, C. and Boya, C. M. (1975) Effects of drug vehicles on ocular contact time. *Arch. Ophthalmol.*, **93**, 42–45

Harte, V. J., O'Hanrahan, M. T. and Timoney, R. F. (1978) Microbial contamination in residues of ophthalmic preparations. *Int. J. Pharm.*, **1**, 165–171

Havener, H. W. (1978) *Ocular Pharmacology*, 4th edn. St Louis: Mosby

Hiratsuka *et al.* (1994) The irreversible corneal epithelial damage presumably due to preservatives in ophthalmic solution. *Jpn. J. Clin. Ophthal.*, **48**, 1099–1102

Hobden, J. A. *et al.* (1990) Ciprofloxacin iontophoresis for aminoglycoside-resistant pseudomonal keratitis. *Invest. Ophthalmol.*, **31**, 1940–1944

Kaufman, H. E. *et al.* (1994) Collagen-based drug delivery and artificial tears. *J. Ocul. Pharmacol.*, **10**, 17–27

Kecik, T. *et al.* (1993) Studies of releasing rate of pilocarpine hydrochloride from hydrogel ointments. *Klin. Oczna*, **95**, 263–264

Linden, C. and Alm, A. (1990) The effect of reduced tear drainage on corneal and aqueous concentrations of topically applied fluorescein. *Acta Ophthalmol.*, **68**, 633–638

Marquadt, R. and Schubert, T. (1991) Effects of preservative free beta blocking eye drops on break up time. *Klin. Monatsbl. Augenheilkund*, **199**, 75–78

Mattila, M. J., Idapaan-Heikkila, J. E. and Takki, S. (1968) Effect of eyedrop adjuvants on the response of the human eye to some autonomic drugs. *Farmuseuttinen Aikakausleti*, **10**, 205–213

Miller, S. J. H. (1978) *Parson's Diseases of the Eye*, 16th edn., pp. 141–150. London: Churchill Livingstone

Patton, T. F. and Francoeur, M. (1978) *Am. J. Ophthalmol.*, **85**, 225

Reidy, J. J., Limber, M. and Kaufman, H. E. (1990) Delivery of fluorescein to the anterior chamber using the corneal collagen shield. *Ophthalmology*, **97/9**, 1201–1203

Robin, J. S. and Ellis, P. P. (1978) Ophthalmic ointments. *Surv. Ophthalmol.*, **22**, 335–340

Schoenwald, R. D., Ward, R. I., De Santis, L. M. and Roehus, R. E. (1978) Influence of high viscosity vehicles on miotic effect of pilocarpine. *J. Pharm. Sci.*, **67**, 1280–1283

Scruggs, J., Wallace, T. and Hanna, C. (1978) Route of absorption of drug and ointment after application to the eye. *Ann. Ophthalmol.*, **10**, 267–271

Simsek, N. and Kozer-Bilgin, L. (1994) Collagen bandage lenses. *Turk. Oftalmol.*, **24**, 396–400

Smith, S. A., Smith, S. E. and Lazare, R. (1978) An increased effect of pilocarpine on the pupil by application of the drug in oil. *Br. J. Ophthalmol.*, **68**, 314–317

Snibson, G. R. *et al.* (1992) Ocular surface residence times of artificial tear solutions. *Cornea*, **11**, 288–293

Spraul, C. W., Lang, G. E. and Lang, G. K. (1994) Corneal stromal ulceration in chronic graft-versus-host disease: Treatment with collagen shields. *Klin. Monatsbl. Augenheilk*, **205**, 161–166

Wheatcroft, S., Sharma, A. and McAllister (1993) Reduction in mydriatic size in premature infants. *Brit. J. Ophthal.*, **77**, 364–365

Willey, D. E. *et al.* (1991) Ocular acyclovir delivery by collagen discs. A mouse model to screen anti-viral agents. *Curr. Eye Res.*, **10** (suppl.), 167–169

5 Factors affecting the choice of diagnostic drugs

Unlike nearly every other group of pharmaceuticals, the range of available ophthalmic diagnostic products has declined significantly over recent years. In most pharmaceutical sectors, as some products are discontinued they are more than replaced by new ones. Many of the presently used ophthalmic diagnostic drugs have been in use for some time, and new ones are rarely introduced. The scarcity of new ophthalmic diagnostic drugs is a consequence of the high cost of introducing novel compounds onto the market. Of the drugs that remain, the choice of concentrations is more limited than it was as product rationalization leads to the discontinuation of old drugs.

It is, however, difficult to bemoan the loss of many of the drugs which are now no longer available or can only be obtained by special manufacture. Many of them were historical oddities, with actions which are no longer appropriate for modern day optometry and, as a result, without a clinical indication for their use.

Classification of ophthalmic drugs

1. Cycloplegics – this group has suffered some attrition and from the seven agents available for use by optometrists under the Medicines Act only four agents remain commercially available, and one of these has little to recommend it.
2. Mydriatics – from a long list of agents that have been used to dilate the pupil only two are seriously considered for optometric use. More potent ones are used prior to surgery.
3. Miotics – the greatest losses have occurred from this group. Miotics have a dual use – therapeutic and diagnostic – and because of a reduction in both uses, there is no longer a need for a large range of agents.
4. Local anaesthetics – despite the use of non-contact tonometers, the range of local anaesthetics has remained fairly steady. Only cocaine (which was never an option as far the optometrist was considered) is rarely used medically, as better agents are available.
5. Stains – this is one area which at one time appeared to have growth. Two stains are routinely used and the use of one far exceeds the other.

Advantages and disadvantages of using diagnostic drugs

There are three possible advantages in using diagnostic drugs, and if none of these apply the optometrist should seriously question whether it is necessary to use a drug at all.

1. Easier on the patient – this certainly applies when the clinical procedure involves a local anaesthetic, but for other agents, if the use of a diagnostic drug will allow the examination to be carried out more quickly and efficiently, then this will be to the patient's advantage.
2. Easier for the practitioner – the use of an agent will often facilitate the examination, especially in the case of mydriatics and cycloplegics.
3. Better examination – again in the case of mydriatics and cycloplegics, the results obtained will often be more valuable.

Against these advantages must be weighed several disadvantages.

1. The eye is in an artificial state – this must be allowed for when carrying out certain tests.
2. The latent period – this can be short (e.g. local anaesthetics), but it can be long enough to inconvenience the patient and in the case of atropine require the drug's administration at home.
3. Prolonged duration of action – prolonged cycloplegia for a child at school or mydriasis for a driver may seriously inconvenience the patient. The use of a reversing drug, if available, may produce problems which are different in nature to those of the cycloplegic but are equally troublesome.
4. Local adverse effects – these can be as mild as stinging on instillation or as severe as angle closure glaucoma. Only acute problems need be considered as the drugs are not used chronically.
5. Systemic adverse effects – many diagnostic drugs are potent modifiers of the autonomic nervous system and are capable of causing effects on autonomically innervated structures.

Ideal properties of diagnostic drugs

In light of the preceding discussion, the ideal diagnostic drug would have the following properties:

1. It should be available- excellent drugs such as thymoxamine are no longer commercially produced.
2. It should produce the desired depth of effect – for some indications the maximum effect would be excessive and inconvenience the patient unnecessarily.
3. Its action should be fast in onset – time waiting for the drug to become effective is time wasted for both the patient and practitioner.
4. Its action should be short in duration.
5. The drug should have no unwanted pharmacological effects.
6. It should have no local or systemic toxic effect.
7. It should be pleasant and easy to use.
8. It should be capable of being produced in a stable and sterile ophthalmic form which is appropriate to the use for which it is intended – a cycloplegic ointment would make retinoscopy difficult if it were used immediately prior to the examination.

Selection of patient

Each patient is unique and the advantages and disadvantages of the drug which it is proposed to use must be weighed in every case. In particular the following questions should be addressed.

1. Will the patient benefit from the use of a particular diagnostic drug?
2. Has the particular drug been applied to this patient before? If so, were there any adverse reactions or allergic responses?
3. Is the patient suffering from any ocular condition that would make the use of this drug inadvisable?
4. Are there any systemic conditions which would be contraindications for the drug's use?
5. Is the patient currently taking any medicine which could interact with the diagnostic drug?

Selection of drug and concentration

Based on the information gained from the patient's history and the practitioner's knowledge, a choice can be made as to the most appropriate drug and concentration. Because of the imprecise method when drugs are applied in topical ophthalmic dosage forms, the commonly used drug concentrations represent supramaximal doses. When lower concentrations of drugs have been made available in the past, their use has been poor and production has been discontinued. If there is any doubt as to which concentration to use, then the lower one should always be employed. Similarly, in choosing between two drugs, the weaker one with the shorter duration will often be the drug of choice.

6

Cycloplegics

Cycloplegics are drugs that paralyse the ciliary muscle by blocking the muscarinic receptors normally stimulated by the release of acetylcholine from the nerve endings of the parasympathetic system. Since the parasympathetic nervous system also innervates the pupil sphincter muscle, cycloplegia must be accompanied by mydriasis. It should be noted that mydriasis is not always evidence of an accompanying cycloplegia and merely indicates paralysis of the pupil sphincter. Cycloplegics are used to prevent or reduce accommodation during refraction, thus making latent refractive errors manifest.

Indications for cycloplegic examination

Cycloplegic examination may be desirable in some children and young adults but is most unlikely to be necessary in presbyopic adults. Use of a cycloplegic is indicated in the following cases:

1. in children with constant or intermittent esotropia, on initial presentation and sometimes subsequently
2. in children and young adults with asthenopia and esophoria, especially when a latent refractive error is suspected
3. when retinoscopy suggests that accommodation is fluctuating significantly
4. when the retinoscopy findings differ significantly from the results of subjective refraction
5. in cases of anomalies of accommodation such as accommodative insufficiency, accommodative fatigue, accommodative inertia and spasm of accommodation
6. in cases where retinoscopy along the visual axis is very difficult due to lack of patient co-operation or mental handicap (Amos, 1978).

Ideal properties of cycloplegics

1. Quick in onset (the delayed onset of atropine puts special requirements on its dosing).
2. Adequate depth of cycloplegia.
3. Adequate duration of cycloplegia (a static level of cycloplegia must be achieved).
4. No mydriasis (as mentioned earlier, this is unattainable so the mydriasis that invariably accompanies cycloplegia must be considered an unwanted side effect which can cause photophobia).
5. No other pharmacological effect.
6. No local toxicity.
7. No systemic toxicity.
8. Stable.

9. Capable of presentation in single use eye drops.
10. No adverse subjective complaints such as 'stinging'.

Cycloplegic refraction – advantages

Under cycloplegia, full static refraction can be estimated without interference from a tonic or clonic (fluctuating) contraction of the ciliary muscle. This is particularly important in the very young because of their large amplitude of accommodation, the latency resulting from this masking a large part of their full refractive error if it is of the hypermetropic type. The unreliability of subjective findings in the very young makes the retinoscopy results of paramount importance.

The full cycloplegic correction found is not necessarily given in any subsequent prescription which is deemed to be necessary. Knowledge of the cycloplegic findings is nevertheless of great importance, especially in young people and particularly where intermittent or constant strabismus, medium to high heterophoria or pseudomyopia are present, or where marked accommodative asthenopic symptoms exist.

Cycloplegic refraction – disadvantages

Refraction under cycloplegia is unnatural because the shape of the lens has been changed. As this will resume its normal form when the effects of the drug have worn off, cycloplegic findings must be compared with those obtained at either a pre- or postcycloplegic test, whichever is appropriate in a given case. The optical aberrations present with the widely dilated pupil are then very much reduced. This procedure normally necessitates the inconvenience of a further visit. Additional disadvantages include making an allowance for the dependent tone of the ciliary muscle, and the dangers of cycloplegia, but as these can be successfully overcome (see later) the advantages of cycloplegic refraction (when it is indicated) far outweigh the disadvantages.

Precycloplegic examination

Since the routine use of cycloplegia is unnecessary in children and young adults, an initial noncycloplegic examination will be made, the results of which may indicate the need for cycloplegia. It will include the following:

1. Symptoms, and ocular and medical history. If the need for cycloplegia is anticipated, enquire about any current or previous drug therapy and any adverse reactions to medications. Establish any history of allergy.
2. Manifest refraction with vision and visual acuity at distance and near.
3. Determine binocular status with tests appropriate to patient's age. In all cases, these will include prism/cover test and a test of ocular motility.
4. External eye examination including tests of pupil function, using slit lamp microscope or hand-held slit lamp and loupe (as appropriate to patient's age).
5. Internal ocular examination (if cycloplegia is to be undertaken, ophthalmoscopic findings can be verified later with the benefit of the dilated pupil).
6. Test of accommodative function.

In those cases in which the noncycloplegic examination has indicated the need for cycloplegia it is helpful to offer advice to the patient or the parent of a young child on the following:

1. How long it will take before near vision becomes clear again.
2. That associated mydriasis can cause photophobia which can be alleviated by the temporary use of sunglasses.
3. In the case of adult patients, they should be advised that because distance visual acuity may be slightly reduced (as a consequence of the mydriasis) it would be advisable to avoid riding a motorcycle or driving a car immediately after the cycloplegic examination.

Cycloplegic examination

The essential components of the cycloplegic examination are retinoscopy, subjective refraction (where possible) and ophthalmoscopy.

Retinoscopy

To confirm that adequate cycloplegia has been achieved in order to undertake retinoscopy, the level of residual accommodation can be determined either objectively, using dynamic retinoscopy, or subjectively. In the latter method, a pair of plus spheres usually +2.50D are placed in the trial frame or phoropter and the push-up method used to measure the assisted accommodation. Residual accommodation is calculated by deducting 2.50D from this measured value.

In all cases, retinoscopy will be undertaken. The use of a streak instrument can facilitate accurate location of cylinder axis, but the use of a spot retinoscope has been advocated by Edgar and Barnard (1996) for paediatric use on the grounds that it is preferable for the techniques of dynamic and near retinoscopy which they describe.

Two essential practical precautions should be observed when undertaking retinoscopy under cycloplegia. First, due to the pronounced mydriasis present it is essential to observe the movement of the light reflex in the central 3–4 mm pupillary area only, ignoring the light movement in the periphery, which may be either in the same or the opposite direction.

Movement of the light reflex in the peripheral parts of the dilated pupil may show positive or negative aberrations due to the differing refractive conditions in this area as compared to the central 'axial' region. In positive aberration (four or five times more common than negative aberration) the peripheral area is more myopic or less hypermetropic than the central area, and thus an 'against' movement still persists in the periphery when the central axial zone is neutralized.

A negative aberration causes the opposite effect. Regardless of any peripheral movement, the central 3–4 mm diameter zone alone must be neutralized and the outer area reflex ignored. Due to peripheral aberrations a scissor movement of the light reflex may be observed on occasion, usually near the neutralization point. Movement of the refractionist's head forwards and backwards over a range of about 25 cm, giving first a 'with' then an 'against' movement, is a useful check that neutralization has been attained. It can readily be seen that, with positive aberration, if the peripheral zone is erroneously corrected, too little plus or too much minus power will be recorded and vice versa when negative aberration is present.

These retinoscopy rules concerning peripheral aberrations apply in all cases of dilated pupils whether drugs have caused the mydriasis or not.

If too bright a light source is used when performing a retinoscopy with dilated pupils it is difficult to differentiate clearly the central from the peripheral light reflex and, therefore, the minimum light retinoscopic reflex that can be seen easily is desirable.

A second precaution is to encourage the patient to look directly at the retinoscopy light, which should be an easy request to obey in the darkened consulting room. In the presence of heterotropia it is of course necessary to occlude the fixing eye in order to undertake retinoscopy along the visual axis of the deviating eye.

With an infant or very young child, it may be convenient to seat the child upon a parent's lap and to hold lenses before the child's eyes instead of using a trial frame. The parent can be asked to cover the fixing eye in the case of a squinting child. Most young children will, however, tolerate a lightweight paediatric trial frame.

If a spot retinoscope is used, two alternative techniques can be employed to verify cylinder axis and the following method has been described by Duke-Elder (1978). An undercorrection (preferably by 0.50 DC) when using plus cylinders or an overcorrection (by the same amount) when using negative cylinders should be made, in order to create a 'with' movement. Move the retinoscopy light exactly at right angles to the cylinder axis in the trial frame. If the cylinder axis, as set in the trial frame, is correct, the edge of the retinoscopic light reflex will move exactly parallel with this axis across the central pupil. Alternatively, if the cylinder axis in the trial frame has been set in error, the edge of the light reflex in the pupil will move along a different axis, not parallel to the cylinder axis in the trial frame but making an angle (with the cylinder axis) which is approximately six times greater than the angle of error in the setting of the cylinder axis in the trial frame. For example, if the correct cylinder axis is $85°$, but the cylinder in the trial frame has been set in error with its axis at $90°$, the edge of the light reflex will then lie very neatly along the $60°$ meridian, as it gives a 'with' movement. The cylinder axis in the trial frame should be reset, tilting it approximately one sixth of the difference between its original position and the position occupied by the edge of the light reflex, and towards the latter position. This adjustment is repeated until light edge reflex and cylinder axis are parallel as the retinoscopy light is tilted.

A similar, alternative method of checking the cylinder axis is that of Lindner, which has been described by Hodd and Freeman (1955) as follows. Observation is made along the meridians approximately $45°$ to either side of the axis of the trial cylinder. If the trial cylinder is slightly off axis, a 'with' shadow movement will be noted in one oblique meridian and an 'against' shadow movement will be noted in the other oblique meridian. To correct the error in setting, locate the meridian showing the 'with' shadow movement and turn the trial cylinder axes slightly towards this position. This procedure is repeated until the oblique movements are eliminated. If the 'with' movement is difficult to locate it may be accentuated by moving forward slightly or by adding −0.25D sphere. The addition should be just sufficient to neutralize the 'against' movement in the other oblique meridian: the refractive error in the first oblique meridian will then be doubled.

The use of a streak retinoscope facilitates axis location.

Subjective refraction

With children from about five years of age it may be possible to undertake some subjective results. Edgar and Barnard (1996) advocate a 'bracketing' technique in which the child's reaction to modification of the retinoscopy findings with ±1.00D spheres is assessed. If sensible responses can be elicited, the practitioner can attempt to refine the refraction using ±0.50D, then ±0.25D spheres. A similar approach can be followed to check cylinder axis and power by the use of crossed cylinders of decreasing power.

Since the subjective refraction is carried out immediately following the cycloplegic retinoscopy, it must be expected that the sphere power will vary somewhat from that determined objectively because of the presence of spherical aberration caused by mydriasis. Usually, as positive spherical aberration is more common, less plus sphere will be accepted in hypermetropia and more minus sphere in myopia. A further discrepancy under these conditions (also attributable to this aberration) will frequently be the loss of a line or so in the visual acuity.

It is helpful to record all refractive findings obtained under cycloplegia in red ink in order to differentiate them readily from results obtained without its use.

Ophthalmoscopy

Precycloplegic findings can be verified, taking advantage of the dilated pupil.

Choice of cycloplegic
(Table 6.1)

Many antimuscarinic agents have been used in the past but today only three are used regularly. Arranged alphabetically, and in descending order of efficacy, they are: atropine, cyclopentolate and tropicamide.

Of the others, homatropine is still used infrequently, while hyoscine is hardly ever employed at all.

The principle of 'as little as possible but as much as necessary' should apply to the use of drugs by doctors, optometrists and patients alike. Having decided that a particular patient will benefit from a cycloplegic refraction, it is incumbent on the optometrist to use the weakest agent consistent with achieving the required depth of cycloplegia. Antimuscarinic drugs can affect the whole body, and the stronger the cycloplegic the stronger will be the side effects. Additionally, stronger agents will produce longer effects and the inconvenience to the patient of dilated pupils and the inability to read or do close work will be prolonged.

The popularity of atropine has declined significantly over the past three decades, principally due to the disadvantages of slow action and long duration in comparison to alternative drugs. Indeed, it now tends to be used only when cyclopentolate has failed to achieve satisfactory cycloplegia. Ingram and Barr (1979) consider that atropine is absolutely contraindicated in the first three months of life because of the danger that its prolonged action could result in stimulus deprivation amblyopia. The use of atropine cycloplegic refraction in cases of intermittent squints

Table 6.1 Cyclopegics

Official name	Trade name	Strengths % w/v	Single dose?	Cyclopegic onset	Cyclopegic duration	Residual accommodation	Adverse effects
Atropine sulphate	—	1.0	Yes	36 h	Up to 7 days	Nil	Allergic reactions, general CNS side effects
Cyclopentolate hydrochloride	Mydrilate	0.5	Yes	60 min	24 h	1.00D	Hallucinations CNS side effects
Homatropine hydrobromide	—	1.0	2% only	90 min	24 h	1.00D	As for atropine
Tropicamide	Mydriacil	1.0	Yes	30 min	6 h	2.00D	Occasional hallucinations

and high heterophorias was rejected long ago on the grounds that there is a possible danger of converting these conditions into constant squints. The shorter acting but less complete effects of cyclopentolate are preferable in these conditions, regardless of age. Zetterton (1985) compared atropinization with the use of a phenylephrine-cyclopentolate combination and found that the cycloplegia produced by the latter was adequate for all clinical purposes.

Amos (1978) considers five years to be the maximum age for the use of atropine and this view should be respected since the long duration of action of atropine would either cause serious disruption of school work in the case of older children or its use would have to be restricted to school holidays. The preceding considerations demonstrate that, despite the efficacy of its action, atropine should no longer be regarded as the cycloplegic of first choice.

It is difficult to be rigid about which drug should be used on which patient. One cannot rely on age as the only determining factor. For example, heavily pigmented eyes may require a stronger cycloplegic than light coloured ones of the same age. The following are recommendations, not hard and fast rules.

Cyclopentolate will suffice for all cases irrespective of refractive and binocular states. Up to the age of 12 years, 1% is the recommended strength with 0.5% for older children and adults.

Tropicamide may be used as a less effective alternative cycloplegic, especially when a quick reversal of the cycloplegia is desirable, but it is unsuitable for use with young children. In the main 1% is used as a cycloplegic with older children and adults; the results with 0.5% are too variable.

Atropine

Atropine is an alkaloid extracted from a variety of plant species such as *Atropa belladonna*, and *Hyoscyamus niger*. It was the first antimuscarinic agent used in medicine and is the most toxic substance available for use by optometrists. It is available as 1% eyedrops, both in multidose and single use units. Because of the systemic toxic reactions that can occur, the ointment form is most often favoured. However, Auffarth and Hunold (1992) carried out refractions on 90 strabismic children 90 minutes after administering two drops of atropine eyedrops (0.5 or 1.0% depending on age), and found that there were small differences between results obtained by this method and those after a three day atropinization, the latter producing only an extra 0.5D of cycloplegia. Similar results were obtained by Nagayama *et al.* (1991).

When atropine is used as an ointment, it is usually applied in the child's eyes by the parent at home twice a day for three days prior to refraction (Sowden, 1974) but not on the day of refraction because the unabsorbed ointment may interfere with refractive procedures. The technique for application of eye ointment (as described in Chapter 4) should be carefully demonstrated to the parent by the practitioner either using a simple eye ointment or the first dose of atropine. Parents must be warned that very great care must be taken in handling atropine and that hands must be washed thoroughly before and after its application. They must try to ensure that the child does not wipe an eye with a finger which is then placed in the mouth. The verbal instructions should be accompanied by a written handout which can include diagrams illustrating the procedure. If there is any doubt about the parent's ability to follow these instructions strictly, then the use of atropine is contraindicated in this case. Attention is drawn to the fact that the standard three gram tube contains an amount of atropine which could prove fatal to a young child. The parent should be asked to bring the remaining ointment to the practice on the day of the cycloplegic examination. This request will enable the practitioner to verify that the correct amount of ointment has apparently been used and to ensure the surplus is disposed of safely.

Time scale

After one instillation of the usual 1% strength solution, mydriasis commences in 10–15 minutes and is maximal in 30–40 minutes. Recovery from mydriasis following a single instillation may take as much as three to seven days, but as it is usual to require complete cycloplegia when atropine is used in children, and this necessitates twice daily application for three days, pupillary recovery then usually takes from 10 to 14 days. Cycloplegia commences in half an hour, the action is slow and full recovery may take seven to ten days, although adequate accommodation for near work has usually returned within four to five days (after the usual six applications). Even with one application full ciliary muscle recovery may take three to seven days; the resulting cycloplegia reached in one to three hours, although marked, is not complete.

Because of the different time courses of mydriasis and cycloplegia, the size of the pupil is a poor indicator of cycloplegic effect (Amos, 1978). Wide dilation of the pupil causes photophobia and sometimes the patient complains of micropsia. Normal pupillary reflex constrictions to light and to accommodation–convergence are completely abolished.

Very powerful miotics (such as ecothiopate 0.3%) will overcome the mydriatic effects of atropine 1% but this drug is not readily available in the United Kingdom. It has been withdrawn and is now available on a limited basis.

Tonus allowance

The ciliary muscle, like all other smooth muscles in the body, has both a dependent and an independent tone, the former being conditional on an intact nerve supply while the latter is not. The independent tone in the ciliary muscle is very small and does not give rise to symptoms, neither is it affected by cycloplegics. On the other hand, the dependent tone of the ciliary muscle is totally abolished by complete atropine cycloplegia, but not by the full effects of other cycloplegics.

An allowance therefore has to be considered only in the case of complete atropine cycloplegia for the return of the dependent tone of the ciliary muscle on its recovery from the effects of atropine paralysis. This tonus allowance is an adjustment of the spherical element only of the retinoscopic findings in such cases, to take into account the fact that the eyes, when fully returned to normal, will once more usually have their overall refractive power increased slightly in a positive direction by the constant effect of the (dependent) tone of the recovered ciliary muscle.

The quantitative effect of this tone will vary slightly depending on the nature of the refractive condition of the eye being considered. Traditionally, it has been suggested that −1.00D should be added as an allowance in all refractive errors up to one dioptre whereas a smaller modification is made for higher amounts of myopia. At −3.00D or more, zero allowance might be made. In practice, any prescription issued should not be based on an arbitrary modification to the cycloplegic retinoscopy findings but must take into account factors such as any previous spectacle correction and the binocular status of the patient.

Use of atropine as an 'occluder'

Atropine cycloplegia of the fixing eye of strabismic infants and children has been used in order to encourage the use of the amblyopic eye in near vision. Louis Javal has been credited as the first to use atropine as an occluder at the end of the nineteenth century and Claud Worth became an ardent advocate of its use (Revell, 1971). Use of this technique, which is sometimes described as penalization, during the period of visual immaturity may induce amblyopia in the eye subjected to cycloplegia. Three such cases have been reported by von Noorden (1981). Experiments in monkeys raised with unilateral cycloplegia have demonstrated shrinkage of cells in the lateral geniculate nucleus and loss of cortical binocularity and of neurones responding to stimulation of the atropinized eye. The results of such animal experiments and the occurrence of atropine-induced amblyopia in children point to the need to exercise the greatest caution in the application of this technique.

Cyclopentolate

Cyclopentolate is the most widely used cycloplegic today and is now the one of choice. The paralysis of accommodation is not complete but it gives a depth of cycloplegia which is sufficient for the majority of cases. Havener (1978) aptly sums up the great value of cyclopentolate when he describes its effects in the field of cycloplegia as superior to homatropine (even the 5% concentration of the latter) in its rapidity of onset, shortened duration of action and greater intensity of effect.

Cyclopentolate is available in single dose form ('Minims') and in multi-dose containers in two strengths for cycloplegia – 0.5% and 1.0%. An interesting alternative application method for cyclopentolate has been evaluated by Ismail et al. (1994). They used a spray application to the closed eye and compared it with conventional eyedrop administration. They found that the resulting refractions using the two applications were not significantly different, but the spray application was easier to administer and was more acceptable to the patient.

Aged up to 12 years

Usually only one drop of the 1% solution is necessary, but a further drop should be instilled if little effect is measurable after 15 minutes. A further factor in determining the appropriate concentration is the degree of iris pigmentation, and when this is very light the 0.5% solution may be suitable. Retinoscopic refraction may then be performed in 40–60 minutes (or sooner if desired, when the maximal cycloplegic effect is obtained earlier than this).

Aged 12 years and above

One drop of the 0.5% solution, only repeated if within 15–20 minutes there is no significant measurable reduction in the amplitude of the accommodation. This second drop is sometimes necessary in fair skinned patients with dark hair and irides. Where it is considered necessary to administer two drops of cyclopentolate, it has in the past been accepted procedure to allow a five minute interval between drops so that the conjunctival sac can drain and allow space for the second drop. This has been challenged by Stolovitch *et al.* (1994) who found that an interval of one minute was sufficient.

For dark skinned adults, one drop of the 1% solution should be instilled, and the dose only repeated if the amplitude of accommodation is not falling at a satisfactory rate. Again, retinoscopy is generally carried out in 40–60 minutes, that is, the average time taken for the maximum effect of the drug to reduce the accommodation to less than 2.00D.

Time course

One or two drops of the cyclopentolate solution instilled into the conjunctival sac produces a cycloplegia commencing in a few minutes and becoming maximal in 30–60 minutes, but sometimes as rapidly as in 15 or (on rare occasions) even in 10 minutes, especially in patients with light irides (Manny *et al.*, 1993). Because of the variation in the time taken to produce maximum cycloplegia and also in view of the fact that the duration of this condition varies from 10 to 60 minutes (averaging about 40 minutes), the amplitude of accommodation should be measured every 10 minutes after a time lag of 20 minutes following instillation, until no further fall in the accommodation is recorded (Mitchell *et al.*, 1958). In very young children and others unable to respond to this test, the accommodative state can be assessed using dynamic retinoscopy. Like most drugs which affect accommodation and the pupil, the time course of the mydriasis is different to that of the cycloplegia and pupil diameter should not be relied upon to give a measure of the remaining accommodation.

Depth of cycloplegia

As in nearly all cases the residual accommodation is 1.50D or less around 40–60 minutes after instillation (although not infrequently a second drop of the solution may be necessary to reduce the accommodation level to this), a period during this interval is the most usual time for retinoscopic refraction. Priestley and Medine (1951) considered that cyclopentolate (then known as Compound 75 G.T.) more closely approximated their ideal criteria for a cycloplegic or mydriatic than any other drug discovered up to that time.

Priestley and Medine compared the depth of cycloplegia reached after one hour following instillation of two drops of a 0.5% solution of cyclopentolate with the same dosage of a 5% solution of homatropine in a group of over 50 patients which included children and young adults. The cyclopentolate was instilled in the right eye and the homatropine in the left eye.

Their results showed that the residual accommodation for cyclopentolate ranged between 0.50 and 1.75D, with an average of 1.25D, whereas with homatropine this range was between 1.00 and 3.00D, with an average of 2.00D. In an endeavour to ensure that any anisocycloplegia present did not vitiate their findings, the series was later repeated using cyclopentolate in both eyes. Anisocycloplegia, a term originated by Beach (1942), who found it a phenomenon of fairly frequent occurrence, is the difference that may occur in the residual accommodation between the two eyes of the same patient to the same dose of a cycloplegic (often it amounts to about 0.5D, but exceptionally as much as 10.0D).

Rosenfield and Linfield (1986) proposed the use of what they termed 'a distance accommodation ability' measurement, in which negative spherical lenses are introduced until the patient is no longer able to clearly read a line of Snellen letters, as a measure of the degree of cycloplegia. They considered it an easier test to perform than apparent near point, especially on young children. It is interesting that the average minimum near and distance accommodation were not significantly different for 1% cyclopentolate as compared with 0.5%.

The residual accommodation was found again invariably to be less in these eyes than the homatropine recordings, whereas anisocycloplegia might well occur in either eye.

Stolzar (1953), in a further series (this time of 80 patients) using two drops of a 0.5% solution of the original American proprietary brand of cyclopentolate hydrochloride (Cyclogyl), found an average residual accommodation after one hour of 1.03D. His results (with average residual accommodation measured after correction of any distance refractive error) were as shown in Table 6.2. Further analysis of this range of residual accommodation is also interesting (Table 6.3).

Full recovery of the accommodation without the instillation of a miotic usually occurred between 4 and 12 hours, but in a few cases this was delayed for 24 hours. Reading, in practice a more important consideration than full restoration of accommodation, was usually possible after three to four hours. Recovery from mydriasis was shown as occurring between 24 and 48 hours, in all instances without the aid of a miotic. Stolzar, in his investigations (presumably carried out on normal eyes), found no increase in intraocular pressures. He made no direct comparisons of residual accommodations against those encountered using a homatropine–hydroxyamphetamine combination, the latter formerly being one of the most popular combinations of cycloplegic and sympathomimetic drugs used by American ophthalmologists, but considered that the cycloplegic effect obtained with cyclopentolate was either equal to or more profound

Table 6.2

Age group (years)	Number of cases	Residual accommodation (D)
1–20	28	1.14
20–30	29	0.97
30–40	23	0.97

Table 6.3

Residual accommodation (D)	Percentage of cases
0.50	2.5
0.75	13.7
1.00	55.0
1.25	27.5
1.50	1.3

than that of this combination. Gettes and Leopold (1953) actually confirmed this view. Mitchell *et al.* (1958) made such a comparison with the comparable homatropine-ephedrine combination used at that time by optometrists in Great Britain and came to much the same conclusions. They confirmed the more rapid onset and shorter duration of cyclopentolate cycloplegia.

As with all other cycloplegics with the exception of atropine, distance fixation during retinoscopy is necessary to relax as much of the residual accommodation as possible. Measuring of the latter before and after examination may be carried out with reasonable accuracy using a +3.00D sphere monocularly with the near point rule.

Where children under the age of seven years who have previously shown allergic reactions to atropine require cycloplegic refraction, one or two drops of cyclopentolate hydrochloride eyedrops 1% may be substituted.

Therapeutic uses

Cyclopentolate may be used in the treatment of corneal ulceration, iritis, iridocyclitis and keratitis, one or two drops of the 0.5% solution being instilled every six to eight hours, to prevent the formation of posterior synechiae and 'rest' the painful ciliary and pupil sphincter muscles. For long term treatment in these conditions, cyclopentolate does not compare favourably with the longer acting drugs such as atropine and homatropine. When breaking down lenticular adhesions, one or two drops of the 0.5% solution are instilled, followed six hours later by one or two drops of a 2% solution of pilocarpine nitrate; this alternating treatment is repeated daily.

Tropicamide (Bistropamide) (Proprietary preparation: *Mydriacyl*, USA)

Tropicamide is another rapidly acting synthetic antimuscarinic drug. It is used as a mydriatic in a 0.5% solution and a cycloplegic in a 1.0% solution.

As a mydriatic, two drops of the weaker solution instilled into the conjunctival sac produce a full mydriasis in about 15 minutes, the pupil returning to normal in eight to nine hours if no miotic is used to counteract the pupillary dilatation.

To produce cycloplegia, two drops of the 1% solution are instilled into the eye allowing a five minute interval between each drop. The full cycloplegic effect is achieved in about 30 minutes, when the retinoscopy is performed. If the latter examination has to be delayed beyond 35 minutes, because of the very brief maximal effect of the cycloplegia a further (third) drop of the 1% solution should be used. Complete recovery of the accommodation usually occurs within six hours and reading is generally possible after two to four hours from the time of the initial instillations.

Excellent cycloplegia (with residual accommodation below 2.00D) is usually obtained, according to Gettes and Belmont (1961), following the procedures outlined above, but due to the very brief duration of maximum effect the third drop is not infrequently necessitated in routine practice. In a series of 193 patients, Gettes and Belmont (1961) were only able to examine 60% of these during the interval of 20–35 minutes (when cycloplegia was maximal) and 40% had to receive the third drop. However, as Havener (1978) emphasizes, the great advantage of tropicamide is its rapid action and short duration, the patient having fully recovered from cycloplegia in two to six hours, and these very qualities also make it a most useful mydriatic in its weaker concentration of 0.5% (Smith, 1971).

The speed of onset allowed Harding (1970) to see more patients in his working day and the short duration of action allowed patients to return to work within two hours.

On the other hand, Milder (1961) did not find when using two drops of the 1% solution that it was as satisfactory a cycloplegic as the same number of drops of a 1% cyclopentolate or a 5% homatropine solution. He instilled tropicamide in one eye and cyclopentolate or homatropine in the other. In a series of 50 consecutive cases (100 eyes) he found better cycloplegia produced by the cyclopentolate in 23 out of the 25 cases and homatropine in 20 out of 25 cases in comparison to the tropicamide instilled in the second eye in each case. Thus, in only seven eyes (five with homatropine in the other eye and two with cyclopentolate in the other eye) out of the 100 eyes was tropicamide superior in its cycloplegic effect to these other drugs. In children in particular, his results indicated a poor paralysis of the ciliary muscle; in the six cases in this series up to the age of nine years an average of 6.25D of residual accommodation was present after 30 minutes, and in 20 cases from 10 to 14 years this reading was still averaging 3.65D. Tropicamide would therefore appear to be a relatively inadequate cycloplegic for use with children. This is confirmed by Hiatt and Jenkin (1983) who found that tropicamide was less effective as a cycloplegic for pre-school esotropia.

In some countries, a mixture of tropicamide and phenylephrine is marketed as a fast acting cycloplegic and mydriatic. Lovasik and Kergoat (1990) compared this mixture with tropicamide alone and found that although a deeper cycloplegia was obtained with the mixture, the residual accommodation present after 20 minutes was too much for most refractive purposes.

Other cycloplegics
Homatropine

Homatropine is a semisynthetic alkaloid prepared from atropine; the base tropine obtained by hydrolysis of atropine is chemically combined with mandelic acid. Homatropine Hydrobromide Eyedrops BP, the standard solution, contains up to 2% w/v homatropine hydrobromide.

At one time this drug was quite popular as a routine mydriatic and cyclo-plegic, but its use has declined. It does not produce as satisfactory a cyclo-plegia in children. Its use for this purpose is therefore usually restricted to the over 15 years age groups. Conventional dosage of the eyedrops is one drop of the 2% solution repeated twice at ten minute intervals (that is, a total of three drops).

Mydriasis commences in 15 minutes and is maximal in about 30–40 minutes, with complete abolition of pupillary reflex to light and accom-modation. Complete recovery of the pupil may take between 24 and 48 hours, depending on dosage. The amplitude of accommodation begins to fall in 15 minutes and is usually at its lowest between 45 and 90 minutes. Therefore, cycloplegic retinoscopic refraction should not commence until about 60 minutes after instillation, and the residual accommodation should be measured to ensure that it is below 2.00D. Refraction should be completed before 90 minutes has elapsed from the time of instillation of the drops.

Not infrequently the depth of cycloplegia in the under 20 years age group is not reduced much below 2.00D, but if a lower amount is recorded (the first reading being taken after half an hour and then every ten minutes until no further fall of accommodation is noted) cycloplegic retinoscopy can usually be adequately performed with the patient gazing at a distant target to relax the small amount of accommodation left unparalysed. No tonus allowance is made as the dependent tone of the ciliary muscle has not been affected.

Koyama *et al.* (1995) used a combination of homatropine (4%) and cyclopentolate (1%) to examine myopic children and compared the refrac-tions obtained under cyclopentolate (1%) alone. Not surprisingly they found no difference between the two cycloplegic drops.

Lachesine and hyoscine

These are two antimuscarinic compounds which at one time had a limited use as mydriatics and cycloplegics. However, because of the development of newer drugs with properties closer to the ideal, they have fallen out of use and production. This prevents further research being carried out using them (Morrison and Reilly, 1989).

Prescribing following cycloplegia

When cycloplegia discloses a significant difference in refractive findings compared to the precycloplegic examination, it will be beneficial to arrange a further postcycloplegic visit. At this further consultation, it is particularly important to assess the effect of the proposed correction on the patient's binocular status. Each prescription issued will be determined by the individual circumstances of the case, and it is therefore only pos-sible to offer general guidelines on prescribing. In the case of esophoria accompanied by hyperopia, the aim would be to prescribe the minimum plus which would allow this heterophoria to become compensated.

In esotropia accompanied by hyperopia, the ideal is to prescribe that plus power which permits binocular fixation as demonstrated by the cover test. Both esophoria and esotropia may be of the convergence excess type, and since the degree of plus power required at near is greater than that for distance it is likely to impair distance visual acuity. In such cases, bifocal or multifocal spectacles lenses may be appropriate.

It is unlikely that cycloplegia would be considered necessary in patients with exophoria or exotropia. Generally, the aim in these cases is to pre-scribe the minimum plus correction or a full minus correction. In some younger patients, a minus over-correction may allow the compensation of the heterophoria or the attainment of binocular fixation in exotropia.

In every case, consideration must be given as to whether the patient will be able to tolerate the proposed prescription when it is compared to the present correction, if any.

Adverse effects of cycloplegics

Antimuscarinic drugs are potent agents which can produce effects on several structures in the body. Atropine was a favourite of the medieval professional poisoners and is probably the most toxic compound that is used routinely as a diagnostic agent. Other cycloplegics also have the potential to produce marked side effects.

Toxic effects from topical ophthalmic use have been known for a long time (Wise, 1904). These consisted of a high temperature and the central nervous system effects of hallucinations and ataxia. Daly (1959) and Harel et al. (1985) also reported psychotic reactions to atropine eye drops.

Hoefnagel (1961) reported confusion, hallucinations, ataxia and rest-lessness after the use of atropine. Death from the use of atropine has been reported by Heath (1950).

CNS effects represent an advanced stage of atropine poisoning. Milder effects can be seen at earlier stages of poisoning. These affect peripheral tissues, including exocrine glands such as the salivary glands and the sweat glands. Patients suffering from atropine poisoning are said to be:

blind as a bat;
dry as a bone;
red as a beetroot;
mad as a hatter.

Patients are as blind as a bat because of the effect on accommodation. They are as dry as a bone because of the inhibition of the sweat glands and salivary glands. A dry mouth is one of the earliest signs of atropine poisoning. The inhibition of sweat glands deprives the body of one of its methods of losing heat and in order to compensate for this there is a dilation of skin blood vessels, giving the patient the appearance of being as 'red as a beetroot'. When CNS effects occur patients become as 'mad as a hatter'.

CNS effects have also been reported following the use of cyclopento-late. In the majority of cases these effects followed the administration of a higher than recommended dose or a combination with other drugs. CNS effects manifest themselves as confusion, difficulty in speaking, hallucinations and ataxia. Fortunately there have been no fatal reports following these effects of cyclopentolate, and the patient is back to normal in a matter of hours.

These effects would appear to be dose related, as Cher (1955) used two drops of 0.5% with a ten minute interval between applications on 159 patients without producing CNS problems. Beswick (1962) used 2% cyclopentolate (not available in the UK) and noted hallucinations in a nine year old child. Binkhorst *et al.* (1963) found that 2% cyclopentolate elicited reactions in four patients out of 40. One case has been reported in which CNS effects were seen after the use of 0.2% cyclopentolate (Carpenter, 1967) but the patient had a history of chronic dementia.

From the above, it would appear that 0.5% cyclopentolate should be used whenever possible and cyclopentolate 1% should be used sparingly.

Problems in the gastrointestinal tract following the use of cyclopento-late in premature babies have been reported (Isenberg *et al.*, 1985). It was found that cyclopentolate 0.5% decreased gastric acid secretion while 0.25% did not. Bauer *et al.* (1973) had earlier reported necrotizing enterocolitis following the use of cyclopentolate.

Homatropine, although less toxic than atropine, has produced problems in the past. Hoefnagel (1961) reported CNS effects such as ataxia and hallucinations in four children who had received six drops of homa-tropine 2% at ten minute intervals. Such a dose must be considered excessive and it is not surprising that problems arose.

Tropicamide in comparison with other cycloplegics is relatively free from adverse reactions. Wahl (1969) reported unconsciousness and pallor following one drop of 0.5%. As there have been no similar reports, it would appear that the reaction is probably not drug related.

Allergic reactions can occur to many compounds. Atropine is probably the most notorious for producing reactions but cyclopentolate has also been implicated. It may appear that the use of cycloplegics is potentially hazardous. If the precautions mentioned in this chapter are observed by the practitioner, then the risk of an adverse effect is minimized and will be a very rare occurrence.

The optometrist who has maintained knowledge of and practice in the application of current first aid procedures is clearly better equipped to recognize and deal with adverse reactions.

References

Amos, D. M. (1978) Cycloplegics for refraction. *Am. J. Optom. Physiol. Opt.*, **55**, 223–226

Auffarth, G. and Hunold, W. (1992) Cycloplegic refraction in children single dose atropinization versus three day atropinization. *Doc. Ophthal.*, **80**, 353–362

Bauer, R., Trepannier Trottier, M. C. and Stern, L. (1973) Systemic cyclopentolate (Cyclogyl) toxicity in the new born infant. *Paediatr. Pharmacol. Ther.*, **82**, 501–505

Beach, S. J. (1942) Anisocycloplegia. *Am. J. Ophthalmol.*, **26**, 522

Beswick, J. A. (1962) Psychosis from cyclopentolate. *Am. J. Ophthalmol.*, **53**, 879–880

Binkhorst, R. D., Weinstein, G. W., Baretz, R. M. and Clahane, A. C. (1963) Cyclopentolate toxicity in paediatric patients. *Am. J. Ophthalmol.*, **55**, 1243–1246

Carpenter, W. T. (1967) Precipitous mental deterioration following cycloplegia with 0.2% cyclopentolate. *Arch. Ophthalmol.*, **78**, 445–447

Cher, I. (1959) Experiences with Cyclogyl. *Transact. Ophthalm. Soc. UK.*, **79**, 665–670

Daly, P. J. (1959) Psychotic reactions to atropine poisoning. *Br. Med. J.*, **2**, 608

Duke-Elder, S. (1978) *Practice of Refraction*, 9th edn., pp. 39, 41, 51, 71, 77, 119. Edinburgh and London: Churchill Livingstone

Edgar, D. and Barnard, S. (1996) Refraction. In *Pediatric Eye Care*. (Barnard, S. and Edgar, D., eds). Oxford: Blackwell Science

Gettes, B. C. and Belmont, O. (1961) Tropicamide. Comparative cycloplegic effects. *Arch. Ophthalmol.*, **661**, 336

Gettes, H. C. and Leopold, I. H. (1953) Evaluation of five new cycloplegic drugs. *Arch. Ophthalmol. N. Y.*, **49**, 24

Harding, R. (1970) Benefits for office practice using tropicamide – A short acting mydriatic cycloplegic. *Eye, Ear Nose and Throat Monthly*, **49**, 75–76

Harel, L., Frydman, M. and Kauschansky, A. (1985) Prolonged parasympathetic paralysis and psychosis caused by atropine eye drops. *J. Paedriatr. Ophthalmol. Strabis.*, **22**, 38–39

Havener, W. H. (1978) *Ocular Pharmacology*, 4th edn., pp. 253–256. St Louis: Mosby

Heath, W. E. (1950) Death from atropine poisoning. *Br. Med. J.*, **2**, 608

Hiatt, R. L. and Jenkin, G. (1983) Comparison of atropine and tropicamide in esotropia. *Ann. Ophthalmol.*, **15**, 341–343

Hodd, F. A. B. and Freeman, H. (1955) Comparative analysis of retinoscopic and subjective refraction. *Br. J. Physiol. Optics*, **12**, 31–33

Hoefnagel, D. (1961) Toxic effects of atropine and homatropine eye drops in children. *N. Engl. J. Med.*, **264**, 168–171

Ingram, R. M. and Barr, A. (1979) Refraction of one year old children after cycloplegia with 1% cyclopentolate: comparison with findings after atropinization. *Br. J. Ophthalmol.*, **63**, 348–352

Isenberg, S. J., Abrams, C. and Hyman, P. E. (1985) Effects of cyclopentolate eyedrops on gastric secretory function in pre-term infants. *Ophthalmology*, **92**, 698–700

Ismail, E. E., Rouse, W. and De Land, P. N. (1994) A comparison of drop instillation and spray application of 1% cyclopentolate hydrochloride. *Optom. Vis. Sci.*, **71**, 235–241

Koyama, R. *et al.* (1995). Cycloplegia with 4% homatropine and 1% cyclogyl in children with low grade myopia. *Rinsho-Ganka*, **49**, 469–472

Lovasik, J. V. and Kergoat, H. (1990) Time course of cycloplegia induced by a new phenylephrine-tropicamide combination drug. *Optom. Vis. Sci.*, **67**, 352–358

Manny, R. E. *et al.* (1993) 1% Cyclopentolate hydrochloride: Another look at the time course of cycloplegia using an objective measure of the accommodative response. *Optom. Vis. Sci.*, **70**, 651–665

Milder, B. (1961) Tropicamide as a cycloplegic agent. *Arch. Ophthalmol.*, **66**, 70

Mitchell, D. W. A., Linfield, J. A. and Francis, J. L. (1958) A comparison of the effects of cyclopentolate with those of homatropine and ephedrine in the eye. *Optician*, **135**, 3

Morrison, J. D. and Reilly, J. (1989) The effects of 0.025% hyoscine hydrobromide eye drops on visual function in man. *Ophthalmic Physiol. Opt.*, **09**, 41–45

Nagayama, M. *et al.* (1991) Study of one percent atropine cycloplegia. *Folia Ophthalmol. Jpn.*, **42**, 1827–1831

Priestley, B. S. and Medine, M. M. (1951) A new mydriatic and cycloplegic drug. *Am. J. Ophthalmol.*, **34,** 572

Revell, M. J. (1971) *Strabismus: a history of orthoptic techniques*. London: Barrie and Jenkins

Rosenfield, M. and Linfield, P. B. (1986) A comparison of the effects of cycloplegics on accommodation ability for distance vision and the apparent near point. *Ophthalmol. Physiol. Opt.*, **6**, 317–320

Smith, S. L. (1971) Mydriatic drugs for routine fundal inspection, *Lancet*, **2**, 837

Sowden, A. S. (1974) The preschool child: indications for cycloplegic examination. *Aust. J. Optom.*, **57**, 215–218

Stolovitch, C., Alster, Y., Loewenstein, A. and Lazar, M. (1994). Influence of the time interval of two drops of cyclopentolate 1% on refraction and dilation of the pupil in children. *Am. J. Ophthalmol.*, **119**, 639

Stolzar, I. H. (1953) A new group of cycloplegic drugs. *Am. J. Ophthalmol.*, **36**, 110

Von Noorden, G. K. (1981) Amblyopia caused by unilateral atropinisation. *Ophthalmology*, **88**, 131–133

Wahl, J. W. (1969) Systemic reactions to tropicamide. *Arch. Ophthalmol.*, **82**, 32–321

Wise, C. H. (1904) A case of poisoning from atropine eye drops. *Br. Med. J.*, **11**, 189

Zetterton, C. (1985) A cross-over study of the cycloplegic effects of a single topical application of cyclopentolate-phenylephrine and routine atropinization for 3.5 days. *Acta Ophthalmol.*, **63**, 525–529

7

Mydriatics

Mydriatics are drugs which dilate the pupil to facilitate a more thorough examination of the fundus, lens periphery and vitreous. They are mostly used on elderly patients, as their pupils are usually smaller and lens opacities and abnormal retinal conditions are not uncommon. Their use may be essential in any age group, especially where the macula or the peripheral areas of the retina need particularly careful observations, for example suspected macular cyst or hole, location of a penetrating foreign body, intraocular tumours, peripheral detachments, etc. Martin-Doyle (1967) considers the instillation of a mydriatic indispensable for an adequate examination of the macula. Siderov et al. (1996) examined patients' attitudes to pupil dilatation during optometric examination and found that the majority were in favour although a large proportion suffered adverse effects such as glare and blurring of vision.

Ideal properties of mydriatics

1. Quick in onset.
2. Adequate duration.
3. Fast recovery after examination.
4. Light reflex abolished.
5. No cycloplegia.
6. Capable of quick reversal in an emergency.
7. No rise in intraocular pressure.
8. No other pharmacological effect.
9. No local toxic reaction.
10. No systemic toxic reaction.
11. No adverse subjective complaints such as 'stinging'.

The indications and contraindications for mydriatic examination have been admirably summarized by Havener (1975).

Indications for mydriatic examination

The occasions where there is a special need for a thorough fundus inspection through a dilated pupil, where the latter does not already exist, include the following.

1. Recent onset of floating opacities in the vitreous.
2. A relatively sudden decrease in visual acuity, necessitating a careful study of the macula.
3. Unexplained loss of visual field.
4. Unexplained ocular pain, not accompanied by raised intraocular tension.
5. Redness of the eye not attributable to superficial infection, allergy, or raised intraocular tension.
6. After contusion, to rule out eye damage.

7. Cloudiness of the vitreous or lens, when good mydriasis will reveal fundus detail hidden by a small pupil.
8. Annual examination of the diabetic patient.

Obviously only some patients need mydriatic examination. If none of the specific ocular signs or symptoms enumerated above is present, or if the patient has a (systemic) disease not known to produce eye manifestations, a reasonable view of the optic disc and retinal vessels through the undilated pupil may be considered an adequate examination. Spontaneously large pupils are commonly found in many young people conveniently permitting a relatively thorough fundus examination. It is usually with the older age-groups, with their smaller pupils, that mydriatics are on occasion necessary. In his typically succinct style Havener aptly compares 'the view of a fundus through a small pupil or a dilated pupil with the view of a room as seen through a keyhole or with the door open'!

Adequate dilation of the pupils reveals small details of great diagnostic significance, for example, diabetic micro-aneurysms, hypertensive arteriolar attenuation, early signs of macular degeneration, small traumatic retinal holes, peripheral retinal lesions etc. Newell (1969) emphasizes an important clinical principle when he comments that 'there is more danger of missing significant ocular or systemic disease by failing to dilate than there is of precipitating glaucoma by dilatation'. This 'approach' is reflected in Havener's remark that 'a physician who dilates many eyes may expect to precipitate not more than one case of acute glaucoma in a lifetime'. It is to be hoped that such views expressed by eminent authorities, taken in conjunction with the precautions listed in the following contraindications, will give the optometric student and practitioner a balanced attitude to the use of mydriatics in appropriate cases. It is the optometrist's moral and legal duty to refer pathological conditions (ocular or systemic) for medical attention; he will obviously be unable to do this unless he can 'see' such conditions in the first instance.

Siderov et al. (1996) conducted a survey in a suburban optometric practice in order to establish the patients' perception of pupillary dilation. Most of them reported that the mydriasis resulted in blurry vision and increased sensitivity to glare which had interfered with some aspects of their everyday life, notably driving a motor vehicle. These authors considered that patients should be informed about the visual disturbances which may be associated with mydriasis. It is especially helpful to provide information on the following:

1. the probable duration of the mydriasis (commonly four to six hours) and any expected blurred near vision
2. the benefit of using sunglasses and/or the wearing of a broad-brimmed hat to alleviate photophobia
3. the desirability of avoiding riding a motorcycle or driving a car immediately after the mydriatic examination.

Contraindications for a mydriatic examination

Before instillation of any mydriatic (whether of the antimuscarinic or sympathomimetic group) the optometrist must first confirm (as indicated in the previous chapter for cycloplegia in older patients) that no contraindications to the dilatation of the pupil(s) are present. Contraindications will include the following.

1. The known presence of glaucoma, which is being treated with pilocarpine, as ascertained from the case history and inspection of the eyes for signs of 'therapeutic miosis'.
2. The presence of an abnormally shallow anterior chamber, which is almost invariably associated with a narrow anterior angle. In such a case, the examiner should believe that the potential benefit of mydriatic examination exceeds the risk of inducing an episode of angle closure glaucoma.

Not only will full mydriasis in predisposed eyes result in an increased intraocular tension by mechanical blockage of the angle by the iris, but a state of semidilation of the pupil may initiate this rise by producing pupillary block. This may occur in these eyes, with their shallow anterior chambers and anteriorly placed lens, the iris being more closely opposed to the lens capsule over a much wider area than in the normal deep chamber where the pupillary iris margins lightly touch the anterior lens surface. The passage of aqueous between the posterior and anterior chambers is then hindered and, with the semidilated pupil, a physiological iris bombe results. The peripheral iris bulges forward to come in contact with the posterior corneal surface, thus impeding the drainage of the aqueous via the filtration channels of the angle.

Two simple techniques have been described which permit estimation of the depth of the anterior chamber. In the flashlight or oblique illumination test, a pen light is held parallel to the iris plane and temporally to direct a beam of light nasally. It is inferred that if the entire iris appears to be illuminated then the angle is deep, but if only the temporal iris appears illuminated, then the angle is shallow (Fig. 7.1). The grading scheme used by Pophal and Ripkin (1995) is illustrated in Table 7.1.

Van Herick (Van Herick et al., 1969) and subsequently Polse (1975) and Stone (1979) described how a very narrow slit lamp microscope beam is directed perpendicularly to the corneal surface at the temporal limbus to form an optic section. Observation is made with the microscope, using a magnification of about ×16 to 20, placed at an angle of 60° to

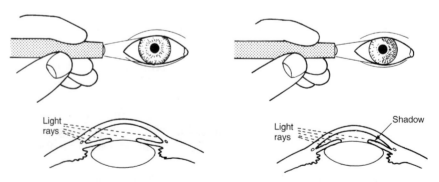

Figure 7.1 Penlight screening for shallow anterior chamber. Left, normal anterior chamber. Right, shallow anterior chamber.

Table 7.1 Grading of anterior chamber based on the flashlight and Van Herick methods, interpretation of results and corresponding decision on the use by the optometrist of a mydriatic

Flashlight or oblique illumination test (extent of illumination of nasal iris)	Van Herick test (Numerator is dark space, denominator is optic section)	Grade	Interpretation of angle of anterior chamber	Decision
Full	>1	4	Wide open	Can dilate
$\frac{2}{3}$ to full	$\frac{1}{4}$ to $\frac{1}{2}$	3	Moderately open	Can dilate
$\frac{1}{3}$ to $\frac{2}{3}$	$\frac{1}{4}$	2	Moderately narrow	Do NOT dilate Gonioscopy indicated
$<\frac{1}{3}$	$<\frac{1}{4}$	1	Extremely narrow	Do NOT dilate Gonioscopy indicated

the illumination system. A fixation target is selected such that the patient's gaze is directed in the primary position. An assessment is made of width of the dark space representing the interval between the iris and the posterior corneal surface, relative to the width of the corneal section. A fraction is recorded in which the numerator is the width of the dark space and the denominator is the width of the optic section (Fig. 7.2). The nasal depth of the anterior chamber can be similarly assessed. In some cases, the presence of arcus senilis may make it difficult to determine whether the illumination system has been correctly positioned at the limbus. The corresponding grading system is also shown in Table 7.1.

There are conflicting estimates of the sensitivity and specificity of these two tests (Table 7.2). The variation may reflect different levels of experience of the observers, different patient samples and other experimental variables (such as the comparison of Van Herick either with measured

Table 7.3 The sensitivity and specificity of the flashlight or oblique illumination test and the Van Herick test

Authors	Sensitivity (%)		Specificity (%)	
	Oblique illumination test	Van Herick test	Oblique illumination test	Van Herick test
Vargas et al. (1973)	89	82	88	84.6
Pophal and Ripkin (1995)	90.9	81.8	76.2	95.8
Thomas et al. (1996)	45.5	61.9	82.7	89.3

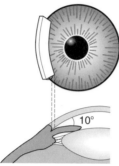

Grade 1:
The width of the anterior chamber interval is less than 1/4 of that of the corneal section. The angle is extremely narrow and with full pupil dilation closure is probable.

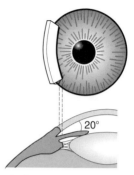

Grade 2:
The width of the anterior chamber interval is approximately 1/4 of that of the corneal section. The angle is narrow and closure is possible.

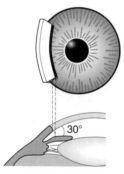

Grade 3:
The width of the anterior chamber interval is between 1/4 and 1/2 of that of the corneal section. Closure of the angle is unlikely.

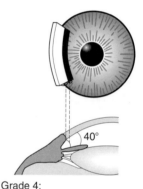

Grade 4:
The width of the anterior chamber interval is equal to, or greater than, that of the corneal section. The angle is wide open.

Figure 7.2 Van Herick angle estimation.

anterior chamber depth or with gonioscopic findings). While the use of gonioscopy is mandatory prior to the dilation of known or suspected closed angle glaucomatous patients, it is not used routinely on all other patients who are deemed to require mydriatic examination.

With regard to the prevalence of very narrow anterior chamber angles, Van Herick *et al.* (1969) reported that 'Narrowing of the anterior chamber angle progresses during ageing but Grade 1 angles are found in only 0.64% of an ageing population and Grade 2 angles in only 1%'. Their study was based on an unselected group of 2185 patients.

Notwithstanding the low prevalence of anterior chambers which are very narrow, the fear of precipitating acute angle closure glaucoma has tended to deter non-ophthalmologists from dilating pupils. The incidence of angle closure glaucoma secondary to pupil dilation has been the subject of a study by Patel *et al.* (1995). Of 4870 subjects whose pupils were dilated, none developed this complication despite the fact that 38 patients were subsequently judged to have occludable angles on the basis of gonioscopic examination. It follows that identification of patients as having a potentially occludable angle means that their pupils should be dilated with caution and not that the angle will occlude as a result of a single dilated examination.

It was acknowledged by Patel *et al.* that their subjects were predominantly of either European or African descent and their findings might not be generalized to the Asian population, in whom angle closure glaucoma is reportedly more common.

Patel *et al.* made the significant comment that 'the potential risk to the patient of dilated ophthalmoscopic examination is low, and the benefits may include preservation of sight or even life'.

Mode of action
(Table 7.3)

Because of the presence of the two opponent muscles, the pupil sphincter and dilator muscles, there are two different modes of action of mydriatics.

The pupil dilator muscle is innervated by the sympathetic nervous system and sympathomimetic drugs will cause a contraction of the dilator muscle causing mydriasis. The parasympathetic system is largely unaffected by such drugs and thus the pupillary light reflex remains active. Sympathomimetic drugs also have little effect on accommodation.

On the other hand, the pupil sphincter muscle, which is innervated by the parasympathetic system, can be paralysed by the same class of drugs which cause cycloplegia, the antimuscarinic agents. With this type of drug the pupillary light reflex is reduced or abolished.

Irrespective of the type of mydriatic employed, when a mydriatic is applied unilaterally the light reflex in the other eye is unaffected and the mydriasis in the treated eye is accompanied by a consensual miosis. That this miosis is a result of the light reflex is confirmed by the fact that the consensual miosis is not manifest when the pupil diameters are measured in darkness (Theofilopoulos *et al.*, 1988). It is usual practice to dilate both eyes and this effect will have little significance unless the clinician is trying to assess the amount of anisocoria.

Antimuscarinic mydriatics

By using weak concentrations of 'strong drugs' (for example, homatropine) or 'weak drugs' (for example, tropicamide) of the antimuscarinic group, mydriasis can be produced with a much less profound cycloplegia, with the latter's attendant incapacitating effect on near vision thereby considerably reduced, as the pupil sphincter is more susceptible than the ciliary muscle to these substances.

Tropicamide

Tropicamide is the antimuscarinic mydriatic of choice today. Normally available in 0.5% and 1.0% strengths, it is the weaker of the two that is used most often for mydriasis. Davidson (1976) states that the mydriatic effect is greater than the cycloplegic effect and that this propensity for mydriasis is of clinical value. The 1% strength is used for cycloplegia. Tropicamide is quick in onset and short in duration, and the depth of mydriasis is adequate for most examinations since the pupil light reflex

Table 7.3 Mydriatics

Official name	Strengths % w/v	Single dose?	Mode of action	Mydriatic onset	Mydriatic duration	Reversed by	Adverse reactions	Notes
Atropine sulphate	1.0	Yes	Antimuscarinic	40 min	7 days	Ecothiopate	Allergic reactions CNS toxic effects	Too strong for routine use
Homatropine hydrobromide	1.0 2.0	1.0 only	Antimuscarinic	40 min	48 h	Physostigmine	As for atropine	Rarely used
Cyclopentolate	0.1 0.5 1.0	Yes	Antimuscarinic	30 min	24 h	Physostigmine	CNS effects	No longer available
Tropicamide	0.5 1.0	Yes	Antimuscarinic	15 min	8–9 h	Physostigmine	Some CNS effects	Mydriatic of choice
Phenyl-ephedrine	2.5 10.0	Yes	Sympathomimetic	30 min	12–24 h	Pilocarpine	Systemic hypertension	

is depressed. Pollack *et al.* (1981) investigated the dose/response relationships of tropicamide's mydriasis and cycloplegia under two levels of illumination. They found that the mydriatic effect was independent of dose (range 0.25–1.0%) and level of illumination, whilst the cycloplegic effect was greater for the stronger concentrations.

This finding confirms that 0.5% should be used for mydriasis and 1% for cycloplegia. Pollack *et al.* used patients with a range of eye colours, but did not collate the findings for different degrees of pigmentation. Hence it is possible that the strength may need to be varied with the level of pigmentation. The mydriasis caused by tropicamide can be reversed if necessary with weak solutions of physostigmine.

Other antimuscarinic mydriatics

All cycloplegics can be used as mydriatics but the effect is usually too long lasting. The following have been used in the past.

Cyclopentolate

The mydriatic concentration of cyclopentolate is 0.1% (compared with 0.5% and 1.0% for cycloplegia). However, this strength is no longer available and if cyclopentolate is used as a mydriatic then significant cycloplegia will accompany its use. Mydriasis commences in about 10 minutes and is maximal in about 30 minutes. The effect may last up to 24 hours (Davidson, 1976). It produces similar mydriasis but more cycloplegia than homatropine. Cyclopentolate 1% is sometimes used preoperatively to produce maximal mydriasis.

Homatropine

At one time homatropine was the principal mydriatic and was often used in mixtures such as homatropine and cocaine or homatropine and ephedrine. The mydriatic effect commences in 10–20 minutes and is maximal in 30–40 minutes. At 30 minutes both light and accommodative reflexes are absent and an examination may be carried out. Recovery takes the same time as cyclopentolate if a miotic is not used, but may be as prolonged as three days (Davidson, 1976). It can be employed as 0.25% or 0.5%, but these concentrations are not available commercially. As would be expected, the higher strength produces a slightly larger pupil but a much more marked effect on the ciliary muscle in reducing accommodation.

Eucatropine

Eucatropine is no longer available in any pharmaceutical form.

Sympathomimetic mydriatics
Phenylephrine

This is the only sympathomimetic mydriatic in regular use and the only one available in single use units. Phenylephrine is available in a variety of strengths but 2.5% and 10.0% are the ones most often used. Mydriasis commences in about 10 minutes and is maximal in 30 minutes. The mydriasis lasts for several hours. Phenylephrine has been compared with ephedrine, which it has replaced as the most commonly used mydriatic.

Phenylephrine is an alpha agonist and as well as producing mydriasis it causes vasoconstriction of the conjunctiva. In low concentrations (0.125%) it is used as a vasoconstrictor in some over the counter eye brightening drops. There is little doubt that sympathomimetic amines produce less effect on accommodation than antimuscarinics, and some authors (Kanski, 1969) suggest that phenylephrine produces mydriasis without any cycloplegic effect at all. On the other hand, larger decreases in near point accommodation than can be attributed to the increase in the size of the pupil have been reported (Garner et al., 1983). Phenylephrine, like other sympathomimetics, will also cause a widening of the palpebral fissure (Munden et al., 1991).

Phenylephrine like all sympathomimetics is less effective in highly pigmented patients and will allow the light reflex to remain.

There has been some discussion of the effectiveness of the 2.5% strength of phenylephrine relative to the 10% strength. Although Duffin et al. (1983) found a greater effect from 10% phenylephrine than from 2.5%, it must be pointed out that they were using a viscolized 10% solution against an aqueous 2.5% and this difference in vehicles could have had an influence on the mydriatic action. The disparity in mydriasis was greater for darkly pigmented eyes as opposed to lightly coloured eyes. Neuhaus and Hepler (1980) found similar mydriatic effects with 2.5% and 10% phenylephrine and recommend 2.5% for routine dilation. Another comparison of the two strengths was carried out by Glatt et al. (1990) but in this study it was the Müller muscle induced elevation of the upper eyelid which was recorded. The stronger solution produced a slightly greater elevation which was significant statistically but not important in the context of the test being carried out. It is likely that in spite of the good reports on the use of 2.5% solution, the use of the stronger solution will predominate in the future.

Another possible future development is the use of a prodrug which would enhance the mydriatic effect and reduce the possibility of side effects. Miller-Meeks et al. (1991) evaluated the mydriatic effects of phenylephrine oxazolidine prodrug by comparing the mydriasis it produced after 30 minutes with that produced by viscolized solutions of phenylephrine. A 1% solution of the prodrug produced a markedly greater mydriasis than the 10% solution of phenylephrine.

Cocaine

This alkaloid derived from the leaves of the *Erythroxylum coca* is a colourless, crystalline substance, the official salt being the hydrochloride; maximum therapeutic dose 15 mg. Solubility of the alkaloid is 1 in 300 in water, and 1 in 10 in castor oil; solubility of the salt is 2 in 1 in water. Cocaine is a powerful local anaesthetic, blocking nerve conduction on topical application to sensory nerve endings, for example those in the corneal epithelium. The ophthalmic use of cocaine has declined very markedly along with most other medical uses because of its toxicity.

Hydroxyamphetamine hydrobromide (*Paredrine*, USA)

This is a white crystalline powder, soluble one in one in water; it is a sympathomimetic agent with direct and indirect effects on adrenergic alpha and beta receptors. It may be given in a single dose of up to 60 mg by mouth, 20 mg by intramuscular injection and 10 mg by intravenous injection.

In general medicine its main use is in nasal sprays as a decongestant, by intramuscular or intravenous injection to maintain blood pressure in spinal anaesthesia, and for its direct stimulatory effect on the heart in the treatment and prevention of bradycardia due to excessive carotid sinus irritability. When used as a mydriatic in 1–3% eyedrops full mydriasis occurs in about 30–45 minutes and lasts two to three hours. It is of little clinical interest as it is not commercially available and there are superior drugs.

Ephedrine hydrochloride

Ephedrine is a colourless crystalline alkaloid obtained from species of Ephedra, or prepared synthetically. Both the alkaloid and the official hydrochloride salt, which may occur as a colourless crystalline substance or as white crystalline powder and has a maximum therapeutic dose of 60 mg, are soluble in water (1 in 36 and 1 in 4, respectively).

The mydriatic effect of ephedrine is unreliable especially in patients with darkly pigmented irides and this has led to its lack of present day use for this purpose.

Antimuscarinic or sympathomimetic

In selection of a mydriatic, the optometrist will no doubt invoke some personal preference. With the demise of many traditional mydriatics, the probable choice will be between phenylephrine and tropicamide. Cyclopentolate should only be considered if the other drugs produce insufficient depth of mydriasis.

Tropicamide is the more effective mydriatic, especially if photography is contemplated, as the pupillary light reflex will be abolished. However, Mordi et al. (1986) when comparing 0.1% cyclopentolate and 10% phenylephrine as mydriatics concluded that neither were ideal, since both caused a loss of accommodation signified by a recession of near point and a slowing of the accommodation response.

Tropicamide has the ability to cause a rise in intraocular pressure in eyes with a deep anterior chamber, as opposed to phenylephrine which causes a fall (like all sympathomimetics). However, the rise in IOP is likely to be small and transient and unlikely to cause a problem.

Phenylephrine can have effects on blood pressure (see below) and is contraindicated in patients with cardiovascular problems and patients taking certain drugs.

In summary, it would appear that tropicamide 0.5% is the first choice as a mydriatic, but special conditions require special considerations. Huber et al. (1985) found that diabetic patients responded poorly to tropicamide and recommended a combination of this agent with phenylephrine to give adequate mydriasis with a minimum of accommodative paralysis. Chang et al. (1985) found that phenylephrine produced better sector pupil dilation than tropicamide. Sector pupil dilation (in which the pupil becomes oval or pear-shaped) is recommended for dilating eyes with narrow filtration angles because it reduces the risk of acute angle closure glaucoma.

Mixed mydriatics

When the mydriasis produced by one or other of the two types of mydriatic will not produce sufficient depth of mydriasis, mixtures of an antimuscarinic and a sympathomimetic may be used. The following mixtures are some of the ones that have been employed:

homatropine and cocaine
homatropine and ephedrine
tropicamide and phenylephrine
cyclopentolate and phenylephrine

The strengths of the compounds in the mixtures can be varied according to the degree of mydriasis required. Apt and Hendrick (1980) investigated the mydriatic effect of three combinations:

cyclopentolate 0.5% and phenylephrine 2.5%
tropicamide 0.5% and phenylephrine 2.5%
tropicamide 1.0% and phenylephrine 2.5%

and found no significant difference between the mixtures. They recorded dilation of around 7 mm within 60 minutes, which must be approaching maximal effect. The light reflex was abolished. Unfortunately they did not report on the duration of effect.

Cases in which dilation is difficult

The two principal conditions which make pupils less responsive to the action of a mydriatic are dark iris pigmentation and diabetes mellitus. Inevitably, a number of patients present both problems.

Iris pigmentation

Phenylephrine, like all sympathomimetics, is less effective in highly pigmented patients and will allow the light reflex to remain. When mydriasis is necessary with pupils that are obviously going to be difficult to dilate, one of the more powerful antimuscarinic mydriatics should be the drug of choice without hesitation. It is a waste of the patient's and practitioner's time to attempt to dilate such pupils with one of the weaker sympathomimetic drugs; for example, Barbee and Smith (1957) concluded that phenylephrine is a relatively ineffective mydriatic when used on Afro-Caribbean patients. They found that only the antimuscarinic drugs (and these in cycloplegic concentrations) were really adequate in these patients, and even then cyclopentolate 1% produced only a 1.5 mm mean increase in pupillary diameter compared to the approximately 3.0 mm increase obtained with atropine 1%, hyoscine 0.2% and homatropine 4%. Phenylephrine 10% actually proved slightly more effective than the cyclopentolate, giving an average 1.75 mm increased pupil width. As Havener (1978) remarks, the eyes of Afro-Caribbeans are only dilated with great difficulty, especially when using phenylephrine, cyclopentolate or hydroxyamphetamine as the mydriatic.

Priestley and Medine (1951) have also carried out a comparative study of the mydriatic responses to various drugs of subjects from different races. They found that after 20 minutes the speed of mydriasis with cyclopentolate 0.5% was surpassed by homatropine (2%) and phenylephrine (neosynephrine) 10% and at the end of 60 minutes the latter ranked first. Nevertheless, after this time the cyclopentolate drops did produce an average 7.0 mm pupil in the Afro-Caribbean subjects compared to 7.5 mm in the white subjects.

Diabetes mellitus

Huber *et al.* (1985) found that diabetic patients responded poorly to tropi-camide and recommended a combination of this agent with phenyl-ephrine to give adequate mydriasis with a minimum of accommodative paralysis.

Sector dilation

In the presence of a narrow angle anterior chamber, localized dilation of the pupil can be undertaken to reduce the risk of inducing an acute angle closure glaucoma. Following instillation of one or two drops of topi-cal anaesthetic, the tip of a cotton-tipped applicator is moistened with two or three drops of 2.5% phenylephrine and then held against the limbus for 15 to 20 seconds (Fingeret *et al.*, 1990). Oval or pear-shaped dilation ensues. Chang *et al.* (1985) found that phenylephrine produced better sector pupil dilation than tropicamide.

Mydriatics for diagnosis of Horner's syndrome

Sympathetic denervation of the iris dilator muscle will lead to a slightly miosed pupil. The iris will be supersensitive to sympathomimetic amines but subsensitive to parasympathomimetics such as pilocarpine or carbachol. Colasanti *et al.* (1978) demonstrated these phenomena in rabbits. As a differential diagnostic test, a weak sympathomimetic mydria-tic may be used. Adrenaline 0.1% or phenylephrine 0.125% is instilled, and if the muscle is sympathetically denervated it will be hypersensitive to the mydriatic and dilate. Normally innervated irides will not respond.

As a further test, indirectly acting sympathomimetics can be used to determine the site of the lesion giving rise to the anisocoria. If the damage to the sympathetic nerve supply has occurred distal to the gang-lion, i.e. in the postganglionic nerve, then the stores of catecholamines normally found at the nerve terminals will not be present and indirectly acting sympathomimetics will have little effect. However if the damage has occurred to the preganglionic nerves, the postganglionic nerve will be intact and thus will be able to respond to such agents as hydroxy-amphetamine (Cremer *et al.*, 1990a and b).

Adverse effects of mydriatics

With any topically applied ophthalmic drug there is a possibility of pro-ducing an undesirable effect, either on the eye or on the body as a whole. Mydriatics have the ability to do both.

Angle closure glaucoma

The use of a mydriatic causes pupil dilation which in turn introduces the possibility of angle block. The danger will be dependent on the degree of dilation, not on the mydriatic employed. The probability of inducing an attack of closed angle glaucoma is remote (figures vary from 0.06% to 0.09% of the population): (Lowe, 1967; Hollows and Graham, 1966) and it can be made even more remote by careful prior examination of the patient and detailed history taking. Keller (1975) concludes that, pro-viding proper precautions are taken, the risk of precipitating angle closure is virtually nil. Prevention is better than cure, and the time to find out that the patient has a shallow anterior chamber depth is before the mydriatic is instilled, not after.

Obviously it is important that the optometrist is aware of the signs and symptoms of such an attack, which can occur not only from the use of a mydriatic, but also spontaneously. An optometrist may expect to see an attack of closed angle glaucoma about once in 40 years.

The classical symptoms of closed angle glaucoma are well known but are worth repeating here. The patient experiences intense pain which may be severe enough to induce vomiting. The conjunctival blood vessels are dilated, giving an appearance to the inexpert eye of conjunctivitis, and the cornea loses transparency slightly because the high intraocular pressure causes it to imbibe water and swell. The patient may report this as seeing haloes around lights. Through the hazy cornea the pupil can be seen, often mid-dilated (Chandler, 1952) and probably noncircular. The pupil will not constrict to light, accommodation or to the action of miotics. The intraocular pressure is very high. The situation is an emergency one, but does not require panic measures. Providing the intraocular pressure is reduced over the ensuing period, there should be no long lasting damage.

A wise precaution is to issue patients with a note which explains that if they experience symptoms such as decreased vision, eye pain or redness, nausea or vomiting, then they should contact the practitioner immediately so that prompt referral to an ophthalmologist can be arranged.

Other complications

Angle closure glaucoma is not the only adverse reaction which can be induced by the use of mydriatics and the optometrist should be alert to other problems. The other side effects of antimuscarinics have been dealt with under cycloplegics (Chapter 6), but as it is usual to use lower concentrations of mydriatics, they should be less likely to occur.

Other local toxic effects from topical sympathomimetic drugs include a toxic epithelial desquamation of the cornea similar to that seen with local anaesthetics (Havener, 1978) and a case of allergic conjunctivitis following the use of phenylephrine (Shoji and Watanabe, 1991).

Liberation of iris pigment into the anterior chamber has been reported by Aggarwal and Beveridge (1971) following the use of 10% phenyl-ephrine. The pigment appeared as aqueous floaters within 45 minutes of the drug being instilled, causing an aqueous flare which could be confused with anterior uveitis. There were apparently no symptoms.

Sympathomimetic mydriatics like any other topically applied drug can produce systemic effects, and the cardiovascular system is the one most sensitive to their effects. The problem with sympathomimetics is exacerbated by the high concentration of active agent that is used relative to the normal systemic dose. Topically administered drugs may gain access to the vascular system either by direct absorption through the conjunctival blood vessels or via the nasolacrimal system to the alimentary tract. Absorption can be very quick, with maximum levels being reached 10–20 minutes after instillation (Kumar et al., 1985). Absorption can be markedly reduced by reducing the volume of the drugs solution in the conjunctival sac. This in turn can be achieved by reducing the volume of the drop administered. The principal determinant of drop size is the diameter of the dropper from which the drop is expelled. Craig and Griffiths (1991) found that the reducing the tip size reduced the drop size but not the mydriatic effect, thus confirming the fact that normal droppers deliver a substantial overload to the conjunctival sac, thereby increasing the possibility of systemic effects.

There are several predisposing risk factors which will increase the possibility of severe systemic reaction (Hopkins and Lyle, 1977). These are:

1. Prior use of a local anaesthetic.
2. Conjunctival disruption and/or bleeding.
3. Patients with high blood pressure, heart disease or thyrotoxicosis.
4. Multiple applications.
5. Concomitant medication.

Fraunfelder and Scafidi (1978) reviewed 33 cases of adverse reactions following the topical ocular use of 10% phenylephrine. There were no cases following 2.5% phenylephrine. Fifteen patients suffered myocardial infarcts which could not definitely be attributed to the use of phenylephrine, but seven patients showed significant increases in systemic blood pressure. They recommend the use of 2.5% phenylephrine in infants and the elderly. Accordingly, the use of sympathomimetic mydriatics in patients with cardiac disease, hypertension, aneurysms, advanced arteriosclerosis and patients receiving monoamine oxidase inhibitors or tricyclic antidepressants should be avoided.

Apparently healthy patients may also be at risk, a case of coronary artery spasm having been reported in a healthy 28 year old patient (Alder et al., 1981).

When used properly, the incidence of a blood pressure rise from the use of phenylephrine should be low. Epstein and Murphy (1981) found that only two patients out of 62 responded with a change in blood pressure of more than 20 mmHg to the use of phenylephrine 10% with cyclopentolate 1%. Brown et al. (1980) failed to find significant changes in patients who had received 10% phenylephrine.

References

Aggarwal, J. C. and Beveridge, B. (1971) Liberation of iris pigment in the anterior chamber after instillation of 10% phenylephrine hydrochloride solution. Br. J. Ophthalmol., 55, 544–545

Alder, A. G., McElwain, G. E. and Martin, J. H. (1981) Coronary artery spasm induced by phenylephrine eyedrops. Arch. Int. Med., 141, 1384–1385

Apt, I. and Henrick, A. (1980) Pupillary dilatation with single eyedrop mydriatic combinations. Am. J. Ophthalmol., 89, 553–559

Barbee, R. F. and Smith W, O. (1957) A comparative study of mydriatic and cycloplegic agents. Am. J. Ophthalmol., 44, 617

Brown, M. M., Brown, G. C. and Spaeth, G. (1980) Lack of side effects from topically administered 10% phenylephrine eyedrops. Arch. Ophthalmol., 98, 487–489

Chandler, P. (1952) Narrow angle glaucoma. Arch. Ophthalmol., 47, 695–716

Chang, F. W., McCann, T. A. and Hitchcock, J. R. (1985) Sector pupil dilatation with phenylephrine and tropicamide. Am. J. Optom. Physiol. Optics, 62, 482–486

Colasanti, B. K., Chui, P. and Trotter, R. R. (1978) Adrenergic and cholinergic drug effects on rabbit eyes after sympathetic denervation. Eur. J. Pharmacol., 47, 311–318

Craig, E. W. and Griffiths, P. G. (1991) Effect on mydriasis of modifying the volume of phenylephrine drops. Br. J. Ophthalmol., 75, 222–223

Cremer, S. A. et al. (1990a) Hydroxyamphetamine mydriasis in normal subjects. Am. J. Ophthalmol., 110, 66–70

Cremer, S. A. *et al.* (1990b) Hydroxyamphetamine mydriasis in Horner's syndrome. *Am. J. Ophthalmol.,* **110**, 71–76

Davidson, S. I. (1976) Mydriatic and cycloplegic drugs. *Trans. Ophthalmol. Soc. UK,* **96**, 327–329

Duffin, R. M., Pettit, T. H. and Straatsma, B. R. (1983) 2.5% vs 10% phenylephrine in maintaining mydriasis during cataract surgery. *Arch. Ophthalmol.,* **101**, 1903–1906

Epstein, D. L. and Murphy, E. (1981) Effects of combined 1% cyclopentolate–phenylephrine eye drops on systemic blood pressure of glaucoma patients. *Ann. Ophthalmol.,* **13**, 735–736

Fingeret, M., Casser, L. and Woodcome, H. T. (1990) *Atlas of Primary Eyecare Procedures.* Norwalk, Connecticut: Appleton and Lange

Fraunfelder, F. T and Scafidi, A. F. (1978) Possible adverse effects from topical ocular 10% phenylephrine. *Am. J. Ophthalmol.,* **85**, 447–453

Garner, L. F., Brown, B., Baker, R. and Colgan, M. (1983) The effect of phenylephrine hydrochloride on the resting point of accommodation. *Invest. Ophthalmol. Vis. Sci.,* **24**, 363–395

Glatt, H. J., Fett, D. R. and Putterman, A. M. (1990) Comparison of 2.5% and 10% phenylephrine in the elevation of upper eyelids and ptosis. *Ophthalmic Surg.,* **21**, 173–176

Havener, W. H. (1975) *Synopsis of Ophthalmology,* 4th edn., pp. 307, 491–494. St Louis: Mosby

Havener, W. H. (1978) *Ocular Pharmacology,* 4th edn, pp. 233, 237. St Louis: Mosby

Hollows, F. C. and Graham, P. A. (1966) Intraocular pressure, glaucoma and glaucoma suspects in a defined population. *Br. J. Ophthalmol.,* **50**, 570–586

Hopkins, G. A. and Lyle, W. M. (1977) Potential systemic side effects of six common ophthalmic drugs. *J. Am. Optom. Assoc.,* **48**, 1241–1245

Huber, M. J. E., Smith, S. A. and Smith, S. E. (1985) Mydriatic drugs for diabetic patients. *Br. J. Ophthalmol.,* **69**, 425–427

Kanski, J. J. (1969) Mydriatics. *Br. J. Ophthalmol.,* **53**, 426–429

Keller, J. T. (1975) The risk of angle closure from the use of mydriatics. *J. Am. Optom. Assoc.,* **46**, 19–21

Kumar, V., Schoenwald, K. D., Chien, D. S., Packer, A. J. and Choi, W. W. (1985) Systemic absorption and cardiovascular effects of phenylephrine eyedrops. *Am. J. Ophthalmol.,* **99**, 180–184

Lowe, R. F. (1967) Primary angle closure glaucoma, a review of provocative tests. *Br. J. Ophthalmol.,* **51**, 727–732

Martin-Doyle, J. L. C. (1967) *A Synopsis of Ophthalmology,* 3rd edn., p. 8. Bristol: Wright

Miller-Meeks, M. J. *et al* (1991) Phenylephrine prodrug: Report of clinical trials. *Ophthalmology,* **98/2**, 222–226

Mordi, J., Tucker, J. and Charman, W. N. (1986) Effects of 0.1% cyclopentolate or 10% phenylephrine on pupil diameter and accommodation. *Optom. Physiol. Optics,* **6**, 221–227

Munden, P. M. *et al.* (1991) Palpebral fissure responses to topical adrenergic drugs. *Am. J. Ophthalmol.,* **111**, 706–710

Neuhaus, R. W. and Hepler, K. S. (1980) Mydriatic effect of phenylephrine 10% vs phenylephrine 2.5% (aq). *Ann. Ophthalmol.,* **12**, 1159–1160

Newell, E. (1969) *Ophthalmology, principles and concepts,* 2nd edn., p. 140. St Louis: Mosby

Patel, K. H., Javitt, J. C., Tielsch, J. M., Street, D. A., Katz, J., Quigley, H. A. and Sommer, A. (1995) Incidence of acute angle closure glaucoma after pharmacologic mydriasis. *Am. J. Ophthalmol.,* **120**, 709–717

Pollack, S. L., Hunt, J. S. and Poise, K. A. (1981) Dose-response effects of tropicamide HCl. *Am. J. Optom. Physiol. Optics,* **58**, 361–366

Polse, K. A. (1975) Technique for estimating the angle of the anterior chamber using the slit lamp. *Optom. Weekly,* **66** (22), 524

Pophal, M. D. and Ripkin, D. J. (1995) Assessment of anterior chamber depth. Olique illumination test. *Ann. Ophthalmol.*, **27**, 171–174

Priestley, H. S. and Medine, M. M. (1951) A new mydriatic and cycloplegic drug. *Am. J. Ophthalmol.*, **34,** 572

Shoji, A. and Watanabe, K. (1991) A case of allergic conjunctivitis due to phenylephrine hydrochloride. *Skin Res.*, **33** (Suppl.), 48–52

Siderov, J., Bartlett, J. R. and Madigan, C. J. (1996) Pupillary dilation: the patient's perspective. *Clin. Exp. Optom.*, **79**, 62–66

Stone, J. (1979) The slit lamp biomicroscope in ophthalmic practice. *Ophthal. Optician.*, **19** (12), 439

Theofilopoulos, N. *et al.* (1988) Consensual pupillary responses to mydriatic and miotic drugs. *Brit. J. Clin. Pharmacol.*, **26**, 697–702

Thomas, R., George, T., Braganza, A. and Muliyil, J. (1996) The flashlight test and Van Herick's test are poor predictors for occludable angles. *Aus. and N.Z. J. Ophthalmol.*, **24**, 251–256

Van Herick, W., Shaffer, K. N. and Schwartz, A. (1969) Estimation of width of the anterior chamber: incidence and significance of the narrow angle. *Am. J. Ophthalmol.*, **68**, 626

Vargas, E., Schulzer, M. and Drance, S. M. (1973) The use of the oblique illumination test to predict angle closure glaucoma. *Can. J. Ophthalmol.*, **9**, 104–105

8

Miotics

Miotics are drugs which constrict the pupil. In the hands of the optometrist they are used to reverse the mydriasis produced by drugs such as phenylephrine and tropicamide, but they may also be used in the emergency treatment of closed angle glaucoma.

In medicine their principal use is in the treatment of primary open angle glaucoma. As the ideal properties for a glaucoma treatment vary greatly from those of an antimydriatic miotic, this chapter will only deal with the latter. Antiglaucoma treatments will be dealt with in Chapter 12.

Ideal properties

1. Quick in onset.
2. A length of action appropriate to the mydriatic previously employed.
3. An effect on the ciliary muscle which leaves the patient without cycloplegia or cyclospasm.
4. An effect on the iris which allows a normal pupil light reflex.
5. No other pharmacological effect.
6. No local toxic reaction.
7. No systemic toxic reaction.
8. No adverse subjective complaints such as 'stinging'.

From the above it can be seen that there will be no perfect miotic. Much will depend on the appropriate selection of a miotic to follow the mydriatic.

At one time it was routine to instil a miotic after mydriatic examination in all patients over the age of 40. Nowadays, with the use of short acting mydriatics such as tropicamide, the necessity for their routine use must be questioned and the advantages of the miotic must be carefully weighed against its disadvantages. The view expressed by Gilmartin *et al.* (1995) that if an eye is considered safe to dilate it is normally at little risk from allowing the eye to recover naturally is to be supported, especially if short acting mydriatics are used.

Advantages

The use of a miotic:

1. Reduces the danger of angle closure. Nevertheless it introduces the danger of pupil block and, as previously indicated, all patients should have their angles assessed before a mydriatic is instilled.
2. Avoids photophobia, especially on a bright sunny day.
3. Speeds the return of accommodation if the mydriatic has a cycloplegic action.
4. Lowers the intraocular pressure. This should not be too elevated if the anterior chamber is sufficiently deep and some mydriatics, e.g. phenylephrine, actually cause a fall.

Disadvantages

1. The small pupil can lead to dimness of vision. This can be a problem at twilight, especially if the patient is proposing to drive a car.
2. A spasm of accommodation may be caused, leading to pseudomyopia.

Mode of action

Mydriatics can cause mydriasis either by paralysing the sphincter (anti-muscarinics) or by stimulating the dilator (sympathomimetics). Conversely, miotics may cause their effect by either inhibiting the dilator (alpha blocking agents) or by stimulating the sphincter (parasympathomimetics or anticholinesterases).

Miotics acting on the pupil sphincter muscle

The sphincter muscle is stimulated to contract by the action of acetylcholine on muscarinic receptors, so drugs can act by mimicking the action of acetylcholine on the muscarinic receptor (parasympathomimetic) or by preventing the breakdown of acetylcholine by the cholinesterase present at the cholinergic neuroeffector junctions (anticholinesterases).

Miotics acting on the pupil dilator muscle

As the sympathetic innervation to the dilator muscle is stimulatory (motor), it is logical that alpha receptors predominate. The effect of noradrenaline on this muscle can be blocked by an alpha blocking agent. There are many alpha blocking agents available for use in general medicine. They are used in the treatment of hypertension and peripheral vasospastic conditions, but only thymoxamine has been formulated as an eyedrop. Unfortunately, this is no longer available.

Studies have been carried with an alpha blocking drug dapiprazole (Molinari *et al.*, 1994), but whether this will become commercially available remains to be seen.

Parasympatho-mimetic miotics

Parasympathomimetic miotics can be grouped into choline esters which are derivatives of acetylcholine, and cholinomimetic alkaloids which include pilocarpine, arecoline and muscarine. By far the most commonly used parasympathomimetic miotic is pilocarpine.

Pilocarpine

Obtained from the leaves of *Pilocarpus microphyllus* (jaborandi plant) and other species of Pilocarpus, pilocarpine is a colourless, syrupy, liquid alkaloid which is soluble in water. The hydrochloride salt, which is freely soluble in less than one part of water, is now preferred to the nitrate (previously used) in the preparation of eyedrops, because it is compatible with a wide range of antimicrobial preservatives.

Mechanism of action

Pilocarpine is a direct acting parasympathomimetic agent (compare with the indirect acting physostigmine). Like all such agents (including synthetic choline esters such as carbachol and bethanecol) its primary action is the stimulation (or inhibition) of autonomic effector cells in a similar manner to that accomplished by the acetylcholine released by stimulation of postganglionic parasympathetic nerves, that is, it acts primarily at muscarinic receptors of autonomic effector cells. Koelle (1975) also states that in addition it has some nicotinic ganglionic effects, but part of this secondary ganglionic action involves stimulation of muscarinic receptors which are now known also to be present in varying proportions on autonomic ganglion cells. The nicotinic actions of parasympathomimetic drugs refer to their initial stimulation, and in higher dosage to subsequent blockade (as with nicotine) of autonomic ganglion cells and neuromuscular junctions. All the actions of pilocarpine and other parasympathomimetic drugs (as well as ACh) can be blocked by atropine through competitive occupation of the cholinoceptive sites on autonomic effector cells, and on the secondary muscarinic receptors of autonomic ganglion cells.

Bowman and Rand (1980) consider the nicotinic action to be very weak. In this nicotinic action pilocarpine resembles the endogenous mediator acetylcholine, but it does not, like the latter, stimulate the motor endplates of skeletal muscle in normal doses. Its effects systemically are also similar to its fellow cholinomimetic alkaloid muscarine; it slows the heart and pulse, increases peristalsis, constricts the bronchioles, and increases the secretions of the salivary, lacrimal, gastric, pancreatic and intestinal glands, and of the mucous glands of the respiratory tract. Pilocarpine causes marked sweating, due to the drug's direct stimulatory action on the sweat glands and vasodilatation of blood vessels in the skin, this latter effect producing flushing in man. Large doses of pilocarpine at first stimulate then depress the CNS. It will have been noted that physostigmine taken orally produces all these effects, but in this case they are caused by the anticholinesterase prolonging the activity of acetylcholine and not, as with pilocarpine, by the direct excitatory (or inhibitory) action of the alkaloid itself on the cholinoceptive receptor sites.

Ophthalmic preparations   Applied locally to the eye as a 0.5–4% solution (the 1% strength is that most commonly used by practitioners), pilocarpine hydrochloride (or nitrate) causes a miosis which, after commencing in about ten minutes, is maximal within half an hour and gradually decreases over a period of six hours with the 1% solution (Lowenstein, 1956). While the spasm of the ciliary muscle may last for up to two hours, unlike that following physostigmine, once this spasm has worn off it does not return if near work is commenced.

Whilst pilocarpine 1% adequately reconstricts the mydriasis produced by sympathomimetic agents it appears unnecessary to use the more powerful but also more uncomfortable physostigmine, although the latter does appear necessary to satisfactorily reverse the mydriasis following antimuscarinic eyedrops. This is a view which coincides with that of Anastasi *et al.* (1968), who found that pilocarpine 1% counteracted the effects of phenylephrine and hydroxyamphetamine (another sympathomimetic mydriatic) in concentrations usually used in ophthalmology within 30 minutes, but after mydriasis with antiparasympathomimetic agents such as tropicamide and homatropine, pilocarpine did not cause effective miosis.

As with physostigmine, pilocarpine is ineffective in the presence of atropine, the latter successfully competing for the effector cell receptors but not resulting in the excitation of these as does pilocarpine.

The miotic effect of pilocarpine in various patients produces rather marked individual differences in the latent period before miosis in the rate, the degree, and the duration of contraction and the time factor for redilation (Lowenstein and Loewenfeld, 1953). Strength for strength, it is only about half as powerful a drug as physostigmine, and thus a 1% solution does not produce the extreme degree of miosis that the anticholinesterase agent does in the same concentration. Neither is the spasm of accommodation nearly as marked or as painful as when physostigmine is used. However, for a patient with light coloured irides, the amount of pseudomyopia could be sufficient to cause problems driving (Gilmartin *et al.*, 1995).

After pilocarpine has diffused out of the eye, the pupil on recovery remains slightly more dilated than normal because of a diminished response of the pupil sphincter to normal reflex stimulation after the direct action of the pilocarpine. The lack of recurring accommodative spasm on attempting close work together with the absence of pain and discomfort are advantages of pilocarpine over physostigmine, but the latter is a more reliable miotic in counteracting the dilation of the pupil caused by the antimuscarinic mydriatics as the effects of these may outlast those of the pilocarpine, in which case the pupils will redilate.

In addition to the effect of the drug on the ciliary and pupil sphincter muscles, pilocarpine increases the flow of blood through the vasculature of the anterior uvea (Alm and Bill, 1973).

Carbachol (Doryl; Carcholin)

Carbachol (maximum therapeutic dose 0.5 mg by subcutaneous injection or 4 mg orally) occurs as very hygroscopic colourless crystals or as a white crystalline powder. It is used in general medicine to produce motility of the gut in postoperative paralytic ileus, and contraction of the bladder in nonobstructive conditions of urinary retention. Carbachol, a quaternary ammonium parasympathomimetic drug (direct action), has muscarinic and nicotinic properties and is not rapidly inactivated by cholinesterase. It may be used as a miotic in a 3% solution in the treatment of glaucoma, and is a useful alternative to pilocarpine and to other miotics where resistance or intolerance has developed. However, it is not considered a suitable agent in the treatment of accommodative esotropia because of its irregular onset and short duration of action.

The only prepacked proprietary ophthalmic solution (Isopto Carbachol) is 3%. As it is poorly absorbed through the cornea, the drops include a wetting agent such as benzalkonium chloride which also performs the additional role of acting as a bactericide. It is a derivative of, but more stable than, acetylcholine.

Acetylcholine chloride + mannitol (*Miochol*)

Synthetically manufactured acetylcholine chloride has a maximum therapeutic dose of 200 mg subcutaneously or intramuscularly; a white very hygroscopic crystalline powder and very soluble in water, it is a powerful parasympathomimetic agent, but when injected its action is very transient as it is so rapidly hydrolysed by cholinesterase. It has of course the same action as endogenous acetylcholine, but has largely been replaced in medicine by the more stable synthetic parasympathomimetics discussed above. However, a freshly prepared 1% solution incorporating 5% mannitol, a white crystalline powder soluble one in six in water and acting as an osmotic agent in the combination, intensifies the effect of the acetylcholine. This preparation is used in intraocular surgery after cataract extraction to constrict the pupil in seconds. A solution of acetylcholine instilled into an intact eye will not cause miosis as this substance would be hydrolysed by acetylcholinesterase long before it could reach an effective concentration in the anterior chamber aqueous.

Bethanecol chloride (*Urecholine*; *Mecothane*)

Bethanecol chloride, maximum therapeutic dose 5 mg subcutaneously, 30 mg orally, occurs as white hygroscopic crystals or a crystalline powder, soluble one in one in water. It has the same uses in general medicine as carbachol. A quaternary ammonium parasympathomimetic agent that is not inactivated by cholinesterase (Martindale, 1977), it has a muscarinic but (unlike carbachol) no nicotinic action (Koelle, 1975). Bethanecol is used in a 1% solution as a miotic, and like carbachol also needs a wetting agent to help it penetrate the cornea.

As there are no official or proprietary ophthalmic preparations available, eyedrops have to be extemporaneously prepared by the pharmacist if required and if indeed he can obtain the basic compound. In reality this particular miotic must at this stage be considered as historical, and it is included only for completeness.

Methacholine chloride

Methacholine chloride, maximum therapeutic dose 25 mg by subcutaneous injection, occurs as deliquescent colourless or white crystals or a white crystalline powder, soluble in less than one part of water. It has the muscarinic action of acetylcholine but is more stable, and is used in general medicine to terminate attacks of atrial paroxysmal tachycardia when simpler methods have failed. Of the two synthetic parasympathomimetic drugs carbachol and methacholine, although they possess in general the same muscarinic actions as acetylcholine (slowing of the heart, increased peristalsis, dilatation of peripheral blood vessels and increased sweat, salivary and bronchial secretions), there is some selectivity on particular structures; for example, carbachol is relatively more effective on the gastrointestinal tract and bladder, whilst methacholine is relatively more effective on the cardiovascular system. Normal pupils require a 10–20% solution to produce miosis, and this drug has also been used in these strengths for the treatment of simple glaucoma, but other miotics are now generally preferred principally because of availability. Contraindications and precautions are similar to those appertaining to pilocarpine. Methacholine is hydrolysed by acetylcholinesterase, but even alone in an adequate concentration it is successful in producing a marked miosis (and spasm of accommodation and lid twitching) by its direct action, as it has some resistance to this enzyme.

Anticholinesterases

Anticholinesterase agents can be divided into reversible and irreversible agents, depending on their duration of action. Anticholinesterases and acetylcholine are taken up by cholinesterase in the same way. There then follows a series of reactions in which the anticholinesterase or acetylcholine is broken down and the enzyme regenerated. The difference is that the reactions are very fast when acetylcholine is the substrate, while for anticholinesterase they are very slow. If the anticholinesterase is an irreversible one, the regenerating reactions are thought to take place at such a slow rate that they do not effectively occur and the body manufactures new enzyme.

Reversible anticholinesterases

The principal agents in this group are physostigmine (eserine) and neostigmine.

Physostigmine (eserine)

Physostigmine is an alkaloid obtained from the seeds of *Physostigma venenosum* (Calabar beans) and may also be prepared synthetically. It forms large colourless crystals which are sparingly soluble in water (1 in 75), but the official salt, the sulphate, is deliquescent and has a solubility in less than one part of water, and the salicylate (which stings rather less when used in the eyedrops) is soluble 1 in 90 parts water. Because of the greater solubility of the sulphate and its compatibility with a wider range of preservatives, it is now preferred to the salicylate for the preparation of eyedrops.

Physostigmine eyedrops are not now available prepacked by pharmaceutical manufacturers in the United Kingdom, but they may of course be prepared extemporaneously if necessary by the pharmacist, a costly process. Solutions of physostigmine salts, like the alkaloid itself, become pink on exposure to light and air, especially the sulphate, due to oxidation. This results in the formation of rubreserinel, which is more irritating to the eye than eserine even though the miotic effect is maintained. Physostigmine eyedrops usually contain an antioxidant to retard formation of this degradation product. Roger and Smith (1973) have brought this problem into perspective by their investigations into the stability of physostigmine eyedrops. They found that the 0.25%, 0.5% and 1% eyedrops, prepared in accordance with the *BPC*, 1973 formula (pH 3.6–3.8) and sterilized by heating or filtration, retained more than 99% of their activity after storage at 25°C for one year. A faint pink colour appeared after sterilization by heat and was also present in all samples after storage for this time. It would appear from these researches that filtration may be the method of choice to obtain colourless eyedrops from the date of manufacture. On the other hand, despite a faint pink colouration, as long as the date of manufacture is within a year and the interval after first opening the container not more than a month, it would appear to be in order to use these drops.

Mechanism of action

Physostigmine is an anticholinesterase (anti-AChE) drug. The role of this enzyme in terminating the action of the transmitter acetylcholine, liberated by cholinergic nerve impulses at junctions with their effector organs and at synaptic sites, has already been discussed in Chapter 2. Thus the acetylcholine is allowed to accumulate at sites of cholinergic transmission, and as the action of the acetylcholinesterase on the acetyl-choline is being inhibited, the effect will be similar to continuous stimulation of these cholinergic fibres. Physostigmine is an excellent example of this class of drug, but because the chemical complex of drug and acetyl-cholinesterase is only temporary and finally dissociates, its effects are limited to about 12 hours and it is termed a reversible anticholinesterase. This is in contrast to the effects of very much more potent organophosphate compounds, which also act in this manner but for very prolonged periods (from days to weeks); these are called irreversible anticholinesterase drugs, for example Dyflos (see later). The latter are extremely toxic compounds and are never used by optometrists. The irreversible anticholinesterases form extremely stable complexes with the enzyme (acetylcholinesterase), whilst in the case of the physostigmine-enzyme complex slow hydrolysis eventually results in regeneration of the cholinesterase.

Physostigmine, when topically applied to the eye, therefore permits a prolonged stimulation by acetylcholine of the ciliary and pupil sphincter muscles resulting in spasm of accommodation and miosis respectively. Conjunctival hyperaemia also occurs due to the peripheral vasodilatory effects of this miotic.

In the body, the cholinergic fibres of the parasympathetic system slow the heart and pulse rate, increase peristalsis and salivary, bronchial and gastric secretions and dilate peripheral blood vessels. Taken orally, physostigmine enhances these cholinergic effects. It is not surprising that this drug in toxic doses causes slow pulse, vomiting, diarrhoea, intestinal colic, and flushing.

Ophthalmic preparations   Strength for strength, physostigmine is about twice as active as pilocarpine, that other most useful miotic. On instillation of eyedrops of this anticholinesterase drug, constriction of the pupil commences in between five and ten minutes and miosis is maximal in about 30 minutes. The effects last for up to 12 hours or more with a 0.5% solution, and somewhat less with the 0.25% solution.

Physostigmine ointment 0.5% (the *BPC* 1963 eye ointment was 0.125%) causes an intense miosis continuing for 12–36 hours (Havener, 1978), but this is no longer available.

The 1% eyedrops of this drug should not be used by the optometrist even in the emergency produced by a sudden attack of acute glaucoma. Because of the pain and discomfort this concentration causes, this strength is unsuitable for constricting the dilated pupil of the normal eye after mydriatic examination. The marked pupillary contraction resulting from instillation of a 1 % solution (the pupil diameter being less than 2 mm) persists for more than 12 hours, and its normal size may not be regained for a few days. Eyedrops of this concentration of the drug should be reserved for the medical treatment of the later stages of simple glaucoma, when weaker strengths and weaker miotics (for example, pilocarpine) no longer control the rise in tension.

The 0.25-0.5% solutions of physostigmine, particularly the former, are the more usual concentrations of this miotic, and the 0.25% proves to be quite adequate in constricting the pupil in about half an hour following the dilation produced by the mydriatic concentrations of such anti-muscarinic eyedrops as cyclopentolate hydrochloride 0.1%, homatropine hydrobromide 0.25–0.5%, eucatropine 2–5%, and tropicamide 0.5%.

Irreversible anticholinesterases

There are many agents in this group which are chemically related to the organophosphorus compounds. They were originally developed as nerve gases and insecticides but some have found medical uses, e.g. Di-isopropyl fluorophosphonate (Dyflos) (now unavailable) and ecothiopate, which has a restricted supply.

Ecothiopate iodide
(Ecothiophate iodide *USP*)
(*Phospholine Iodide*)

Ecothiopate iodide is an irreversible organophosphorous anticholinesterase miotic, used in 0.06–0.25% solution mainly in the treatment of open angle glaucoma. It considerably improves the facility of outflow in these glaucomatous eyes (Drance and Carr, 1960), but is not without some adverse effects. These include such systemic toxic effects in some patients (frequency of dosage is an important factor here) as diarrhoea, nausea, abdominal cramps and general weakness and fatigue (Humphreys and Holmes, 1963), and locally, iris cysts. It is also used on occasion in the treatment of accommodative esotropia in children. The iris cysts (which also occur with prolonged Dyflos therapy) fortunately disappear when the miotics are discontinued, or may often be prevented from forming by the simultaneous use of phenylephrine (2.5–10.0%) which does not impair the therapeutic effect of the ecothiopate (Abraham, 1964).

Ecothiopate eyedrops must be freshly prepared by the pharmacist in a diluent supplied by the manufacturers, the drops only remaining stable if the solution is kept refrigerated.

Ecothiopate iodide is not available for use by optometrists.

Alpha blocking agents
Thymoxamine

The principal agent in this group is thymoxamine, which is purely an alpha blocker, having little beta blocking activity. Many other alpha blockers have been isolated, e.g. tolazoline, phentolamine and ergotoxine, but only thymoxamine was used ophthalmically. Unfortunately it is no longer available commercially. It causes miosis by relaxing the pupil dilator muscle. Its main indication is the reversal of mydriasis caused by sympathomimetic agents. When a 0.1% solution was used to reverse the mydriasis caused by 2.5% phenylephrine the pupil returned to normal in about two hours compared with five hours for the control eye which received only the mydriatic (Wright *et al.*, 1990). It would also appear to have some activity in overcoming the mydriasis caused by tropicamide. It can be used intraocularly (Grehn *et al.*, 1986). It produces no endothelial damage when used in very dilute concentrations (e.g. 0.02%) and is potentially useful in cataract surgery and penetrating keratoplasty. Its miotic effects are modified by iris pigmentation to such an extent that it is poorly effective on dark brown irides (Diehl *et al.*, 1991).

In addition to its miotic action, thymoxamine paralyses the smooth muscle of the upper lid, causing a slight ptosis. For this effect it has been used in the treatment of exophthalmos. These effects are most notable in patients with thyroid problems and there would appear to be little effect on normal patients (Dixon *et al.*, 1979). Its effects last for about five hours.

There would appear to be little effect on ciliary muscle or on intraocular pressure in eyes with deep anterior chambers. The latter is surprising, as phenylephrine (which it antagonizes) lowers intraocular pressure and thus a small rise would have been expected, but the mydriatic and ocular hypotensive effects of sympathomimetics have separate time courses and probably involve different receptors. Conversely, in closed angle glaucoma thymoxamine does for several reasons appear to have a role in reducing pressure (Halasa and Rutkowski, 1973). First, it is thought that during such attacks the sphincter becomes less effective than the dilator and the latter muscle dominates. Secondly, a relaxed sphincter reduces the possibility of pupil block and Halasa and Rutkowski (1973) explain this by the use of a mathematical model. In pupil block, forces trying to pull the iris back towards the anterior lens capsule should be avoided. If both muscles are relaxed there are no posterior vector forces. Thirdly, it may have an overall synergistic effect with other miotics.

Because thymoxamine reduces the pressure in closed angle but not open angle glaucoma, it can form the basis of a useful differential test. It is effective in concentrations between 0.01% and 1.3% (Lee *et al.*, 1983).

Dapiprazole

Molinari *et al.* (1994) investigated the clinical effectiveness of dapiprazole (an alpha blocking drug) in reversing the effects of 1% tropicamide. Pupillary recovery was faster following the application of the miotic, as was the return of accommodation. The latter effect could have been due to an increased depth of field. However, in a later experiment (Molinari *et al.*, 1995) it was shown that true improvement in accommodation was achieved with the miotic. All patients exhibited conjunctival hyperemia, which would be expected as the agent would cause a vasodilation of the conjunctival blood vessels. It has been instilled experimentally directly into the anterior chamber in rabbits, where it was found to be effective and no more damaging than the saline controls (Bonomi *et al.*, 1989).

Choice of miotic following the use of a mydriatic

In the past, the optometrist had a choice of three miotics; pilocarpine (a parasympathetic), physostigmine (an anticholinesterase) and thymoxamine (an alpha blocker), and would have based the choice on the mydriatic used and the circumstances of the patient during the time taken for the mydriatic to be reversed naturally. Today he or she has to choose between pilocarpine or nothing. Due to the short duration of the action of mydriatics and the recognition of the rarity of the incidence of closed angle glaucoma, most patients can safely be spared the discomfort of a miotic.

Mixed miotics

Just as it has been the practice in the past to use mixed mydriatics containing agents with different modes of action in order to produce synergy, mixtures of miotics have also been employed. Whereas mixed mydriatics always contain an agent acting on the pupil dilator muscle and an agent acting on the pupil sphincter muscle, mixed miotics tended to contain a parasympathomimetic and an anticholinesterase, e.g. pilocarpine and physostigmine, both of which are active on the sphincter. Their use has been based on empiricism rather than pharmacological evidence.

Miotics as aids for the diagnosis of Adie's pupil

Adie's pupil is the parasympathomimetic counterpart of Horner's syndrome. In the differential diagnosis of anisocoria, a weak solution of a directly acting miotic may be used, e.g. 0.125% pilocarpine. Because the sphincter muscle is parasympathetically denervated, it is supersensitive to acetylcholine and other parasympathomimetrics. Because there is no natural release of acetylcholine, anticholinesterases will have no effect.

Bourzon et al. (1978) compared 2.5% methacholine and 0.125% pilocarpine in the diagnosis of Adie's pupil. They found methacholine effective in 64% of patients while pilocarpine was effective in 80%, so the latter can be considered to be the better drug for this differential test.

Miotics in the treatment of strabismus

According to Revell (1971), it was Green of St. Louis who first suggested, in 1870, the use of eserine in cases of subnormal accommodation and later advocated the use of pilocarpine in esotropia. Hiatt (1983) found that miotics were no better than and often not as good as glasses in correcting the deviation and enhancing binocularity in accommodative esotropia and they are little used for this purpose today. A further problem is that the long term use of miotics can be associated with side effects.

Adverse reactions to miotics

In the main, the most serious side effects from miotics arise from their chronic use in glaucoma or from possible overdosage during acute glaucoma treatment rather than the single application used to reverse mydriatics. However, miotics can cause transient effects which may trouble some patients and may therefore discourage the optometrist from using them.

Thymoxamine is irritant on instillation, as are some other miotics. Miotics with a principal action on the pupil sphincter may also cause a spasm of accommodation even in some apparently presbyopic patients.

Abramson et al. (1973) demonstrated an axial thickening of the lens and a decrease in anterior chamber depth in patients between 70 and 80 years of age. Even when this effect has apparently worn off, it may return when close work is attempted. If the miotic is much stronger than the mydriatic, then the patient will have smaller than normal pupils. This dimness of vision can be a problem, especially if combined with a pseudomyopia from the spasm of accommodation.

The blood vessels of the conjunctiva will dilate in response to parasympathomimetic agents and conjunctival injection may result. Additionally, some patients may be allergic to pilocarpine, but this is unlikely to develop after one instillation. Anticholinesterases can have nicotinic as well as muscarinic effects and these will be manifested as lid twitching. Anticholinesterases have been implicated in cataract formation (Pietsch et al., 1972).

The parasympathetic nervous system supplies many of the visceral structures and theoretically these may be affected by topically administered agents. In particular, one could expect effects on the respiratory, cardiovascular and gastrointestinal systems.

Drugs which stimulate muscarinic receptors will cause bronchoconstriction and may cause respiratory embarrassment to asthmatic patients, but this is a theoretical possibility rather than an actual danger. Bradycardia (slowing of the heart) and vasodilation similarly do not appear to be a problem. Anticholinesterase can reduce the level of plasma cholinesterase leading to diarrhoea and adverse interaction with certain muscle relaxants used in surgery, but this is only from chronic use. Few systemic effects should therefore result from the postmydriatic use of miotic.

However, gastrointestinal symptoms such as diarrhoea and vomiting, and respiratory problems, have been reported following large doses of topical pilocarpine (Epstein and Kaufman, 1965).

References

Abraham, S. V. (1964) The use of an ecothiopate-phenylephrine formulation (Ecophenylin-B3) in the treatment of convergent strabismus and amblyopia with special emphasis on iris cysts. *J. Pedriatr. Ophthalmol. Strabis.*, **1**, 68

Abramson, D. H., Franzen, L. A. and Coleman, D. J. (1973) Pilocarpine in the presbyope. *Arch. Ophthalmol.*, **89**, 100–102

Alm, A. and Bill, A. (1973) The effects of pilocarpine and neostigmine on the blood flow through the anterior uvea of the monkey. A study with radioactively labelled microspheres. *Exp. Eye Res.*, **15**, 31–36

Anastasi, I. M., Ogle, K. N. and Kearns, I. P. (1968) Effects of pilocarpine in contracting mydriasis. *Arch. Ophthalmol.*, **79**, 710–715

Bonomi, L. *et al.* (1989) Effects of intraocular dapiprazole in the rabbit eye. *J. Cataract. Refractive Surg.*, **15**, 681–684

Bourzon, P., Pilley, S. F. J. and Thompson, H. S. (1978) Cholinergic supersensitivity of the iris sphincter in Adie's tonic pupil. *Am. J. Ophthalmol.*, **85**, 373–377

Bowman, W. C. and Rand, M. J. (1980) *Textbook of Pharmacology*, 2nd edn. Oxford and London: Blackwell

Diehl, D. L. C., Robin, A. L. and Wand, M. (1991) The influence of iris pigmentation on the miotic effect of thymoxamine. *Am. J. Ophthalmol.*, **111**, 351–355

Dixon, R. S., Anderson, R. L. and Hatt, M. V. (1979) The use of thymoxamine in eyelid retraction. *Arch. Ophthalmol.*, **97**, 2147–2150

Drance, S. M. and Carr, F. (1960) Effects of phospholine iodide (217MI) on intraocular pressure in man. *Am. J. Ophthalmol.*, **49**, 470

Epstein, E. and Kaufman, I. (1965) Systemic pilocarpine toxicity from overdosage. *Am. J. Ophthalmol.*, **59**, 109–110

Gilmartin, B., Amer, A. C. and Ingleby, S. (1995). Reversal of tropicamide mydriasis with single instillations of pilocarpine can induce substantial pseudomyopia in young adults. *Ophthalmol. Physiol. Opt.*, **15**, 475–479

Grehn, F., Fleig, T. and Schwarzmuller, A. (1986) Thymoxamine: a miotic for intraocular use. *Graefe's Arch. Clin. Exp. Ophthalmol.*, **224**, 174–178

Halasa, A. H. and Rutkowski, P. C. (1973) Thymoxamine therapy for angle closure glaucoma. *Arch. Ophthalmol.*, **90**, 177–180

Havener, W. H. (1978) *Ocular pharmacology*, 4th edn., pp. 289, 298–299. St Louis: Mosby

Hiatt, R. L. (1983) Medical management of accommodative esotropia. *J. Pediatr. Ophthalmol. Strabis.*, **20**, 199–207

Humphreys, J. A. and Holmes, J. H. (1963) Systemic effects produced by ecothiopate iodide in the treatment of glaucoma. *Arch. Ophthalmol.*, **69**, 737

Koelle, G. B. (1975) In *Goodman and Gilman's Pharmacological Basis of Therapeutics*, 5th edn., p. 473. New York: Macmillan

Lee, D. A., Rimele, T. J., Brubaker, R. F., Negatki, S. and Vanhoutte, P. M. (1983) Effect of thymoxamine on the human pupil. *Exp. Eye Res.*, **36**, 655–662

Lowenstein, O. (1956) The Argyll Robertson pupillary syndrome. *Am. J. Ophthalmol.*, **42**, 105

Lowenstein, O. and Loewenfeld, I. T. (1953) Effect of physostigmine and pilocarpine on iris sphincter of normal man. *Arch. Ophthalmol.*, **50**, 311

Martindale, W. (1977) *Extra Pharmacopoeia*, 27th edn. London: The Pharmaceutical Press

Molinari, J. F., Johnson, M. E. and Carter, J. (1994) Dapiprazole clinical efficiency for counteracting tropicamide 1%. *J. Optom. and Vis. Sci.*, **71**, 319–322

Molinari, J. F., Carter, J. H. and Johnson, M. E. (1995) Dapiprazole's effect upon accommodative recovery: Is it due entirely to changes in depth of field? *J. Optom. Vis. Sci.*, **72**, 552–556

Pietsch, R. L., Bobo, C. B., Finklea, J. F. and Valloton, W. W. (1972) Lens opacities and organophosphorus cholinesterase-inhibiting agents. *Am. J. Ophthalmol.*, **73**, 236–242

Revell, M.J. (1971) *Strabismus: a history of orthoptic techniques*. London: Barrie and Jenkins.

Roger, A. R. and Smith, G. (1973) Stability of physostigmine eye drops. *Pharm. J.*, **211**, 353

Wright, M. M. *et al.* (1990) Time course of thymoxamine reversal of phenylephrine induced mydriasis. *Arch. Ophthalmol.*, **108**, 1729–1732

9   Local anaesthetics

Local anaesthetics are chemical agents that reversibly block the transmission of nerve impulses along sensory fibres. They will also block motor nerves, but only at higher concentrations than are normally obtained by topical instillation. Different sensations are lost according to the size of axons serving them. Pain (which is carried by the smallest fibres) is lost first, followed by touch and temperature sensitivity. Pressure, which is carried by the largest nerve fibres, is lost last if at all (Table 9.1).

Not all local anaesthetics are suitable for topical ophthalmic use because of the poor absorption characteristics of some agents, for example procaine, an excellent injectable anaesthetic which because of the highly polar nature of the compound has poor lipid solubility and therefore crosses mucous membranes very slowly.

Table 9.1 Local anaesthetics

Official name	Alternative names	Strengths	Single dose	Anaesthetic onset	Anaesthetic duration
Amethocaine	tetracaine	0.5 1.0	Yes	1 min	20 min
Benoxinate	oxybuprocaine	0.4	Yes	1 min	15 min
Proxymetacaine	proparacaine	0.5	Yes	1 min	15 min
Lignocaine	lidocaine	2.0 to 4.0	Yes with fluorescein	1 min	30 min

Ideal properties

Topical anaesthetics should:

1. Be quick in onset of action.
2. Be effective for a reasonable duration of time. (It should allow the practitioner time to carry out the procedure, and then reverse completely, returning to the patient the protection of the sensitive eye.)
3. Not affect the pupil, accommodation or intraocular pressure.
4. Not antagonize or enhance the effects of other drugs, e.g. mydriatics, cycloplegics, antimicrobials etc.
5. Be comfortable to the patient on initial application.
6. Not interfere with the healing process.
7. Be nontoxic, both locally and systemically.
8. Have no adverse subjective complaints such as 'stinging'.

Indications for use

The cornea and conjunctiva are very sensitive and there are several clinical techniques which require contact with the cornea. These are facilitated by the prior use of a topical anaesthetic.

They include:

1. *Foreign body removal*. The blepharospasm which normally accompanies a superficial foreign body makes examination of the eye very difficult, so a drop of local anaesthetic will make location and removal of the offending object much easier.
2. *Tonometry*. Local anaesthetics are required for any form of contact tonometry.
3. *Contact lens fitting*. Some procedures may be more easily carried out if a topical anaesthetic is instilled initially.
4. *Schirmer tests*. The Schirmer I test is performed without topical anaesthesia and measures total reflex and secretory levels of the tears, while in the Schirmer II test a topical anaesthetic is instilled and reflex tear secretion is measured by irritating the unanaesthetized nasal mucosa with a cotton tipped applicator.
5. Gonioscopy.

Topical anaesthesia is also sometimes used prior to the instillation of rose bengal stain, but this may give a slightly false picture if the anaesthetic interferes with the integrity of the corneal epithelium.

Advantages

1. Certain procedures would be impossible without a topical anaesthetic. For example, most simple portable tonometers which can be used for domiciliary visits require a local anaesthetic.
2. Use of a local anaesthetic makes procedures more comfortable for the patient.
3. They correspondingly make procedures easier for the practitioner.

Disadvantages

1. While the surface of the eye is insensitive, it is susceptible to damage from superficial foreign bodies.
2. Some topical anaesthetics cause initial stinging.
3. The effects of other drugs may be enhanced. Where this occurs it is probably due to an effect of the preservatives used in multidose bottles rather than an action of the local anaesthetic itself (Ramselaar *et al.*, 1988). This is yet another reason for using single dose containers.
4. Topical anaesthetics can delay the healing processes in cases where trauma to the corneal epithelium has occurred.

Mode of action

Sensory information passes along nerve fibres as 'electrical impulses' or action potentials. When the nerve is at rest, the interior has a negative charge. An action potential is generated by the influx of sodium ions into the interior of the nerve, causing it to have a positive charge (depolarization). The nerve fibre is returned to its resting potential (negative state) by the efflux of potassium ions (repolarization). The action potential is then generated along the axon by successive depolarizations and repolarizations of adjacent regions, the exact mechanism of action at the cellular level having been the subject of much study. Schoen and Candida (1975) found that the chloride permeability of corneal cells was reduced by the application of local anaesthetics.

Choice of topical anaesthetic

Cocaine is of course the original local anaesthetic against which the newer synthetic agents are assessed. This naturally occurring drug is now better known for its abuse rather than its use as a local anaesthetic, being a CNS stimulant which leads to euphoria and eventual dependence. In addition to its local anaesthetic action, it has a sympathomimetic action which leads to mydriasis on topical application. It has deleterious effects on the corneal epithelium, leading to desquamation and an increased penetration of other substances across the cornea. This is a property which is peculiar to cocaine and not to local anaesthetics in general.

Cocaine is controlled by both the Misuse of Drugs Act and The Medicines Act under which it is available only on prescription (Prescription Only Medicine or POM). It is not legally available to optometrists for use in their practice.

There is, nevertheless, an extensive range of topical anaesthetics which are available to optometrists for professional use, i.e. amethocaine, proxymetacaine, benoxinate and lignocaine. All are available in commercial preparations in multidose and single dose units.

The property in which respect the agents vary most is the initial stinging on instillation. In descending order of comfort, the agents can be listed thus:

Proxymetacaine-most comfortable
Benoxinate
Lignocaine
Amethocaine-least comfortable

Whichever local anaesthetic is selected, the concentration chosen should be as low as possible. Polse *et al.* (1978) plotted the dose-response curves of benoxinate and proxymetacaine. They found benoxinate at concentrations as low as 0.1% and proxymetacaine at 0.125% produced a maximal increase in threshold to touch. Although the concentrations currently employed (0.4% and 0.5%, respectively) are definitely supramaximal with respect to the depth of anaesthesia, the recovery time was found to be proportional to the concentration used. At the lowest concentration the duration of effect was sufficient to carry out normal optometric procedures, so at the normally used concentrations it is plainly excessive.

Draeger *et al.* (1984) similarly found a prolongation of effect when 0.5% was used compared with 0.1%. The vehicle and preservative had little effect on the performance of the local anaesthetic.

Proxymetacaine hydrochloride (Proparacaine Hydrochloride, USP) (*Ophthaine: Alcaine*, Canada, USA: *Ophthetic*, Australia, Canada, South Africa, USA)

Proxymetacaine is a white or almost white crystalline powder soluble 1 in 30 in water. A synthetic topical anaesthetic, it has greater potency than amethocaine but there is little clinical difference. The instillation of one drop of 0.5% solution of proxymetacaine produces anaesthesia lasting about 15 minutes. In ophthalmology deep anaesthesia (as required for cataract extraction) may be obtained by instilling one drop every five to ten minutes until five to seven drops have been administered (Martindale, 1977).

Time of onset of anaesthesia is very similar, 6–20 seconds (average 12.9 seconds), to that with amethocaine, 9–26 seconds (average 14.7 seconds) (Boozan and Cohen, 1953).

In this series using 0.5% solutions of three local anaesthetics, amethocaine, proxymetacaine (proparacaine) and benoxinate, Lin and Vey (1959) found similar duration and intensity of anaesthesia among all three.

Instillation of proxymetacaine is however considerably more comfortable than the use of amethocaine; it causes much less stinging and squeezing of the eyes and is often painless (Boozan and Cohen, 1953).

The eyedrops should be stored protected from light, and when opened kept at a temperature of between 2° and 10°C. Sensitivity reactions are rare and Havener (1978) describes the only case he observed in several years which occurred in a patient where the drug had been used for repeated tonometries. The allergic reaction manifested itself as marked epithelial stippling and slight stromal oedema, with considerable conjunctival hyperaemia and slight puffiness of the lids: pain and profuse lacrimation were severe for some hours. Sensitivity of patients to proxymetacaine is not experienced when amethocaine is used, and vice versa (Havener, 1978).

Recently a single use form (*Minims Proxymetacaine*) has been introduced which has removed the remaining disadvantage of this drug, i.e. that it was only available in multidose form. In this form storage has to be between 2° and 8°C. As proxymetacaine has less intrinsic antibacterial action than the other topical anesthetics, it is particularly useful for taking conjunctival swabs.

Proxymetacaine is a POM.

Oxybuprocaine hydrochloride (benoxinate hydrochloride) (*Novesine*, Australia, South Africa; *Dorsacaine*, USA)

Oxybuprocaine is a synthetic local anaesthetic which occurs as white crystals or a white crystalline powder and is very soluble in water. It is used in a 0.4% solution and has clinical characteristics essentially similar to proxymetacaine, both drugs causing less irritation and stinging than amethocaine (Emmerich *et al.*, 1955). As both cocaine and amethocaine cause more or less punctate epithelial staining which may be confusing during applanation tonometry, this procedure is performed with more accuracy with oxybuprocaine or proxymetacaine than with amethocaine (Havener, 1978). One drop instilled into the conjunctival sac anaesthetizes the surface sufficiently to allow tonometry to be performed in 60 seconds. Three drops instilled over an interval of about four to five minutes will produce sufficient surface anaesthesia after a further five minute interval for an ophthalmologist to remove a foreign body embedded in the corneal epithelium, or for incision of a Meibomian cyst through the conjunctiva (Martindale, 1977). The sensitivity of the cornea after three drops is normal again in about one hour, whereas after one drop (for example, as used for removing a superficial non-embedded corneal foreign body, or tonometry) the effective anaesthesia lasts 10–15 minutes. This topical anaesthetic has an additional advantage in that it possesses bactericidal properties.

Havener (1978) stated that 'In a series of more than 1000 patients anaesthetized with benoxinate, no toxic effects were encountered, either locally or systemically'.

Lignocaine hydrochloride (Lidocaine Hydrochloride, Eur. P., USP) (Xylocaine)

Lignocaine occurs as a white crystalline powder soluble in less than one part of water. Unlike the other three topical anaesthetics (amethocaine hydrochloride, proxymetacaine hydrochloride and oxybuprocaine hydrochloride) which are all of the ester type, lignocaine hydrochloride is a local anaesthetic of the amide type. A 2–4% solution (the latter strength is available as a proprietary preparation) will anaesthetize the cornea. It is an alternative agent in individuals sensitive to ester type local anaesthetics (Ritchie and Cohen, 1975). As a topical eyedrops preparation it is a POM. It is also used in ophthalmology for infiltration analgesia (see below).

Amethocaine hydrochloride (Tetracaine Hydrochloride Eur. P., USP) (Anethaine, Decicain, Australia: Pontocaine, Canada, USA)

Amethocaine hydrochloride, a white crystalline powder soluble in 1 in 7.5 water, is one of the most popular topical anaesthetics and is used in 0.25–1% solutions. Solutions stronger than 1% should be avoided as they may damage the cornea. On instillation patients often complain of an initial burning sensation, but this passes off in about half a minute or less, by which time the anaesthetic effects are well advanced. Employed in these concentrations amethocaine does not normally cause desquamation of corneal epithelial cells. The peculiar numb sensation persists for 10–20 minutes depending on the concentration of the drops, but the patient must be warned (as with all other topical anaesthetics) not to rub his eyes during this time, especially during the initial stinging, as the corneal epithelium can unwittingly be damaged in the process. Within a minute or two of instillation of one drop of 0.5% solution of this drug contact tonometry can be carried out painlessly. The instruction to the patient gently to close his eyes immediately on instillation of these (or any) eyedrops will definitely reduce the amount of stinging experienced. Tears should be patted away from the closed eyes by the practitioner with a fresh paper tissue or cotton wool.

Removal of a non-embedded foreign body should generally not necessitate more than one drop of a 0.5% solution.

Topical anaesthetics, including amethocaine, should not be prescribed even in very dilute concentrations for home use in an attempt to tide a prospective rigid contact lens patient over the more difficult initial stages of wear. Repeated instillations of even very weak concentrations of these drugs will intensify the tiny superficial corneal epithelial lesions commonly seen with the slit lamp microscope after use of these eyedrops. Healing of corneal abrasions is significantly retarded by local anaesthetics, and even removal of a foreign body should be performed (if this is possible without blepharospasm and severe discomfort to the patient) without their use. Epithelial regeneration, both mitosis and cellular migration, have been shown to be affected by their employment (Gundersen and Liebman, 1944), which should therefore be avoided unless absolutely necessary, and even then only the weakest concentration that will adequately suit the specific situation should be instilled.

Sensitivity to amethocaine is extremely uncommon and only likely to occur after repeated use of the drug (which is most unlikely in optometric practice). The lids become red, swollen, then irritated and itching, and this lasts for some days (Havener, 1978).

Amethocaine is relatively stable in solution, but it is affected by light and should therefore be stored in an amber bottle or dark cupboard, as after long periods it hydrolyses in solution.

Adverse reactions to local anaesthetics

As with all topically applied drugs there is a possibility of both local and systemic adverse effects. With their action of modifying transmembrane ionic flow it is inevitable that local effects will be produced on the cells with which it comes in contact. Before the drugs can reach the nerve fibres they must first cross corneal epithelial cells. Sturrock and Nunn (1979) examined the cytotoxic effects of three local anaesthetics, procaine, lignocaine and bupivacaine, and they found an inhibition of cell growth and cell survival of cultured cells. Scanning electron microscopy showed damage to the cell membrane and loss of microvilli as well as accelerated desquamation of the corneal epithelium when amethocaine 0.5% was applied to the human cornea (Bolkja et al., 1994). Tear film stability is unaffected by benoxinate (Cho and Brown, 1995), but not tear flow. Schirmer's test results after the instillation of 0.4% benoxinate were reduced by 47% (Shiono, 1989). Corresponding reductions were recorded in the secretion lysozyme and other enzymes. Oxygen flux was investigated by Augsberger and Hill (1973), who found that while cocaine depressed the uptake of oxygen by corneal epithelial cells, benoxinate (even in multiple applications) did not.

Probably the most common use of local anaesthetics is in the measurement of intraocular pressure, and the reported reduction in tonometric measurements following the use of local anaesthetics is a matter of concern. Baudouin and Gastaud (1994) found that the fall was as much as 8 mm in some patients. However, falls of this value were only seen after 15 minutes, and the reductions after one minute were statistically significant but small enough not to be clinically significant.

Another measurement that may be affected by the use of local anaesthetics is pachometry (Herse and Siu, 1992). An increase in corneal thickness was noted after the use of two drops (but not one!) of proparacaine.

Local anaesthetics in ointment form produced morphological changes in the corneal epithelium, cocaine being the most toxic. Benoxinate and proxymetacaine caused a decrease in microvilli and microplicae. Repeated administration caused changes to the plasma membrane and cytoplasm (Brewitt et al., 1980). Gundersen and Liebman (1944) tested several local anaesthetics including cocaine and amethocaine on the healing of wounds in the guinea pig cornea. All anaesthetics tested caused a delay in wound healing and a similar result was obtained when lignocaine was tested on the healing of skin wounds in rats (Morris and Tracey, 1977).

Dangers of abuse of topical anaesthetics

It is well known that cocaine is subject to abuse for its CNS effects. The other local anaesthetics are subject to abuse for their ability to remove temporarily the feeling of discomfort from the surface of the eye. The people who abuse them, more often than not, are those who should know better, i.e. medical personnel who have access to these agents. Burns and Gipson (1978) warned that paramedical personnel may abuse topical anaesthetics. The irritation which may persist after a foreign body has been removed can lead to someone instilling a local anaesthetic repeatedly. Exposure keratitis is an example of another condition which may lead to the misguided supply of a topical anaesthetic for domiciliary use.

It is recognized that topical anaesthetics can be used incorrectly and that is why they are restricted to use by optometrists in their practice and may not be supplied to patients for use at home under any circumstances. As they are POM drugs, they are not available to the general public.

Unfortunately, this is not the case in all countries of the world. Penna and Tabbara (1986) reported keratopathy following the use of benoxinate which was bought over the counter in Saudi Arabia. Two patients had had exposure keratitis and one a foreign body and they developed disciform keratitis and stromal infiltration. The final best corrected acuity was 6/30 in most eyes, with one eye being reduced to counting fingers at 1.5 m. The patients had all received bottles of benoxinate from a pharmacy and had used the drops continuously. The legislation which covers the use of drugs may be irksome and time consuming, but if it can avoid cases like these then it is worthwhile.

Three similar cases were reported in Holland by Henkes and Waubke (1978), these patients having developed a physical dependence on the drops because of the intense pain in the insensitive cornea. The local anaesthetics in these cases were supplied by an ophthalmologist. Vision in one eye was reduced to counting fingers, and keratoplasty was required.

Jallet et al. (1980) described a case where a solution containing only 0.05% benoxinate when used for the treatment of arc eye led to abuse and keratopathy. This solution (which contains an antiseptic in addition to the local anaesthetic) is available in France without prescription. A dramatic illustration of the problem of local anaesthetic abuse was a patient whose left eye had to be removed due to the corneal ulcer perforation and panophthalmitis which developed in the course of her use of local anaesthetic eye drops with hard contact lenses (D'Haenes, 1984). Other cases which resulted in enucleation were reported by Rosenwasser et al. (1990), who make the point that in the differential diagnosis of chronic keratitis local anaesthetic abuse can be mistakenly diagnosed as acanthamoeba keratitis.

Systemic effects are minimal providing that small volumes are used. Fainting or syncope is known to occur sometimes, but it is not certain to what extent this is related to the drug being used.

References

Augberger, A. R. and Hill, R. M. (1973) Topical anaesthesia and corneal function. *Ophthalmol. Opt.*, 12–18

Baudouin, C. and Gastaud, P. (1994) Influence of topical anaesthesia on tonometric values of intraocular pressure. *Ophthalmologica*, **208**, 309–313

Boljka, M., Kolar, G. and Vidensk, J. (1994) Toxic effects of local anaesthetics on the human cornea. *Br. J. Ophthalmol.*, **18**, 386–389

Boozan, C. W. and Cohen, I. J. (1953) Ophthaine. *Am. J. Ophthalmol.*, **36**, 16–19

Brewitt, M., Bonatz, E. and Honegger, J. (1980) Morphological changes of the corneal epithelium after application of topical anaesthetic ointment. *Ophthalmologica*, **180**, 198–206

Burns, R. P. and Gipson, I. (1978) Toxic effects of local anaesthetics. *JAMA*, **240**, 347

Cho, P. and Brown, B. (1995) The effect of benoxinate on the tear stability of Hong Kong Chinese. *Ophthal. Physiol. Opt.*, **15**, 299–304

D'Haenes, J. D. (1984) Le cas clinique. Complications corneenes par instillations de collyres anesthetiques sur les lentilles de contact. *Contactologica*, **6**, 142–143

Draeger, J., Langenbucher, H. and Bannert, C. (1984) Efficacy of topical anaesthetics. *Ophthalmol. Res.*, **16**, 135–138

Emmerich, R., Carter, G. T. and Berens, C. (1955) An experimental clinical evaluation of Dorsacaine hydrochloride (*Benoxinate, Novesine*). *Am. J. Ophthalmol.*, **40**, 481

Gundersen, T. and Liebman, S. D. (1944). Effects of local anaesthetics on regeneration of corneal epithelium. *Arch. Ophthalmol.*, **31**, 29–33

Havener, W. H. (1978) *Ocular pharmacology*, 4th edn., p. 73. St Louis: Mosby

Henkes, H. E. and Waubke, T. N. (1978) Keratitis from the abuse of local anaesthetics. *Br. J. Ophthalmol.*, **62**, 62–65

Herse, P. and Siu, A. (1992) Short term effects of proparacaine on human corneal thickness. *Acta Ophthalmol.*, **70**, 740–744

Jallet, G., Cleires, S., Girard, E. and Bechetoille, A. (1980) Kératopathie toxique grave à l'oxybuprocaine d'apparition particulièrement rapid. *Bull. Soc. Ophthalmol., France*, **80**, 385–387

Lin, J. G. and Vey, E. K. (1959) Topical anaesthesia in ophthalmology. *Am. J. Ophthalmol.*, **40**, 697

Martindale, W. (1977) *Extra Pharmacopoeia*, 27th edn., p. 871. London: The Pharmaceutical Press

Morris, M. and Tracey, J. (1977) Lignocaine: its effects on wound healing. *Br. J. Surg.*, **64**, 902–903

Penna, E. P. and Tabbara, K. F. (1986) Oxybuprocaine keratopathy: a preventable disease. *Br. J. Ophthalmol.*, **70**, 202–204

Polse, K. A., Keener, R. J. and Jauregui, M. J. (1978) Dose-response effects of corneal anaesthetics. *Am. J. Optom. Physiol. Opt.*, **55**, 8–14

Ramselaar, J. A. M. *et al.* (1988) Corneal epithelial permeability after instillation of ophthalmic solutions containing local anaesthetics and preservatives. *Curr. Eye Res.*, **07**, 947–950

Ritchie, J. M. and Cohen, D. J. (1975) In *Goodman and Gilman's The Pharmacological Basis of Therapeutics*, 5th edn., p. 389. New York: Macmillan

Rosenwasser, G. O. D. *et al.* (1990) Topical anaesthetic abuse. *Ophthalmology*, **97**, 967–972

Schoen, H. F. and Candida, O. A. (1975) Effects of tertiary amine local anaesthetics on ion transport in the isolated bullfrog cornea. *Exp. Eye Res.*, **28**, 199–209

Shiono, T. (1989) Effect of topical anaesthesia on secretion of lysozyme and lysosomal enzymes in human tears. *Japan J. Ophthalmol.*, **33**, 375–379

Sturrock, J. E. and Nunn, J. F. (1979) Cytotoxic effects of procaine, lignocaine, and bupivacaine. *Br. J. Anaesthesiol.*, **51**, 273–281

Further Reading

Burns, R. P., Forster, R. K., Laibson, P. and Gipson, I. K. (1977) Chronic toxicity of local anaesthetics on the cornea. In *Symposium on Ocular Therapy*, **10**, 31–44 (Leopold, L. H. and Burns, R. P., eds.). New York: John Wiley.

10

Stains

Stains are amongst the most useful diagnostic agents, providing information fairly rapidly without producing a pharmacological effect; their usefulness lies in their differential staining characteristics. Important clinical information is provided both by the presence and the absence of staining demonstrated by the use of these agents (Table 10.1).

Many dyes and substances have been investigated in the past for their staining properties. Foster (1980) lists 34 chemical substances which have been used for vital staining of the eye, including such marvellous names as Magadala Red, Safranin, Brilliant Black and Victorian Blue. His bibliography contains a reference to the use of fluorescein by M. Straub in 1888, which indicates how long ago the principle of vital staining of the eye was established. Today only two stains are in regular use, fluorescein sodium and rose bengal.

Table 10.1 Stains

Official name	Strengths	Single dose	Uses	Adverse reactions
Fluorescein sodium	1.0–2.0	Yes	Tonometry, corneal abraisons, contact lens fitting	Supports growth of *Pseudomonas aeruginosa*
Rose bengal	1.0	Yes	Stains dead cells, diagnosis of dry eye	Irritant on application to dry eyes
Alcian blue	1.0	No	Stains mucus	Persistent staining of corneal epithelium
Trypan blue	1.0	No	Stains mucus and dead cells	

Ideal properties

1. They should be water soluble, because vehicles other than water will be toxic and/or interfere with staining patterns.
2. Stains should selectively stain certain cells or structures in the eye.
3. They should not stain skin, clothes, contact lenses or any instrument which is likely to come in contact with the eye when the stain is present.
4. The effect should be reversible, either as a result of tear flow or by use of an irrigating solution.
5. There should be no interference with vision.
6. There should be no other pharmacological effect.

7. They should be nonirritant to the surface of the eye.
8. They should be nontoxic, especially as one is looking for pathological changes.
9. They should be compatible with other stains and any other compound with which they are likely to be used.

Norn (1972a) has laid down an extensive scheme for the testing of dyes for vital staining of the cornea and conjunctiva. In particular, he was concerned how any new stain would fit in with the characteristics of existing dyes.

Fluorescein sodium

Fluorescein is an orange-red dye which fluoresces in high dilution. As well as being used as a topical stain, it can also be used as an injection for fluorescein angiography. Fluorescein does not actually stain tissues, it merely colours the tear film. The normal corneal epithelium is impermeable to the tear film and substances dissolved in it, because the lipid membranes at the surface of the eye are an effective barrier against polar, water soluble substances. If this barrier is breached then the tear film can gain access to deeper layers. There is a pH difference between the surface and the deeper tissues, and this causes a green colour in the area of desquamation. The factors which affect the fluorescence of fluorescein have been extensively reviewed. The pH of the solution not only influences the absorption spectrum (like any other pH indicator) but also determines the intensity of the fluorescence, which is highest at pH 8, and thus the area of defect is shown up. After gaining access to the deeper layers of the epithelium, the fluorescein will diffuse sideways giving a slightly false picture. Defects in the epithelium, whether caused by trauma or disease (e.g. dendritic ulcer), are disclosed by the stain.

Optimum conditions for observation of fluorescein

For dilute concentrations of fluorescein in an aqueous solution, light with a wavelength between 485 and 500 nm is absorbed maximally. This absorbed energy excites the fluorescein molecules and the emitted light is in a lower energy state and of longer wavelength. The fluorescent light appears green, having its highest intensity at a wavelength between 525 and 530 nm.

In order to observe the fluorescein pattern of the fit of a rigid lens, contact lens practitioners have commonly used a Burton type lamp which is generally fitted with a pair of 4 W 'Blacklight Blue' miniature tubular fluorescent lamps. Wavelengths produced by such a source range from approximately 305 to 410 nm, with maximal emission at 350 nm. Some rigid contact lens materials have been formulated to absorb within the UV-A band of long-wave radiation which ranges from 315 to 400 nm. Since a Burton type lamp is unsuitable for evaluation of the fluorescein pattern of such lenses, it is possible to use the blue filter on a slit lamp microscope as a source instead, since its maximum transmission is likely to be in the region of 390–410 nm (Pearson, 1984). Alternatively, a Wratten filter such as a No. 45A could be placed either in the illumination system of the slit lamp or in front of the white fluorescent bulbs fitted in some Burton type lamps. The use of a blue filter which limits illumination to wavelengths maximally absorbed by fluorescein eliminates veiling glare caused by extraneous wavelengths.

It is established practice to mount a dark yellow filter on the camera lens in order to achieve adequate contrast in the photography of contact lens fluorescein patterns (Abrams and Bailey, 1961). Lee *et al.* (1980) have reported that similar incorporation of a barrier filter such as yellow Wratten No. 15 in the observation system of a slit lamp microscope can significantly facilitate the detection of fluorescein staining of the cornea.

Indications for use

1. Detection of defects in the corneal epithelium.
2. Contact lens fitting.
3. Applanation tonometry.
4. Determination of nasolacrimal duct patency.
5. Assessment of tear break up time.
6. Tear flow assessment.

Corneal defects

Fluorescein should be used routinely after foreign body removal to detect any damage caused by the offending object while it is present. If a small foreign body has penetrated the eye, a corresponding green rivulet may be seen issuing from the entry hole.

Although fluorescein will demonstrate corneal ulcers (Plate II), it may be better to use rose bengal, which is more selective.

Epithelial erosions due to trichiasis will be shown up, but fluorescein is of little help in the diagnosis of keratoconjunctivitis sicca or other forms of conjunctivitis, e.g. those infective, allergic or chemical in origin.

Contact lens fitting

In the fitting of rigid contact lenses, the dye is an aid in studying the areas where the lens is clearing (green fluorescence) or touching (purplish-blue) the cornea, in the case of corneal lenses. With scleral lenses the same observations apply to the optic area but a green colouration, or the absence of it, will show where there is clearance or contact respectively of the scleral portion of the lens in relation to the sclera. Textbooks on contact lens practice deal with the interpretation of these observations in the appropriate detail.

Fluorescein sodium should not be used to study the fit of soft contact lenses as it stains them following absorption into the polymer. A high molecular weight fluorescein derivative has been developed in an attempt to overcome this disadvantage, e.g. *Fluorexon* (Refojo *et al.*, 1972). The use of this dye is limited because although it will not enter pHEMA (poly-hydroxyethylmethacrylate), it stains most other lenses, and even a 4% solution is not as fluorescent as 0.5% fluorescein (Ruben, 1978).

Applanation tonometry

In applanation tonometry the visibility of the fluorescein, observed under cobalt blue filter light, again assumes practical significance. The margin of the applanated area is delineated by a solution of the dye; the 'touch' area (purplish-black) has a diameter of 3.06 mm on the cornea (Plate III). The concentration of the fluorescein is very important in this technique and it should not be too low (as occurs with excessive tearing), when the examiner's visibility of it is impaired, or too high. The best results are often obtained when using benoxinate hydrochloride 0.1% as the local anaesthetic, as recommended by Goldmann. A 2% solution of fluorescein is far too strong for this procedure. Grant (1963) suggests a 0.25% concentration and with experience just the right amount may be obtained by employing sterile fluorescein paper strips.

Because Goldmann type applanation tonometers involve contact with the eye, a topical anaesthetic has to be administered with the fluorescein. Unfortunately local anaesthetics are salts of weak bases and strong acids. Sodium fluorescein is a salt of a strong base and weak acid. Mixtures of the two types of compound are thus inherently unstable. A stabilized mixture of lignocaine (4%) with fluorescein (0.25%) is available in single use units. If benoxinate is the preferred anaesthetic, it should be instilled separately or used to moisten the fluorescein strip. For a full description of the technique of accurate applanation measurements of intraocular pressure, the reader is referred to the appropriate literature issued with the instrument, and such papers as those of Grant (1963), Moses (1960) and Spaeth (1978). Considerable practice and experience are necessary before reliable results are routinely obtained, and visual field examinations should always be conducted, whenever possible, in conjunction with Schiötz or applanation tonometry.

Lacrimal patency

To demonstrate the patency of the lacrimal drainage system in patients complaining of frequent and troublesome epiphora, a drop or two of 2% fluorescein sodium eyedrops may be used. Alternatively, the saline moistened fluorescein strip may be used to convey a sufficient amount of the dye to the conjunctiva. A few drops of saline solution are then also instilled into the conjunctival sac to increase the volume of liquid present, and the patient is asked to blow his nose in a white tissue. Yellow staining of the tissue proves patency of the lacrimal drainage of this particular eye, and the procedure is repeated for the other. Absence of staining of the tissue does not necessarily indicate obstruction to the passage of tears down the lacrimal passageway, until observation has shown that the lacrimal punctum is in correct apposition to the globe of the eye.

Assessment of tear break up time

Since fluorescein colours the tear film, it can be used to assess the tear break up time (TBUT), which is the interval after blinking for discontinuities to appear in the precorneal tear film. After a blink, the tear film is formed anew and if the tears are coloured with fluorescein, a uniform fluorescent layer will be seen. After some time (usually much greater than the interblink period), convection currents disrupt the normal trilaminar layer, the surface active effect of the mucin is diluted and holes appear in the film. TBUT can be lengthened by the application of viscous drops. It is very much reduced in tear deficiency syndromes such as keratoconjunctivitis sicca, and Foster (1980) considers TBUTs of less than 10 seconds to be pathognomonic of dry eye. If the tear film breaks up immediately, the eyes are open and breaks appear repeatedly in the same place, there is probably some pathological process at these sites. A short tear break up time can coexist with a normal Schirmer tear test if the eye is mucin deficient.

Tear flow assessment

The halflife of drops in the conjunctival sac is very low. It will depend on the patency of the nasolacrimal duct and the rate of tear production. The rate at which fluorescein disappears from the conjunctival sac can be taken as a measure of the tear flow. Barendsen *et al.* (1979) used fluorescein to estimate the minimum permissible interval between the application of drugs. Predictably, they found that fluorescein concentration in the tear film decreased more quickly in younger patients and thus viscous solutions were cleared at a slower rate than aqueous ones.

Contamination

Contamination of fluorescein eyedrops is a particularly serious risk, even greater than that encountered with the majority of other eyedrops. As these individual drops are liable to become infected with bacteria and at the same time are being used frequently on damaged tissue which is prone to infection, very great care must be taken in their use. *Pseudomonas aeruginosa* is an especially dangerous pathological micro-organism by which fluorescein eyedrops are inclined to become invaded. Phenylmercuric acetate or nitrate at 0.002% strength is the best bactericide for preserving these particular eyedrops, and this is effective against *Pseudomonas* given adequate contact time. However, the safest method for their employment is sterile single dose units or sterile fluorescein impregnated paper strips, both of which are readily available and highly recommended.

Rose bengal

Rose bengal is a brownish-red powder which is soluble in water and is normally used in a 1% solution. Although not yet approved for sale in the UK, rose bengal strips have been prepared. This substance is a derivative of fluorescein but has markedly different staining characteristics, crossing the cell membranes of dead cells but not living ones. Mucus threads will also be stained. Some practitioners prefer to examine the eye after rose bengal staining with a green light.

Rose bengal also differs from fluorescein in its usage. While there is probably no optometric practice which is without ophthalmic fluorescein in some form, rose bengal is comparatively little used. This is probably due to (a) the initial irritation to the surface of the eye (especially, unfortunately, patients with dry eyes) and (b) unfamiliarity with the results of staining. It is useful in the following conditions:

1. Dendritic keratitis.
2. Keratoconjunctivitis sicca.
3. Keratitis neuroparalytica.
4. Exophthalmos.
5. Pressure areas due to contact lens wear.

Dendritic keratitis

Rose bengal will stain the areas of the dendritic ulcer. It is restricted to the processes of the ulcer and does not diffuse to surrounding areas.

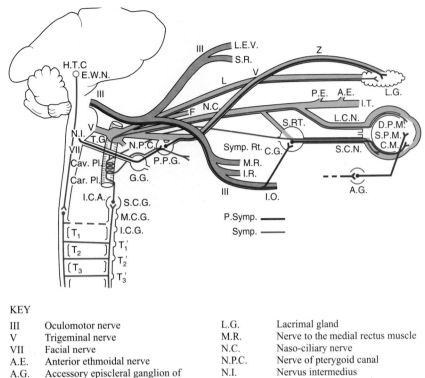

KEY

III	Oculomotor nerve	L.G.	Lacrimal gland
V	Trigeminal nerve	M.R.	Nerve to the medial rectus muscle
VII	Facial nerve	N.C.	Naso-ciliary nerve
A.E.	Anterior ethmoidal nerve	N.P.C.	Nerve of pterygoid canal
A.G.	Accessory episcleral ganglion of Axenfeld	N.I.	Nervus intermedius
		P.E.	Posterior ethmoidal nerve
Car. Pl.	Cartoid plexus	P.P.G.	Pterygo-palatine (sphenopalatine) ganglion
Cav. Pl.	Cavernous plexus		
C.G.	Ciliary ganglion	P. Symp.	Parasympathetic nerves
C.M.	Ciliary muscle	P. Symp. Rt.	Parasympathetic root to ciliary ganglion
D.P.M.	Dilatator pupillae muscle		
E.W.N.	Edinger–Westphal nucleus	S.C.N.	Short ciliary nerves
F.	Frontal nerve	S.P.M.	Sphincter pupillae muscle
G.G.	Geniculate ganglion	S.R.	Nerve to superior rectus muscle
H.T.C.	Hypothalamic centre	S.Rt.	Sensory root from ciliary ganglion
I.C.A	Internal carotid artery	Symp.	Sympathetic nerves
I.C.G.	Internal carotid ganglion	Symp. Rt.	Sympathetic root to ciliary ganglion
I.O.	Nerve to the inferior oblique muscle	T1, T2, T3	1st, 2nd and 3rd thoracic nerves respectively
I.R.	Nerve to the inferior rectus muscle		
I.T.	Infratrochlear nerve	T_1', T_2', T_3'	1st, 2nd and 3rd thoracic ganglia respectively
L.	Lacrimal nerve		
L.C.N.	Long ciliary nerves	T.G.	Trigeminal ganglion
LEV.	Nerve to levator palpebrae superioris	Z	Zygomatic nerve

Plate I Autonomic and sensory nerve supply of the eye (schematic) (based on a drawing by J. B. Davey).

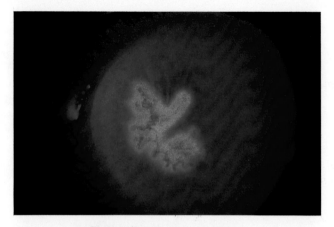

Plate II Small dendritic ulcer.
(Reproduced from Kanski, J.J. (1994) *Clinical Ophthalmology* 3rd edn, Oxford:
Butterworth-Heinemann with permission.)

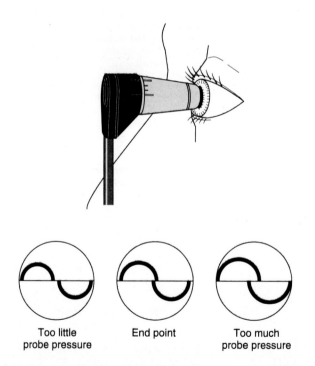

Too little
probe pressure

End point

Too much
probe pressure

Plate III Applanation tonometry with Goldmann tonometer.

Keratoconjunctivitis sicca	The parts which are stained are the exposed triangular areas in the inter-palpebral conjunctiva. Such staining constitutes a better diagnostic indication of dry eye than the Schirmer tear test.
Keratitis neuroparalytica	Extensive staining can occur in the same regions as in KCS.
Exophthalmos	If this is great enough to deny the eye of the normal protection of the lids, drying will occur which will lead to changes in the exposed area.
Pressure areas due to contact lens wear	Contact lens practitioners may use rose bengal during their initial assessment of contact lens patients. It is equally useful in followup visits where stains may be found on the cornea or bulbar or palpebral conjunctiva and although not serious, provide an indication that modification of the lens may be necessary.

Mixtures of fluorescein and rose bengal

A mixed stain containing 1% fluorescein sodium and 1% rose bengal has been investigated by Norn (1964b, 1967), who concluded that it was better than the individual stains alone. He examined normal patients, patients with diseases of the cornea, conjunctiva and lacrimal passages, and contact lens wearers. For the latter, he concluded that these vital stains are suitable for assessing damage in relation to the wearing of contact lenses. He attributed a punctate red crescent on the lower bulbar conjunctiva, but considered that modification was only indicated in the presence of symptoms.

Triple staining with the above mixtures plus alcian blue has also been examined (Norn, 1964a). The three dyes stain different structures – fluorescein stains epithelial lesions, rose bengal stains degenerate cells and alcian blue, mucus.

Other stains

The following stains are seldom used but nevertheless are of interest.

Alcian blue

Alcian blue is a complex copper containing compound which is used in 1% solution and is specific for staining mucus. It is used to counterstain rose bengal which in addition to staining dead cells also stains mucus (Norn, 1972b). If a break in the integrity of the epithelium exists, the exposed deeper layers may be stained a pale blue-green colour which will persist for several months (Norn, 1964b).

Trypan blue

Trypan blue stains mucus and dead cells which have undergone structural changes (Norn, 1972b).

Tetrazolium and iodonitrotetrazolium

These compounds have been used for the vital staining of tumours and assessing corneal grafts (Norn, 1972b). They are by nature pro-stains because the compounds are reduced inside cells to a red dye formazan. The colour takes about four minutes to develop.

Tetrazolium stains degenerate cells, not dead cells. Living healthy cells are not stained because of the impermeability of the cell membrane and dead cells are not stained because the enzymes needed to reduce the dye to formazan are not present. It is a useful dye in the differential diagnosis of chronic simple conjunctivitis.

Bromothymol blue

This is a narrow range pH indicator which changes colour around pH 7 and stains degenerate and dead cells and mucus. It is used to assess the damage caused by chemical agents such as lime.

Methylene blue

Dwyer-Joyces (1967) reported on methylene blue, a bacterial stain which will also vitally stain nerve tissue. Like rose bengal, it will outline an area of ulceration in herpetic keratitis. Hitchen (1971) refers to its ability to 'artistically' stain corneal ulcers when combined with fluorescein, the ulcer appearing as a dark blue area with a green halo.

References

Abrams, B. S. and Bailey, N. J. (1961) Black light photography. *J. Am. Optom. Assoc.*, **32**, 647–648

Barendsen, H., Oosterhuis, J. A. and van Haeringen, N. J. (1979) Concentration of fluorescein in tear fluid after instillation as eye drops. *Ophthal. Res.*, **11**, 73–82

Dwyer-Joyces, P. (1967) Corneal vital staining. *Irish J. Med. Sci.*, **6**, 359–367

Foster, J. (1980) The spectrum of topical dyeagnosis. *Suid-Afrikaanse Argief vir Oftalmologie*, **7**, 23–31

Grant, W. M. (1963) Fluorescein for applanation tonometry. *Am. J. Ophthalmol.*, **55**, 1252

Hitchen, B. (1971) Corneal staining. *Ophthalmic Optician*, **11**, 23

Lee, J., Courtney, R. and Thorson, J. C. (1980) Contact lens application of Kodak Wratten filter systems for enhanced detection of fluorescein staining. *Contact Lens J.*, **9**, 33–34

Moses, R. A. (1960) Fluorescein in applanation tonometry. *Am. J. Ophthalmol.*, **53**, 1149

Norn, M. S. (1964a) Fluorescein vital staining of the cornea and conjunctiva. *Acta Ophthalmol.*, **42**, 1038–1048

Norn, M. S. (1964b) Vital staining in practice. *Acta Ophthalmol.*, **42**, 1046–1053

Norn, M. S. (1967) Vital staining of the cornea and conjunctiva. *Am. J. Ophthalmol.*, **64**, 1078–1080

Norn, M. S. (1972a) Method of testing dyes for vital staining of cornea and conjunctiva. *Acta. Ophthalmol.*, **56**, 809–814

Norn, M. S. (1972b) Vital staining of the cornea and conjunctiva. *Acta Ophthalmol.*, Supplement 113

Pearson, R.M. (1984) The mystery of the missing fluorescein. *J. Br. Contact Lens Assoc.*, **7**, 122–125

Refojo, M. F., Miller, D. and Fiore, A. S. (1972) A new fluorescent stain for soft hydrophilic lens fitting. *Arch. Ophthalmol.*, **87**, 275

Ruben, M. (1978) *Soft Contact Lens Clinical and Applied Technology*, p. 175. London: Bailliere Tindall

Spaeth, G. L. (1978) In *Clinical Ophthalmology* (T. D. Duane, ed.), pp. 26–29. Maryland: Harper and Row

11

Drugs for the treatment of infections and inflammations

Anti-infectives used in the eye
Antibacterials

The successful treatment of an ocular infection will depend on three factors:

1. *The correct choice of antibacterial agent in relation to the infecting organism and the locus of the infection.* It is not possible in most cases to isolate, type and determine the organism's antibiotic sensitivity before commencement of treatment, and an intelligent guess has to be made of the most appropriate agent. If the eye has a surface infection then the absorption characteristics are not important, but if the infection is located inside the eye then an agent capable of penetrating ocular tissues must be used unless a parenteral route is employed.

2. *The most appropriate dosage form – e.g. ointment, drops or more heroic methods.* Drops are the most pleasant form to use, but have the disadvantage of a short halflife in the conjunctival sac. Eye ointments give a longer dwell time but are greasy and can interfere with vision. Techniques such as iontophoresis and direct injection require specialist application and are avoided wherever possible. Successful treatment requires good patient compliance and the choice of dosage form will depend on the site of the infection and factors such as the age of the patient. Ointments are often used with children where frequent dosage is not possible. The use of a viscous eye drop for fusidic acid has combined the ease of use of the drop with the relatively infrequent dosing of an ointment (Sinclair and Leigh, 1988).

3. *The dosage regimen.* The antibacterial effect of an antibiotic will only be maintained as long the infection is exposed to a concentration greater than the minimum inhibitory concentration (MIC), which varies between different bacteria. To increase the level of antibacterial agent requires increasing the frequency of administration. Since aqueous eyedrops have a halflife of about eight minutes, very little will be left after an hour and hourly administration may not be excessive. A three or four times a day administration will result in an effective concentration only being maintained for a very short period. A simplified regimen gives better compliance (Laerum *et al.*, 1994), and with most medical treatments the usual regimen is a compromise between what is desirable and what is possible. It is perhaps fortunate that a high proportion of cases of bacterial conjunctivitis are self resolving (Van Gogh and Smit, 1994).

Propamidine and dibromo-propamidine

Propamidine isethionate

Propamidine isethionate is a white or nearly white granular powder soluble one in five of water, another member of the aromatic diamidine group of compounds. It has good antibacterial properties, being active against *Staphylococcus aureus*, *Streptococcus pyogenes* and certain other streptococci and Clostridia, but not against *Pseudomonas aeruginosa*, *Proteus vulgaris*, *Escherichia coli* or spore forming bacteria. It also has anti-fungal properties. Its antibacterial action is not inhibited by tissue fluids, serum or pus (Martindale, 1977). Propamidine isethionate is available as a proprietary preparation (*Brolene* eyedrops) in a 0.1% concentration, which is used in the treatment (not to exceed a week) of conjunctivitis (particularly that due to Morax-Axenfield and pyogenic cocci), as well as for prophylactic purposes. Dibromopropamidine with neomycin has been successfully used in the treatment of acanthamoeba keratitis (Wright *et al.*, 1985).

The rare possibility of sensitization reaction to *Brolene* preparations is an indication for immediate discontinuation of their use.

Dibromopropamidine isethionate

This is a white or almost white crystalline powder soluble one in two of water. It is a member of the aromatic diamidine group of compounds which possess antibacterial and antifungal properties and is active against pyogenic cocci such as *Staphylococcus aureus* as well as inhibiting certain Gram negative bacilli, including *Escherichia coli*, *Proteus vulgaris*, and some strains of *Pseudomonas aeruginosa*. Dibromopropamidine's antibacterial action is not inhibited by pus or blood (Martindale, 1977).

Dibromopropamidine isethionate is available as a proprietary preparation (*Brolene* eye ointment) in a 0.15% concentration which is used for the treatment of conjunctivitis, blepharitis and other ocular infections, as well as for prophylactic ophthalmic purposes.

Chloramphenicol

Originally isolated from cultures of *Streptomyces venezuelae*, chloramphenicol is by far the most commonly used topical ophthalmic antibacterial agent and is effective against a whole range of bacteria and other organisms such as chlamydiae, rickettsiae (which cause diseases such as typhus and Q fever) and spirochaetes. Of the bacteria against which it is effective, there are many ocular pathogens such as *Corynebacterium*, *E. coli*, *Haemophilus* and Streptococci. It has been recommended for the routine treatment of ophthalmia neonatorum (Pierce *et al.*, 1982). Its effect against chlamydiae has led to its use in trachoma, although its usefulness for this condition is probably in the treatment of secondary infections which are responsible for many of the adverse effects of the infection. It is not effective however against most strains of *Pseudomonas aeruginosa*. The bacteriostatic action of chloramphenicol is due to the inhibition of protein synthesis by interaction with the bacterial ribosomes. It penetrates easily into the cell by a process of facilitated diffusion.

Resistance to chloramphenicol is brought about by the production of inactivating enzymes (chloramphenicol acetyltransferase).

One of the reasons for the popularity of chloramphenicol as an ophthalmic antibacterial is that it is rarely used systemically and thus there is little chance of cross resistance developing. In a study of 738 patients, only 6%

of the organisms cultured were resistant to chloramphenicol. This resistance rate was lower than for any other of the antibiotics tested (Seal *et al.*, 1982), but much higher resistance rates (e.g. 30.9%) against chloramphenicol have been reported by Mahajan (1983).

Apart from its employment in the treatment of life threatening conditions such as typhoid, salmonella infections and bacterial meningitis, the systemic use of chloramphenicol is very restricted today because of the incidence of aplastic anaemia producing agranulocytosis. From systemic treatment the incidence is about 1 in 50 000 patients, and from topical use the incidence is much lower. Trope *et al.* (1979) failed to find systemic absorption after drops were administered every two hours for five to seven days. This has not prevented reluctance by some clinicians to use chloramphenicol. However, McGhee (1996) points out that the theoretical risk of a fatal blood dyscrasia is about the same order as that of fatal penicillin anaphylaxis. He concludes that there is no evidence to suggest that children are more susceptible than adults. Decisions not to use chloramphenicol because of its possible toxicity must take into consideration the increased costs of treatment and the problems that will arise from the overuse of other antibiotics that should be retained for infections that are refractory to chloramphenicol. Chloramphenicol remains the first line treatment for minor infections such as bacterial infections. Titcomb (1997) has reviewed the evidence for the link between chloramphenicol and aplastic anaemia and found the case unproven. Topical use can sometimes lead to irritation.

Apart from the potential to cause this rare blood dyscrasia, chloramphenicol is an excellent topical antibiotic. It is available as a 0.5% solution or a 1% eye ointment. Intramuscular injections have been recommended for the treatment of trachoma (Chastain and Newton, 1954). Chloramphenicol has a high lipid solubility, and in a study on ovine eyes (Ismail and Morton, 1987) was found to be retained in the cornea at higher levels than in the aqueous humour. Ointments gave consistently higher levels in both the cornea and aqueous humour. Solutions of chloramphenicol are not stable at room temperature and must be stored at between 2° and 8°C.

Fusidic acid

Fusidic acid is used extensively as a topical antibiotic as well as (to a lesser extent) internally, in the form of tablets. Internally, the drug is well tolerated but it can cause liver damage and jaundice which is reversible on discontinuation. It is second only to chloramphenicol as the front line treatment of choice for bacterial conjunctivitis, being available in the form of a viscous drop which only requires application twice a day. It has potent bacteriostatic or bactericidal activity against Gram positive bacteria, producing this effect by inhibiting protein synthesis, but unlike other antibiotics it does not bind to ribosomes. This inhibition can be demonstrated in mammalian cells, but luckily the drug is poorly absorbed by them and it has a good therapeutic index. It is effective against *Staphylococcus aureus* (including methicillin resistant *Staphylococcus aureus* – MRSA – 'hospital staph'). Most Gram negative bacteria are resistant but it does have some activity against *Neisseriae* spp. It was compared with

1% chloramphenicol ointment applied every three hours, and produced similar beneficial effects (Sinclair and Leigh, 1988). It is now often used as the front line treatment of conjunctivitis. Compared with chloramphenicol ointment it has a much better compliance (James et al., 1991). Resistant strains can develop quickly. Hovenden et al. (1995) found a large number of resistant strains in isolates from conjunctival swabs.

Gentamicin

Gentamicin is another aminoglycoside antibiotic and has the same toxic effects as neomycin. It is one of the more effective agents in this group and will kill many strains of *Pseudomonas aeruginosa*. It is the treatment of choice for this organism (Seal et al., 1982), although resistant strains of *Pseudomonas* have been found (Insler et al., 1985). Gentamicin is given by injection for serious systemic infections when the nature of the invading organism is not known, and it should be kept for serious infections of the eye where other antibacterial agents are ineffective. Unfortunately there is a large number of topical gentamicin preparations, and gentamicin resistant *Pseudomonas* infections have occurred probably because gentamicin has been used for the treatment of trivial infections such as conjunctivitis.

Absorption across the corneal epithelium is very poor. Hillman et al. (1979) found that after application of gentamicin by drops, very little appeared in the aqueous humour. Subconjunctival injection produced effective corneal concentrations in two hours and these were maintained for 24 hours. Better anterior eye levels were obtained using transcorneal and transscleral iontophoresis in rabbits (Grossman et al., 1990). If a deep infection of the eye occurs, it is best treated by a slow intravitreal injection. Michelson and Nozik (1979) investigated the use of an implantable osmotic minipump for the administration of gentamicin for the treatment of experimental endophthalmitis in rabbits.

Reversible cellular oedema has been reported in the corneal endothelium following anterior chamber injection (Lavine et al., 1979). Systemic injection will not give rise to sufficient ocular levels because of gentamicin's poor ability to cross the blood/aqueous barrier. It is usually applied as a 0.3% solution but more concentrated solutions have been recommended for the treatment of bacterial corneal ulcers (Chaudhuri and Godfrey, 1982). An intense dosing schedule has been suggested in order to achieve high initial levels (Glasser et al., 1985) in the cornea. Loading doses consisting of one drop every minute for five minutes produced significant levels in the cornea of rabbits.

Gentamicin is a very toxic compound and like other aminoglycosides can cause damage to the ears and kidneys. Both functions of the ears are affected, so ataxia due to vestibular damage and deafness from cochlear damage are the results of toxic doses. Hypersensitivity reactions can occur after local use, and when a patient is sensitized to one aminoglycoside he will react to others.

Framycetin

Framycetin is produced by certain strains of *Streptomyces fradiae* or *decaris*. Framycetin is an isomer of neomycin which is used extensively as a topical antibiotic in general.

Neomycin is a mixture of three substances – neomycin A, neomycin B and neomycin C. In fact, neomycin A is an inactive breakdown product of the other two and is normally present at a concentration of 10–15%.

Framycetin is otherwise known as neomycin B, and preparations of framycetin contain not more than 3% neomycin C and not more than 1% neomycin A. It has a broad spectrum of activity against Gram positive and Gram negative bacteria. It is effective against a greater range of bacteria than penicillin or streptomycin, e.g. *Proteus vulgaris*, *Escherichia coli*, *Haemophilus influenzae* and *Klebsiella* spp.

Like all antibiotics, resistance can develop with continued indiscriminate use, but this tends to develop more slowly than to other antibiotics. Of course, there will be a cross resistance between neomycin and framycetin and other aminoglycoside antibiotics.

Neomycin and framycetin are poorly absorbed from the alimentary tract. For this reason neomycin can be used to suppress normal intestinal bacteria prior to alimentary surgery. It is well absorbed from injection but produces toxic reactions, especially to the kidneys and ears. Framycetin will have similar toxicity. Because of the poor systemic absorption and the toxicity, neomycin and framycetin are principally used for topical application. Framycetin is used on gauze dressings, in skin creams, nebulizers and eye preparations.

Neomycin

Neomycin is one of a group of aminoglycoside antibiotics which include amikacin, streptomycin, tobramycin and gentamicin. All aminoglycosides are rapidly bactericidal and inhibit protein synthesis by combining with mRNA, but this does not explain their rapidity of action.

Passage into the cells is dependent on electron transport, which in turn can be influenced by transmembrane potential. The transport of the antibacterial into the cell can be reduced by low pH and aerobic conditions. It will also be decreased by Ca^{2+} and Mg^{2+} ions and hyperosmolarity.

As the antibacterial enters the cell it increases the rate at which further amounts can pass in. This leads eventually to disruption of the cell membrane and rapid death of the cell. Resistance can be brought about by the production of enzymes or low affinity of the ribosomes.

Penicillin will aid the passage of aminoglycosides into the cell and thus these two antibacterials should be synergistic. In an experimental study on guinea pigs (Davis *et al.*, 1979) no additive or synergistic effect was found when penicillin was injected intramuscularly and an aminoglycoside was applied topically; however, the test organism was *Pseudomonas aeruginosa*, and aminoglycosides were found to be the most effective treatment for keratitis produced by this organism.

Neomycin, like chloramphenicol, is favoured as a topical antimicrobial because of the relatively rare systemic use. Neomycin is not absorbed from the gut and is too toxic for parenteral administration. As a result, its use is restricted to either disinfecting the gut prior to surgery or as a topical preparation for skin or mucous membranes.

All aminoglycosides produce nephrotoxicity and ototoxicity but this is not known to occur from topical use. However, keratoconjunctivitis can develop as a result of hypersensitivity to neomycin after ophthalmic use.

Neomycin has a broad spectrum of activity but is not effective against *Pseudomonas aeruginosa*.

Although preparations of neomycin alone (drops or eye ointment) are used, it is most often encountered along with steroids to produce antibiotic cover while treating inflammation.

Tobramycin

Tobramycin is an aminoglycoside antibiotic (see gentamicin) and has similar toxic effects to the others in the group (i.e. nephrotoxicity and ototoxicity). It has a better antibacterial efficacy than gentamicin, being more active against *Ps. aeruginosa in vitro*. It is active against most strains of Staphylococci found on the surface of the eye. Normally it is used as a 0.3% solution, but iontophoresis has been used to treat apparently resistant infections of *Pseudomonas aeruginosa* (Hobden *et al.*, 1989). Collagen shields have also been used as a method of administration in the treatment of Pseudomonal keratitis (Hobden *et al.*, 1988). It produces similar side effects to other aminoglycoside antibiotics but is less nephrotoxic than gentamicin.

Polymixin B

Polymixin shares many of the properties of gentamicin. It is effective against many strains of *Pseudomonas aeruginosa* and is recommended by some authors (Mahajan, 1983) as the best drug for the treatment of infections by this organism. It is also effective against most other Gram negative rods except *Proteus*. It is poorly absorbed from the gut, and passage is slow across the blood/aqueous or blood/brain barriers and the intact corneal epithelium. Kidney damage can result from its systemic use. Polymixin is used topically in combination with either bacitracin in ointment form or trimethoprim as drops or ointment, in which form it is equally as effective as chloramphenicol in treating bacterial conjunctivitis (Behrens-Baumann *et al.*, 1988).

Bacitracin

This bactericidal agent has similar properties to penicillin, especially in its mode of action, and is effective mainly against Gram positive bacteria such as Staphylococci and Streptococci. Most Gram negative organisms are resistant to it. It is mainly used externally in combination with other agents, e.g. polymixin. It penetrates the cornea poorly but is effective for surface infections.

Vancomycin

Vancomycin is another antibacterial which produces its effect by interfering with cell wall production, but it is unrelated to penicillin structurally, being a glycopeptide. It is not absorbed from the gut but this does not preclude it being given by mouth as used to treat some forms of ulcerative colitis. Its action is mainly on Gram positive bacteria, both cocci and bacilli, but it has little effect on Gram negative species as it does not cross the outer membrane of the cell wall. The drug is toxic to the ears and kidneys and can cause hypersensitivity reactions. It also produces the 'red man' syndrome of flushing of the upper body, hypotension and angioedema and pruritus. However, it has successfully been used in the treatment of post cataract endophthalmitis (Doft *et al.*, 1994). Its ability to treat MRSA infections was successfully employed using a topical solution in a case of chronic dacryocystitis caused by such an organism (Tadokoro *et al.*, 1995).

Tetracyclines

Tetracyclines are a group of broad spectrum antibiotics which include chlortetracycline, demethylchlortetracycline, oxytetracycline, tetracycline and minocycline. There is little to choose between them, with the exception of minocycline which has a broader spectrum and more specific indications. Although the rest of the members of the group are quite similar, cross resistance between them does not necessarily occur.

Tetracyclines are effective against Gram positive and Gram negative bacteria as well as spirochaetes, chlamydiae and other organisms, but *Pseudomonas* and *Proteus* are resistant to these agents.

Tetracyclines taken orally may cause stomach upsets (nausea, vomiting and diarrhoea) but are best known for their effect on bone and teeth in children. They permanently colour teeth yellow, and slow bone growth, due to their ability to chelate calcium and magnesium. Adverse effects from topical application are rare due to the low dose of drug that the patient receives in one drop of solution compared with the systemic dose. If a drop of 1% tetracycline solution were to be applied four times a day, it would take four months for the equivalent of one oral dose to be administered.

Penetration across the intact cornea is poor and these compounds are best used for surface infections. Topical tetracycline is used in the treatment of trachoma (normally in ointment form) and is becoming the prophylactic of choice for ophthalmia neonatorum Raucher and Newton (1983) recommend intramuscular penicillin and tetracycline 1% ointment as a prophylactic agent. If the infecting organism is chlamydial, then tetracycline treatment is to be preferred over other antibiotics (Pierce *et al.*, 1982).

Penicillin

The penicillins are a group of bactericidal agents which interfere with the synthesis of cell walls by binding to certain enzymes in the cell membrane which are responsible for the building of the cell wall, producing morphological changes in the bacteria they affect. Long filamentous cells are produced which fail to divide. Lysis of cells can occur due to the antibacterial action of some autolysins which normally only function during cell division. Benzylpenicillin was the first antibiotic to be introduced into medicine. Newer penicillins have been developed which are semisynthetic, but they all share the danger of inducing a possible fatal anaphylaxis in a number of patients. Some of the penicillins are susceptible to breakdown by enzymes (penicillinases) produced by Gram positive bacteria such as Staphylococci. Also, penicillinase producing Gram negative organisms such as the gonococci have been isolated from cases of ophthalmia neonatorum (Dunlop *et al.*, 1980; Pang *et al.*, 1979). More advanced agents have been produced which are resistant to the action of penicillinase. Resistance to penicillins can also be caused by difficulty of the compound penetrating to the site of action. Penicillins pass across the ocular barriers very poorly and products containing them are rarely used in the treatment of ocular infections.

Erythromycin

Erythromycin, a macrolide antibiotic, is often used in the treatment of systemic infections, but for ophthalmic use it is best known for the effect on chlamydiae and other organisms such as Rickettsia, Treponema and Mycoplasma. It can also be used to treat Gram positive infections and a few Gram negative ones such as *Neisseriae gonorrheae*. This has led to its use as a 0.5% ointment for the prophylaxis of ophthalmia neonatorum. It produces its bacteriostatic effect by disrupting protein synthesis which involves binding to ribosomes. Resistance to this antibiotic is brought by modification of the ribosomes and can occur when used widely as a prophylactic. Erythromycin resistant Staphylococci were found in infants on whom it was used to prevent ophthalmia neonatorum (Bloggs *et al.*, 1990). Newer macrolides have been introduced of which clarithomycin is the most commonly used.

Ciprofloxacin

One of the major growth areas for modern antibiotics has the been the development of a group of agents referred to as the fluoroquinolones. The precursor to this group was nalidixic acid which was introduced in the early 1960s. Fluoroquinolones interfere with the production of DNA by inhibiting the enzyme responsible for producing the coils of the nucleic acid in the bacterial cell. The emergence of resistant strains is low and there is no cross resistance with other antibiotic groups such as the aminoglycosides.

Fluoroquinolones are well absorbed after oral administration and are used to treat many common infections, especially those of the upper and lower respiratory tract and the urinary tract, including gonorrhoea. They are effective against a wide range of bacteria, both Gram positive and Gram negative. They are active against *Staph.* spp including those resistant to penicillin and methicillin (MRSA), but less effective against Streptococci. Susceptible Gram negative bacteria include some strains of *Pseudomonas aeruginosa*, even some which are resistant to aminoglycosides (O'Brien *et al.*, 1988). Systemically the fluoroquinolones are well tolerated, with gastrointestinal disturbances being the most common adverse reaction. Other reactions include dizziness and skin reactions.

The antibacterial activity and *in vitro* toxicity of a range of these agents has been tested to discover which of them is most suitable for use ophthalmically (Cutarelli *et al.*, 1991). As a result an ophthalmic form of ciprofloxacin as a 0.3% solution has been introduced, from which absorption into ocular tissues is good, leading to aqueous humour levels which exceed the minimum inhibitory concentrations of many ocular pathogens. It also produced least damage to rabbit corneae experimentally. Tear levels are maintained above MICs for many bacteria up to four hours after instillation in healthy individuals (Limberg and Bugge, 1994). Whether the same levels would be maintained in eyes where tear production and drainage is raised due to inflammation is open to question. It has been shown to be as effective as tobramycin in the treatment of bacterial conjunctivitis (Leibowitz, 1991a), and a safe and effective treatment of bacterial keratitis caused by a wide variety of bacteria both Gram positive and Gram negative (Leibowitz, 1991b). The majority of the former were either Staphylococci (including MRSA) or Streptococci while *Pseudomonas aeruginosa* was the predominant Gram negative bacteria. In treating bacterial conjunctivitis it has proved to be as valuable a drug as chloramphenicol in terms of efficacy and safety (Power *et al.*, 1993). It demonstrates a definite postantibiotic suppression which is more marked than for the other fluoroquinolones (Fuhr, 1995) and was found to be more effective than rifampicin in the treatment of bacterial conjunctivitis and blepharitis (Adenis, 1995). It is also more effective than tobramycin and another fluoroquinolone, norfloxacin, in the treatment of experimental Pseudomonal keratitis in rabbits (Reidy *et al.*, 1991). It has the advantage of not causing aplastic anaemia, but since the occurrence of this effect is very rare from ophthalmic application this may not be sufficient reason for using the newer drug routinely as a first treatment for conjunctivitis.

So far no other fluoroquinolone has been introduced in an ophthalmic form commercially, but ofloxacin has been used in the treatment of chlamydia conjunctivitis (Zhang *et al.*, 1995) and norfloxacin has been compared with gentamicin in the treatment of congenital dacryocystitis (Huber *et al.*, 1991, Huber-Spitzy *et al.*, 1991). Lomefloxacin has a wide antibacterial spectrum and is well absorbed. It demonstrated good antipseudomonal activity in the treatment of experimental bacterial keratitis (Malet *et al.*, 1995).

Sulphonamides

The sulphonamide drugs have a bacteriostatic (rather than a bactericidal) action by virtue of their ability to prevent bacterial utilization of p-aminobenzoic acid (PABA) (Havener, 1978). PABA is required by sulphonamide sensitive bacteria, which use PABA to synthesize the vitamin folic acid. The latter is needed by micro-organisms for normal reproduction and metabolism. The basic structure of PABA is very similar to the sulphonamides which act as competitive antagonists of antimetabolites, substituting for the PABA in the transformation. Preformed folic acid is ingested by man so the sulphonamides do not interfere with its availability to human cells, or bacteria that utilize the preformed vitamin.

The growth of most Gram positive micro-organisms and a variety of Gram negative organisms (including some strains of *Pseudomonas*) is inhibited by sulphonamides. Sulphacetamide sodium in 10–30% solution and a 6% ointment is effective by local application against surface ocular infection from such organisms in a manner which still compares favourably with many of the newer antibiotics.

Generally, however, the antibiotics have replaced the sulphonamides as first choice in the treatment of major infections (Havener, 1978), and few sulphonamide containing products are available today. Sulphacetamide, although possessing a relatively 'weak' bactericidal action compared to some of the other sulphonamides, is suitable for topical application to the eye because of its acceptable pH and its solubility in aqueous solution. A 30% solution has a pH of 7.4% whilst solutions of other sulphonamides are highly alkaline. The drug penetrates into the ocular tissues and fluids in high concentrations, and its solubility in water is approximately 90 times that of sulphadimidine.

Table 11.1 Antibacterials (commercially available in the UK as ophthalmic preparations)

Official name	Trade name	Single dose	Dosage forms	Concentration	Adverse reactions	Notes
Propamidine and dibromopropamide	Brolene*	Unavailable	drops ointment	0.1% 0.15%	Sensitization	Used in the treatment of Acanthamoeba infection
Chloramphenicol	Chlormycetin Sno-phenicol	Available	drops ointment	0.5% 1.0%	Agranulocytes	Requires storage at 4–8°C
Fusidic acid	Fusithalmic	Unavailable	viscous drops	1.0%		
Gentamicin	Genticin Cidomycin Garamycin	Available	drops ointment	0.3% 0.3%	Nephrotoxic and ototoxic	Member of aminoglycoside
Framycetin	Soframycin	Unavailable	drops ointment	0.5% 0.5%	As for gentamicin	
Neomycin	Neosporin	Available	drops ointment	0.5% 0.5%	As for gentamicin	Most ofted used in combination with steroids
Tobramycin	Tobralex	Unavailable	drops	0.3%	As for gentamicin	
Polymixin B	Polyfax Polytrim	Unavailable	ointment drops	10 000 un 10 000 un		
Bacitracin	Polyfax	Unavailable	ointment	500 un		
Ciprofloxacin	Ciloxan	Unavailable	drops	0.3%	Local burning and itching	
Chlortetracycline	Aureomycin	Unavailable	ointment	1%		Used for chlamydial infections
Ofloxacin	Exocin	Unavailable	drops	0.3%		
Trimethoprim	Polyfax	Unavailable	drops ointment	0.1% 0.5%		

* Availabe as an over-the-counter preparation

Antivirals

Because of the intimate relationship of the infecting virus to the host cell, viral infections are more difficult to treat than those caused by bacteria and thus many viral infections still resist treatment with only a few responding to therapy. A lot of research effort has been expended recently in the search for compounds active against viruses, in particular the Human Immunodeficiency Virus. One of the earliest viruses to be treated was Herpes simplex, the causative organism of dendritic ulcers, cold sores and genital herpes. Several agents have been used as topical treatments for these conditions: idoxuridine, vidarabine, trifluorothymidine and acyclovir; the latter is the only one in regular use.

Idoxuridine

This is the oldest antiviral compound and is a derivative of thymidine, one of the organic bases which are incorporated into the nucleic acids. The viral metabolism incorporates the idoxuridine into the nucleic acid, inhibiting further synthesis or leading to mutations. The virus is thus prevented from infecting other host cells. Idoxuridine competitively inhibits the uptake of thymidine and thus an excess of thymidine will antagonize its action (compare sulphonamides and PABA). It is specifically antiviral and has no effect on bacteria.

It is used as 0.1% eyedrops and 0.5% eye ointment. Penetration into the eye is poor but normally the infection is on the surface of the cornea and clinically effective concentrations can be achieved by topical administration.

Idoxuridine is very selective and does not inhibit epithelial growth when applied topically (Foster and Pavan-Langston, 1977). The compound is generally nontoxic although if used systemically it has mutagenic and teratogenic properties. It does however inhibit stromal healing and causes a reduction of wound strength, and cannot therefore be used after corneal transplants.

The antiviral agent is only active while it is present, and during treatment it must administered intensively, i.e. every hour. Resistant strains can sometimes develop.

Vidarabine

Vidarabine, otherwise known as adenine arabinoside, is a nucleoside which stops the growth of the nuclear chain. Since its mode of action is different from idoxuridine, it can be used in patients who are allergic to this compound or to treat idoxuridine resistant cases.

Used in 3% ointment form, it is absorbed to a greater extent than is idoxuridine and can be used topically for herpetic uveitis, but it is often given by injection for this condition. Vidarabine drops of the same concentration have been tested but they showed up as being significantly poorer than liquid preparations of idoxuridine and trifluorothymidine (Pavan-Langston et al., 1979). Vidarabine is effective against both strains of H. simplex (I and II), but does not seem to affect the course of infections with adenovirus. Like idoxuridine it does not interfere with the healing of corneal epithelial defects but will slow the rate of repair of stromal injuries.

The monophosphate derivative of vidarabine – adenine arabinoside monophosphate, otherwise known as AraAMP – has been tested (Falcon and Jones, 1977) as an antiviral in herpetic eye disease. It was found to be better than vidarabine in inhibiting lesions but had similar effects in the treatment of established lesions. It significantly retarded closure of epithelial wounds in rabbits and induced toxic changes in the epithelium (Foster and Pavan-Langston, 1977).

Trifluorothymidine

As the name indicates, trifluorothymidine (TFT F3T) is a thymidine derivative and inhibits the replication of DNA viruses. It is a potent reversible inhibitor of thymidine synthetase and this accounts in part for its mode of action. TFT can also be incorporated into viral DNA to produce defective new virus particles. It has a short halflife when given systemically and is also very toxic when given by this route. Originally designed as an anticancer agent, TFT is lipid soluble and crosses the corneal epithelium. It passes into the eye more readily than vidarabine and idoxuridine and produces levels in the aqueous humour which are effective against deeper viral infections (Pavan-Langston and Nelson, 1979) and therefore it can produce results where idoxuridine (Gilbert and Work, 1980) and vidarabine have had no effect. Like idoxuridine it does not significantly retard the closure of epithelial wounds (Foster and Pavan-Langston, 1977).

Trifluorothymidine was found to be significantly superior to idoxuridine in a study of 78 patients (Wellings *et al.*, 1972) on the grounds that the healing time was significantly shorter and the percentage of treatment failures in patients receiving trifluorothymidine was less. Pavan-Langston and Foster (1977) also found a significant difference in the percentage of successfully treated patients. In a coded study 96% of all TFT patients were successfully healed, compared with 75% for idoxuridine.

McKinnon *et al.* (1975) compared trifluorothymidine with vidarabine. Although they found no significant differences, there were trends which suggested that the former drug produced quicker healing, especially in amoeboid ulcers. There were fewer failures and a smaller incidence of further ulceration with this treatment. Slightly different results were found by van Bjisterveld and Post (1980). TFT was found to be slightly slower than vidarabine in producing healing. The healing time was also found to be dependent on the interval between the onset of symptoms and the onset of therapy. Similarly, McNeill and Kaufman (1979) found in an experimental stromal keratitis model that the effectiveness of therapy with trifluorothymidine depended on early treatment. It was also shown be significantly faster than bromovinyldeoxyuridine in treating corneal herpetic lesions (Power *et al.*, 1991).

TFT's superiority in treating amoeboid ulcers was confirmed by Coster *et al.* (1979). Several reasons for this superiority have been suggested. It may be due to superior antiviral activity of the drug in the corneal epithelium or stroma. It may also be due to better absorption across the epithelium or better uptake by the stroma.

It was found to be of little benefit in the treatment of epidemic keratoconjunctivitis (Ward *et al.*, 1993).

Acyclovir

Acyclovir (acycloguanosine) only affects virus infected cells because it utilizes an enzyme, thymidine kinase, the structure and function of which is slightly different in viruses to that in cells. Viral thymidine kinase can metabolize acycloguanosine while cellular thymidine kinase cannot. Some viral mutants have modified genes for the production of thymidine kinase, but these tend to have low pathogenicity and virulence. Nevertheless, a variant which produces a thymidine kinase with modified specificity has been found (Darby *et al.*, 1981) which is resistant to acyclovir. The nucleoside is phosphorylated into a triphosphate nucleoside which is incorporated into the viral DNA molecule, arresting further development. It is effective against infections with strains of Herpes simplex which are resistant to idoxuridine (Trousdale *et al.*, 1981). Acyclovir is significantly more effective than the other antivirals, even on drug sensitive strains. Acyclovir treated eyes showed less corneal epithelial involvement and conjunctivitis and exhibited less iritis and corneal clouding. McGill *et al.* (1981) compared acyclovir and vidarabine and found that the former had a much better rate of healing and reduction in symptoms but Coster *et al.* (1980) found no difference between acyclovir and idoxuridine. Because of its very selective action it does not interfere with corneal wound healing, whether epithelial or stromal. Lass *et al.* (1979) compared the effect of acyclovir on wound healing with that of idoxuridine. Acyclovir had no significant effect on the regenerating epithelium or re-epithelialization of surface wounds or on the collagen content of stromal wounds. It is effective on its own against dendritic and small amoeboid ulcers, but larger ones require the addition of a topical steroid for complete resolution (Vajpayee *et al.*, 1989).

Acyclovir is now used extensively for the treatment of Herpes zoster infections, both orally and topically. The eye ointment can be used when the eye is affected (*Herpes zoster ophthalmicus*).

Newer agents

Concern about the effects of HIV infection led to the search for antivirals that could cope with the virus in patients with compromised immune systems. One of the first of these to gain widespread use was azidothymidine (AZT, zidovudine) which inhibits the action of reverse transcriptase, which brings about the DNA copy of the viral RNA. The copy DNA is then incorporated into the host genetic material. It is highly toxic and causes bone marrow suppression in a high proportion of patients.

The other virus that has led to new drugs is the cytomegalovirus (CMV). Ganciclovir, a close relative of acyclovir, has marked activity against this agent and has been used in the treatment of CMV retinitis in AIDS patients (Heinemann, 1989). It is more toxic than acyclovir, causing bone marrow suppression as well as being hepatotoxic, teratogenic and mutagenic.

Antifungals

The number of antifungals in routine medical use is low relative to antibacterial agents. The human body is fairly resistant to fungal infection, although some superficial infections are fairly common such as *Tinea pedis* (athlete's foot) and *Candida albicans* (thrush). Deeper infections usually only occur after some form of trauma and can be very serious and potentially life threatening.

Likewise, fungal infections of the eye are much rarer than those caused by bacteria, but nonetheless can be very serious when they do occur and require prompt and effective treatment if loss of an eye is to be avoided. They have been reported following local anaesthetic abuse (Chern *et al.*, 1996). Suspected cases of fungal infection should be referred to specialists in this area.

To cope with fungal infections a range of antifungal agents has been developed; these include nystatin, amphotericin, natamycin, flucytosine, clotrimazole and miconazole. The list is by no means as extensive as the list of antibacterial agents. Fungal cells are eucaryotic like host cells, and therefore will possess many similar enzyme systems which makes it difficult to produce compounds which are toxic to the invading fungal cells without adversely affecting the host cells.

Nystatin

Chemically related to amphotericin, nystatin is probably the oldest and best known antifungal agent. It is produced by a strain of Streptomyces and is fungistatic rather than fungicidal. It is effective against a wide range of fungi but has little effect on other micro-organisms. Nystatin, like the other polyenes, produces its effect by binding to sterols in the cell membrane, causing a loss of K^+ and Mg^{2+} ions and a subsequent interference with the cell's metabolism. The compound is poorly absorbed by the cornea, so topical treatment is only effective for surface fungal infection with organisms such as *Candida albicans*. Suspensions are used for the treatment of oral thrush, but apart from this it is little used today although it has minimal side effects. Deep infections require directly injected therapy.

Amphotericin

Amphotericin is also a product of a Streptomyces species and like nystatin is not effective against bacteria and viruses. Similarly, its mode of action is to increase permeability of the cell membrane by binding to sterols. It is selective for ergosterol (found in fungal cell membranes) as opposed to cholesterol (present in mammalian cell membranes), making it less toxic to the host cell than to the infecting cell. The effect on the cell membranes allows other antifungal agents used in combination to become more effective, and sometimes antifungal agents and antibiotics are combined. Amphotericin was combined with rifampicin (an antibiotic normally associated with the treatment of tuberculosis) in the treatment of experimental *Candida albicans* keratitis and was found to be better than amphotericin alone (Stern *et al.*, 1979). Rifampicin, which is ineffective on its own, passes much more easily through a membrane made more permeable by amphotericin, and inhibits RNA synthesis. Host cells can be similarly affected and this leads to toxicity. Patients' reactions to the drug vary and the dose has to be carefully titrated.

Treatment of fungal infections is much slower than that of bacterial infections, and therapy must often be continued for months. Amphotericin, which is fungistatic, is poorly absorbed and its marked toxicity restricts its use to topical infections. Not all strains of *Candida albicans* are equally susceptible to amphotericin *in vitro* and *in vivo* (O'Day *et al.*, 1991), and sensitivity tests may be required. Patients may experience chills and headaches with elevated temperatures initially, followed by renal toxicity which is dose related.

Natamycin

This fungicidal compound is very effective against a whole range of fungi but not bacteria. Like many other antifungals it penetrates the eye very poorly and was found to be inferior to amphotericin in the treatment of Candida keratitis in rabbits (O'Day et al., 1987). It is used as eye drops (5–10%) or eye ointment (1%).

Flucytosine

Flucytosine, which has a narrow spectrum of activity and is only active against yeast, is used as eye drops (1.5%). It is a synthetic compound which is well absorbed by the gut and, being distributed to all parts of the body including the CSF after oral administration, is used to treat systemic infections of Candida albicans and Aspergillus species. In susceptible organisms it is converted to fluorouracil which inhibits RNA function and inhibits DNA synthesis. The converting enzyme (cyosine deaminase) is not present in mammalian cells and thus the compound has a good therapeutic index. Serious side effects do occasionally occur which affect the blood, causing anaemia and thrombocytopenia. Fungal cells which lack the converting enzyme will be resistant to flucytosine and it is therefore sometimes used in combination with amphotericin, with which it is synergistic.

Clotrimazole

There is a whole group of modern antifungals referred to as the imidazoles and probably the most widely used is clotrimazole. Depending on the concentration, imidazoles are either fungistatic or fungicidal, producing their effect by inhibiting the incorporation of ergosterol into the cell membrane and interfering with cell respiration. It is poorly absorbed and is only used topically. It is therefore most commonly used for fungal infections of the skin, e.g. athlete's foot and ringworm, and vagina, e.g. thrush. In the eye, a 1% solution was shown to penetrate the corneae of rabbits experimentally infected with Candida albicans (Behrens-Baumann et al., 1990). The drug significantly reduced the effects of the infection.

Miconazole

Another imidazole, this broad spectrum antifungal agent produces its effects by acting on the cell membrane and blocking the production of ergosterol. It rivals clotrimazole in its use in skin and genital fungal infections.

Absorption takes place across the intact cornea but if the epithelium is removed much greater absorption takes place.

Fluconazole

Unlike the previous two compounds, fluconazole is active by mouth, being rapidly absorbed after oral administration, and is well distributed throughout the body fluids. It is available as an over the counter preparation for the treatment of vaginal thrush and has an action similar to the other imidazoles. Being used systemically it is more likely to cause side effects which can range from unpleasant nausea and vomiting to the very serious liver damage that can occur with long term use. This condition can lead to jaundice and death.

Terbinafine

This compound is an allylamine antifungal which is active against certain filamentous and dimorphic fungi and is used in the oral treatment of surface fungal infections. It produces its effect by inhibiting an enzyme present in the cell membrane.

Anti-inflammatory agents

Inflammation is the response of the body to a variety of stimuli, e.g. infection, allergy and trauma. There are many processes involved in inflammation, but they result in a characteristic reaction which is typified by a reddening of the area (as a result of vasodilation), oedema, loss of function and pain. The process is brought into play to combat and destroy invading organisms, but sometimes the body's own cells are attacked and destroyed and damage to tissues occurs. This is particularly true for the eye, where the delicate, transparent structures are susceptible to damage by scar formation. Permanent loss of vision can be the result of an ocular inflammation and sight can only be preserved if steps are taken to limit the extent of the inflammatory process.

The inflammatory response involves the following processes:

1. *The increased production of prostaglandins and leukotrienes.* Arachidonic acid is produced by the action of phospholipase and this in turn is converted by the enzyme cyclo-oxygenase to one of the variety of prostaglandins which have effects on smooth muscle and mediate some of the inflammatory reactions. For example, a mixture of prostaglandins called irin can induce an atropine resistant miosis which occurs in uveitis. Lipoxygenase converts arachidonic acid to leucotrienes which bring about an increase in permeability and oedema.
2. *The liberation of histamine from mast cells.* This is caused by the allergen-antigen reaction causing an increase in the influx of calcium ions into the mast cells. Histamine, in addition to its ability to stimulate pain and itch nerve fibres, is best known for the production of the 'triple response'. If a small amount of histamine is injected into the skin, a small red area appears at the point of injection which is due to a direct effect of the histamine on blood vessels causing vasodilation. The permeability of the capillaries is increased, causing loss of cells and proteins. The effect of the protein loss is to raise the osmotic pressure of the fluid, causing increased loss of water into the tissues and consequent oedema. The third component is a diffuse vasodilation, causing a more diffuse red area (flare) around the site of injection.
3. *Vascular effects.* In addition to the action of histamine, other locally active agents can induce vasodilation and increase capillary permeability. In the eye, the permeability of the blood/aqueous barrier is increased, leading to a turbid aqueous which contains more protein than normal. Outflow is impaired and an inflammatory form of secondary glaucoma may ensue.
4. *Fibroblastic activity.* Because of its role in trauma, part of the inflammatory response is to stimulate the mechanism of wound repair (e.g. fibroblast and collagen forming activity) which can sometimes lead to scar formation and, in the cornea, opacity.

5. *Increased leucocyte activity*. Leucocytes normally migrate into the site of inflammation in order to attack and kill invading cells. They contain lysosomal vacuoles which can bring about the destruction of cells including the host inflamed cells.

Because the effects of inflammation can sometimes be excessive and, in the eye, lead to discomfort and loss of vision, it is often desirable to limit the extent by the use of appropriate drugs.

Nonsteroidal anti-inflammatory drugs (NSAIDs)

As their name suggests, these compounds were developed as an alternative to steroids in the treatment of inflammatory disease. Steroids were hailed as wonder drugs when they were first introduced into medicine. Certainly they are very effective and reduce many of the symptoms of inflammation. Unfortunately, they produce many side effects, e.g. cataracts and raised intraocular pressure. Alternative agents were therefore developed which it was hoped would have equal anti-inflammatory effects with fewer adverse reactions.

One of the mechanisms involved in the inflammatory response is the conversion of fatty acids to prostaglandins, which in the eye produce an atropine resistant miosis. Prostaglandins increase the permeability of the ciliary epithelium, allowing larger amounts of protein to pass into the aqueous humour which gives rise to aqueous flare and an increase in intraocular pressure. This rise is followed by a fall some two hours later. Prostaglandins have been implicated in corneal neovascularization.

Indomethacin

There are many inhibitors of prostaglandin formation. The oldest, best known and cheapest is aspirin (acetylsalicylic acid). It has been tested for the prevention of cystoid macular oedema following cataract extraction.

The first of the new generation of NSAIDs was indomethacin, a compound which has been tested in topical formulation for cystoid macular oedema and for the treatment of noninfectious conjunctivitis (Kishore *et al.*, 1994). Eye drops containing 0.1% indomethacin have been used following cataract surgery to reduce surgically induced miosis and postoperative inflammatory response. Indomethacin has produced comparable results to dexamethasone in the treatment of acute anterior uveitis (Sand and Krogh, 1991). It is related to diclofenac, being an acetic acid derivative, and produces its effect by inhibiting the lipoxygenase pathway which converts arachidonic acid to prostaglandins.

Oxyphenbutazone

Oxyphenbutazone is a white crystalline powder almost insoluble in water. It is a derivative of phenylbutazone, with similar anti-inflammatory, analgesic and antipyretic effects, and belongs to the group of NSAIDS known as the pyrazolones. It is given in general medicine, usually by mouth, for the treatment of rheumatic and allied disorders. Oxyphenbutazone may be used in a 10% concentration in a greasy eye ointment base for nonpurulent inflammatory anterior segment eye conditions. Where other conjunctival decongestants are contraindicated, a single application of this ointment provides a useful alternative for the optometric practitioner. This compound has been withdrawn from systemic use.

Ibuprofen

Perhaps one of best known of the modern NSAIDS, ibuprofen is freely available over the counter in preparations for producing analgesia and relieving inflammation. Although not available yet as a topical ophthalmic preparation it has been tested on artificially induced ocular inflammation in rabbits and was found to be effective (Tilden *et al.*, 1990).

Diclofenac

Diclofenac is a potent inhibitor of cyclo-oxygenase, reducing the production of prostaglandins, and while not inhibiting lipoxygenase directly it apparently reduces the amount of arachidonic acid available to it thus preventing the synthesis of leucotrienes. It is used for the inhibition of intra-operative miosis (Bonomi *et al.*, 1987; Erturk *et al.*, 1991; Fabian *et al.*, 1991) and the suppression of postoperative inflammation. For the latter it has been used alone (Vickers *et al.*, 1991) or in combination with prednisolone (Struck *et al.*, 1994) or with dexamethasone (Ronen *et al.*, 1985). In other studies, it has been shown to be as effective as dexamethasone for this purpose (Avci *et al.*, 1993; Ilic *et al.*, 1984) It has also been used in the prevention and treatment of cystoid macular oedema. Its use in the treatment of more everyday inflammations such as vernal conjunctivitis, giant papillary conjunctivitis and seasonal allergic conjunctivitis is less proven and presently undergoing study. Leibowitz *et al.* (1995) found that 0.1% diclofenac relieved the symptoms of acute seasonal allergic conjunctivitis.

NSAIDs have analgesic properties as well as anti-inflammatory ones and they have been used to treat eye pain and reduce photophobia after radial keratotomy (Sher *et al.*, 1992; Sher *et al.*, 1993) and in patients with episcleritis.

Because the mechanism of action is different from that of steroids, it is possible that given together the drugs could have additive if not synergistic actions. Topical solutions are well tolerated

Diclofenac has been compared with prednisolone in topical use (Hersh *et al.*, 1990) and was found to have similar effects on corneal wound healing but a superior performance in treating the accompanying iritis.

Sodium cromoglycate (cromolyn sodium)

Sodium cromoglycate was originally indicated for the treatment of asthma and it produces its effect by stabilizing the membranes of mast cells, thus preventing the release of histamine. A topical preparation of this compound has been prepared for the prophylaxis of vernal conjunctivitis and other allergic reactions. It has to be given as a course of treatment and will prevent the symptoms occurring, but will not act as an antihistamine and thus once the histamine is released produces no effects. It is available over the counter under several trade names.

Nedocromil sodium

Nedocromil sodium is a new mast cell stabilizer which appears to be superior to cromoglycate especially in its action against the mucosal type of mast cell *in vitro*. It is also effective against other cells involved in the inflammatory process such as macrophages and eosinophils, inhibiting the release of chemotactic and inflammatory mediating sub-stances. It is presented as a 2% solution which is normally administered twice daily in cases of seasonal allergic conjunctivitis (Blumenthal *et al.*, 1992; Melamed *et al.*, 1994), but when used in the treatment of perennial conjunctivitis it may require treatment four times a day (Kjellman and Stevens, 1995). In clinical trials it has been shown to be as effective as cromoglycate in controlling seasonal allergic conjunctivitis (Leino *et al.*, 1992) and vernal keratoconjunctivitis (Hennawi, 1994), and superior to it in some cases of perennial allergic conjunctivitis (Van Bijsterveld *et al.*, 1994). The eye drops are effective on their own with no apparent benefit accruing from the concomitant use of an oral antihistamine (Miglior *et al.*, 1993). There are few side effects with a small percentage of patients complaining of initial burning and stinging and some referring to a distinctive taste in the mouth

Lodoxamide

Lodoxamide is another mast cell–eosinophil inhibitor which has been for-mulated for ophthalmic use in the treatment of giant papillary conjuncti-vitis, vernal conjunctivitis and other forms of noninfective conjunctivitis. Cerquen *et al.* (1994) tested its efficacy on patients suffering from seasonal allergic conjunctivitis using a 0.1% solution three times a day (the data sheet states that a four times a day treatment is recommended) and found that the patients benefited from the treatment. In some treatment parameters it has been found to be superior to cromoglycate (Fahy *et al.*, 1988).

Antihistamines

The alternative method of antagonizing the action of histamine is by using a pharmacological antagonist – an antihistamine. Histamine receptors have been divided into two types, H1 and H2. The former are involved in the well known triple response to histamine. When histamine is injected, a local vasodilation occurs which is due to a direct effect of histamine on the blood vessels and is manifested as a bright red spot. Changes in the permeability of the blood vessels cause a loss of plasma protein into the extracellular space. This leads to an area of oedema, causing a bump which becomes red because of reflex vasodilation, with stimulation of pain and itch fibres.

H1 receptors are found on the surface of the eye as well as other mucous membranes, e.g. nasal cavities. They are blocked by antihistamines such as antazoline. H2 receptors mediate gastric acid secretion and are blocked by drugs such as cimetidine which are used for the treatment of gastric ulcers. H2 receptors have been found on the surface of the eye. These receptors are thought to be involved in the dilation of episcleral, conjunc-tival and perilimbal blood vessels (Havener, 1978).

H1 antagonists such as antazoline (*Antistine*) have been used in combi-nation with sympathomimetic vasoconstrictors since this is more effective than each component on its own. By utilizing two forms of antagonism (pharmacological and physiological) an additive effect is produced. The usual symptoms of histamine mediated allergy are lacrimation, redness, itching, pain and photophobia. Antazoline would appear to relieve the itching, while naphazoline (a vasoconstrictor) is more effective on the blood vessels and in reducing the redness. Such a combination under the trade mark *Vasocon-A* was found to be superior to either component used on its own in the treatment of acute allergic conjunctivitis (Abelson *et al.*, 1990).

Levocabastine is a new potent H1 receptor blocker that has been tested for its effect on allergic conjunctivitis (Laerum *et al.*, 1994; Zuber and Pecaud, 1988). Eye drops containing this agent were well tolerated and have a faster onset than some antihistamines taken orally in the treatment of allergic conjunctivitis (Drouin *et al.*, 1995).

Many antihistamine agents also have antimuscarinic activity. Some agents are able to antagonize both histamine and acetylcholine equally. Topical application can reduce tear flow by this atropine-like effect. It is a reported side effect of systemic use of antihistamines that contact lens tolerance may be reduced.

Corticosteroids

The adrenal cortex produces a mixture of steroid hormones which fall into three main groups: glucocorticoids, mineralocorticoids and sex hormones. Mineralocorticoids are necessary to maintain the electrolyte balance of the body, whilst glucocorticoids affect glucose, protein and bone metabolism and have anti-inflammatory properties. The naturally occurring ones include corticosterone and hydrocortisone which have sodium retention properties, and in order to separate this latter effect from the anti-inflammatory effects newer, synthetic and more potent steroids have been developed. Betamethasone and dexamethasone, for example, are 25 times more potent in producing anti-inflammatory effects.

No other group of drugs deserves the title of a 'two edged sword' as much as the corticosteroids. They are known on the one hand for their useful and sometimes sight saving effects in the treatment of inflammation, and on the other for the very serious adverse effects which can arise from their use. For example, corticosteroids can assist in the reduction of intraocular pressure when used to treat uveitic secondary glaucoma but can cause a rise in intraocular pressure if used topically in patients who are 'steroid responders'.

Corticosteroids inhibit the inflammatory response to noxious stimuli, whether radiation, mechanical, chemical, infectious or immunological, affecting the inflammatory process in many ways. They reduce the vasodilation that is responsible for the redness that accompanies inflammation, and stabilize mast cells, thereby reducing the release of histamine. Their use maintains the normal permeability of blood and prevents the development of oedema. Part of their mechanism of action involves the inhibition of the production of prostaglandins, which mediate some of the effects of inflammation. Prostaglandins are produced by conversion of arachidonic acid by cyclo-oxygenase, and steroids prevent the release of this acid. Corticosteroids not only reduce the early signs of the inflammatory process but also the late manifestations, e.g. proliferation of capillaries and scar formation.

Apart from providing symptomatic relief, corticosteroids are important in ophthalmology in preventing scar formation and loss of transparency of the cornea.

Table 11.2 Other anti-inflammatory agents

Official name	Trade name	Mode of action	Dosage form	Concentration	Notes
Antazoline	Otrivine Antistin	Antihistamine	drops	0.5%	Over-the-counter preparation
Diclofenac	Voltavol Ophtha	NSAID	single use drops	0.1%	Limited indication
Flurbiprofen	Ocufen	NSAID	drops	0.3%	Limited indication
Ketorolal	Acular	NSAID	drops	0.5%	Limited indication
Levocabastine	Livostin	Antihistamine	drops	0.05%	
Lodoxamide	Alomide stabilizer	Mast cell	drops	0.1%	
Nedocromil	Rapitil stabilizer	Mast cell	drops	2.0%	
Sodium cromoglycate	Opticrom	Mast cell	drops ointment	2.0% 4.0%	

Cortisone and hydrocortisone were the first corticosteroids discovered. The use of cortisone is now limited to replacement therapy in cases of adrenal insufficiency. It has anti-inflammatory properties but has marked mineralocorticoid properties as well. Hydrocortisone is so widely used as a topical skin treatment that it is now classed as a pharmacy medicine in this form, providing that the indications are strictly controlled.

The introduction of hydrocortisone was followed by prednisolone, which is five times as potent in terms of its anti-inflammatory activity but has less mineralocorticoid action. It is used extensively in the treatment of chronic obstructive pulmonary disease. This drug has itself been superseded by drugs such as dexamethasone and betamethasone, which are even more effective (50 times the potency of hydrocortisone). They have a better therapeutic ratio than hydrocortisone, being proportionately less sodium and water retentive and causing less potassium loss, and are longer acting.

Steroids have many other adverse effects in addition to causing an imbalance in electrolyte levels. When taken systemically they cause weight gain because of increased appetite, exacerbation of peptic ulcers, a deposition of fat leading to the appearance of moon face and cataract (see Chapter 17).

Corticosteroids also have marked side effects when applied topically and their adverse effects must always be balanced against their beneficial ones. For example, they inhibit wound healing and reduce the body's response to infections. If the invading organism is a virus or a non-pyogenic bacteria, then providing the antimicrobial agents are applied at the same time the steroids will have a beneficial effect by reducing the tissue destruction due to the inflammatory process. If on the other hand the infecting organism is pyogenic, it will cause tissue damage itself and steroids will delay resolution of the infection. Corticosteroids are definitely contraindicated in the treatment of fungal keratitis and should be used with great caution in acanthamoeba keratitis (Stern and Buttross, 1991).

The effect on wound healing is brought about by changes in the relationship of collagen and cells. Corticosteroids impair fibroblastic and keratocytic activity. They normally inhibit collagenase activity, but on some occasions this can be potentiated, leading to a rapid destruction of the stroma (melting cornea). Wounds have reduced tensile strength as a result of the actions of steroids.

Another adverse reaction to topical therapy is a rise in intraocular pressure, termed steroid glaucoma, in a number of individuals, caused by an increased resistance to the outflow of aqueous humour by causing morphological and biochemical changes (Clark, 1995). This effect is not limited to humans and can be demonstrated in other animals such as rabbits, cats, dogs and other primates. Patients vary in their responsiveness to this effect of corticosteroids but they are more likely to exhibit a rise in intraocular pressure with prolonged treatment with higher doses. There are many similarities between development of steroid induced ocular hypertension and primary open angle glaucoma and it has been postulated that there is a causal relationship between the higher than normal cortisone levels sometimes noted in such patients.

Newer agents such as clobetasone and fluoromethalone are claimed to produce fewer effects on the intraocular pressure, possibly due to differences in absorption.

Prednisolone

Prednisolone, in comparison with cortisone and hydrocortisone, has marked anti-inflammatory activity with low mineralocorticoid effects. The halflife in blood plasma is intermediate between that of the natural corticosteroids and the long acting dexamethasone, betamethasone triamcinolone. It is extensively used in the treatment of bronchial asthma and other respiratory diseases.

Betamethasone

Betamethasone has minimal mineralocorticoid activity along with marked anti-inflammatory action. The halflife is much longer than that of prednisolone.

Clobetasone

Clobetasone is a steroid which has the advantage of causing less rise in intraocular pressure than other topical steroids. Dunne and Travers (1979) found it less effective in reducing the ocular signs of uveitis than dexamethasone, although it was as effective in reducing the subjects' symptoms. The beneficial reduced rise in intraocular pressure was demonstrated in known steroid responders and ocular hypertensive patients. Following cataract surgery it was found to be equally as effective as prednisolone (Ramsell *et al.*, 1980) and as effective as betamethasone in treating patients with ocular inflammation.

The difference in the effect on intraocular pressure is probably not due to any pharmacological difference but to a pharmacokinetic one. Clobetasone is absorbed into the aqueous humour at a much lower level than other steroids such as betamethasone (Debnath and Richards, 1983).

Table 11.3 Corticosteroids currently employed in ophthalmic treatment

Official name	Trade name	Dosage form	Concentration
Betamethasone	Betnesol	drops	0.1%
	Vistamethasone	ointment	0.1%
Clobetasone	Cloburate	drops	0.1%
Dexamethasone	Maxidex	drops	0.1%
	Maxitrol	ointment	0.1%
Fluoromethalone	FML	drops	0.1%
Hydrocortisone		drops	1.0%
		ointment	0.5%
Prednisolone	Pred forte	drops	0.5 to 1.0%
	Predsol		
	Minims		

References

Abelson, M. B. *et al.* (1990) Effects of *Vasocon A* in the allergen challenge model of acute allergic conjunctivitis. *Arch. Ophthalmol.*, **108**, 520–524

Adenis, J. P. *et al.* (1995) Ciprofloxacin ophthalmic solution versus rifamycin ophthalmic solution for the treatment of conjunctivitis and blepharitis. *Eur. J. Ophthalmol.*, **5**, 82–87

Avci, R., Erturk, H. and Ozcetin, H. (1993) The effect of diclofenac sodium on post-operative inflammation. *Eur. J. Implant Ref. Surg.*, **5**, 68–70

Behrens-Baumann, W. *et al.* (1988) Trimethroprim-polymixin B sulphate ophthalmic ointment in the treatment of bacterial conjunctivitis: a double blind study versus chloramphenicol ophthalmic ointment. *Curr. Med. Res. Opin.*, **11**, 227–231

Behrens-Baumann, W., Klinge, B. and Uter, W. (1990) Clotrimazole and bifonazole in the topical treatment of Candida keratitis in rabbits. *Mycoses*, **33**, 567–573

Blumenthal, M. *et al.* (1992) Efficacy and safety of nedocromil sodium ophthalmic solution in the treatment of seasonal allergic conjunctivitis. *Am. J. Ophthalmol.*, **113**, 56–63

Bonomi, L. *et al.* (1987). Prevention of trauma-induced miosis during cataract extraction by diclofenac eye drops. *New Trends in Ophthalmology*, **II**, 513–519

Cerquen, P. M. *et al.* (1994) Lodoxamide treatment in allergic conjunctivitis. *Int. Archives of Allergy and Immunology*, **105**, 185–189

Chastain, J. B. and Newton, L. K. (1954) Intramuscular chloramphenicol treatment of trachoma. *Rocky Mountain Medical Journal*, March, 191–194

Chaudhuri, P. R. and Godfrey, B. (1982) Treatment of bacterial corneal ulcers with concentrated eye drops. *Trans. Ophthalmol. Soc., UK*, **102**, 11–14

Chern, C. C. *et al.* (1996) Corneal anesthetic abuse and Candida keratitis. *Ophthalmology*, **12**, 37–40

Clark, A. F. (1995) Steroids ocular hypertension and glaucoma. *J. Glaucoma*, **04**, 354–369

Coster, D. J., Jones, B. R. and McGill, J. I. (1979) Treatment of amoeboid herpetic ulcers with adenine arabinoside or trifluorothymidine. *Br. J. Ophthalmol.*, **63**, 418–421

Coster, D. J., Wilhelmus, K. R., Michaud. R. and Jones, B. R. (1980) A comparison of acyclovir and idoxuridine as treatment for ulcerative herpetic keratitis. *Br. J. Ophthalmol.*, **64**, 763–765

Cutarelli, P. E. *et al.* (1991) Topical fluoroquinolones. Antimicrobial activity and *in vitro* corneal epithelial toxicity. *Curr. Eye Res.*, **10**, 557–563

Darby, G., Field, H. J. and Salisbury, B. A. (1981) Altered substrate specificity of herpes simplex virus thymidine kinase confers acyclovir-resistance. *Nature*, **289**, 81–83

Davis, S. D., Sarff, L. D. and Hyaduik, R. A. (1979) Experimental *Pseudommona* keratitis in guinea pigs: therapy of moderately severe infections. *Br. J. Ophthalmol.*, **63**, 436–439

Debnath, S. C. and Richards, A. B. (1983) Concentration of clobetasonein aqueous humour. *Brit. J. Ophthalmol.*, **07**, 203–205

Doft, B. H. *et al.* (1994) Treatment of endophthalmitis after cataract extraction. *Retina*, **14**, 297–304

Drouin, M. A., Yang, W. H. and Horak, F. (1995) Faster onset of action with topical levocabastine than with oral cetirizine. *Mediators Inflamm.*, **4** (Suppl.)., s5–s10

Dunlop, E. M., Rodin, P., Seth, A. D. and Kolator, B. (1980) Ophthalmia neonatorum due to B-lactamase producing gonococci. *Br. Med. J.*, 16th August, 483

Dunne, J. A. and Travers, J. P. (1979) Double blind clinical trial of topical steroids in anterior uveitis. *Br. J. Ophthalmol.*, **63**, 762–767

Erturk, H., Ozcetin, H. and Avci, R. (1991) Diclofenac sodium for the prevention of surgically induced miosis. *Eur. J. Implant Ref. Surg.*, **3**, 55–57

Fabian, E., Dennfer, R. and Wertheimer, R. (1991) Diclofenac eye drops to maintain mydriasis during extracapsular cataract extraction. *Ophthalmo-Chirurgie*, **03**, 115–119

Fahy, G. *et al.* (1988) Double masked efficacy and safety evaluation of Iodoxamide 0.1% ophthalmic solution versus opticrom 2% – a multicentre study. *Ophthalmology Today*, 341–342

Falcon, M. G. and Jones, B. R. (1977) Antivirals for the therapy of herpetic eye disease. *Transact. Ophthalmol. Soc., UK*, **97**, 331–332

Foster, C. S. and Pavan–Langston, D. (1977) Corneal wound healing and antiviral medication. *Arch. Ophthalmol.*, **95**, 2062–2067

Fuhr, B. (1995) Ciprofloxacin for topical use at the eye. *Contactologica*, **17**, 146–153

Gilbert, P., and Work, K. (1980) Trifluorothymidine in the treatment of herpes simplex corneal ulcers. *Arch. Ophthalmol.*, **58**, 117–120

Glasser, D. B., Gardner, S., Ellis, J. G. and Pettit, T. H. (1985) Loading doses and extended dosing intervals in topical gentamicin therapy. *Am. J. Ophthalmol.*, **99**, 329–332

Grossman, R. E., Chu, D. F. and Lee, D. A. (1990) Regional ocular gentamicin levels after transcorneal and transscleral iontophoresis. *Invest. Ophthal. Vis. Sci.*, **31**, 909–916

Havener, W. H. (1978) *Ocular Pharmacology*, 4th edn., pp. 172–194. St Louis: Mosby

Heinemann, M. H. (1989) Long term intravitreal ganciclovir therapy for cytomegalovirus retinopathy. *Arch. Ophthalmol.*, **107**, 1767–1772

Hennawi, M. (1994) A double blind placebo controlled group comparative study of ophthalmic sodium cromoglycate and nedocromil sodium in the treatment of vernal keratoconjunctivitis *Br. J. Ophthalmol.*, **18**, 365–369

Hersh, P. S. *et al.* (1990) Topical nonsteroidal agents and corneal wound healing. *Arch. Ophthalmol.*, **108, 577–583**

Hillman, J. S., Jacobs, S. I., Garrett, A. J. and Kheskani, M. B. (1979) Gentamicin penetration and decay in human aqueous. *Br. J. Ophthalmol.*, **631**, 794–796

Hobden, J. A. *et al.* (1989). Tobramycin iontophoresis into corneas infected with a drug resistant *Pseudomonas aeruginosa*. *Curr. Eye Res.*, **8**, 1163–1169

Hobden, J. A. *et al.* (1988) Treatment of experimental *Pseudomonas* keratitis using collagen shields containing tobramycin. *Arch. Ophthalmol.*, **106**, 1605–1607

Hovenden, J. L., Phillips, G. and MacEwan, C. (1995) An *in vitro* study of fusidic acid susceptibility amongst isolates from conjunctival swabs. *Acta Ophthalmol. Scand.*, **73**, 325–328

Huber, E., Steinkogler, F. J. and Huber-Spitzy, V. (1991) A new antibiotic in the treatment of dacryocystitis. *Orbit*, **10**, 33–35

Huber-Spitzy, V. *et al.* (1991) Norfloxacin in the treatment of congenital dacryocystititis. *Orbit*, **101**, 37–40

Ilic, J., Gigon, S. and Leuenberger, P. M. (1984) Comparison of the anti-inflammatory effects of dexamethasone and diclofenac eye drops. *Klin. Monatsbl. für Augenheilk*, **184**, 494–498

Insler, M. S., Cavanagh, H. D. and Wilson, L. A. (1985) Gentamicin resistant *Pseudomonas* endophthalmitis after penetrating keratoplasty. *Br. J. Ophthalmol.*, **69**, 189–191

Ismail, B. and Morton, D. J. (1987) Ophthalmic uptake of chloramphenicol from proprietary preparations using an *in vitro* method of evaluation. *Int. J. Pharm.*, **37**, 1113

James, M. R., Brogan, R. and Carew-McColl, M. (1991) A study to compare the use of fusidic acid viscous eye drops and chloramphenicol eye ointment in an accident and emergency department. *Arch. Emerg. Med.*, **8**, 125–129

Kishore, K., Panda, A. and Gupta, S. K. (1994) Prospective placebo controlled clinical trial in the management of chronic noninfectious conjunctivitis with indomethacin. *Afro-Asian J. Ophthalmol.*, **133**, 69–70

Kjellman, N.-I. M. and Stevens, M. T. (1995) Clinical experience with tilavist: An overview of efficacy and safety. *Allergy*, **50** (Suppl.), 21, 14–22

Laerum, E. *et al.* (1994) Chloramphenicol eye drops in the treatment of acute bacterial conjunctivitis. A comparison of two dose regimens in general practise. *Tidsskr-Nor Laegeforen*, **114**, 671–673

Lass, J. H., Pavan-Langston, D. and Park, N. H. (1979) Acyclovir and corneal wound healing. *Am. J. Ophthalmol.*, **88**, 102–108

Lavine, J. B., Binder, P. S. and Wickham, M. G. (1979) Antimicrobials and the corneal endothelium. *Ann. Ophthalmol.*, **11**, 1517–1528

Leibowitz, H. L. (1991a) Antibacterial effectiveness of cipropfloxacin 0.3% ophthalmic solution in the treatment of bacterial conjunctivitis. *Am. J. Ophthalmol.*, **21**, 29S–33S

Leibowitz, H. L. (1991b) Clinical evaluation of ciprofloxacin 0.3% ophthalmic solution for the treatment of bacterial keratitis. *Am. J. Ophthalmol.*, **21**, 34S–47S

Leibowitz, H. L.*et al.* (1995) Safety and efficacy of diclofenac sodium 0.1% in acute seasonal allergic conjunctivitis. *J. Ocul. Pharmacol. and Therap.*, **11, 361–368**

Leino, S. *et al.* (1992) Double blind group comparative study of 2% nedocromil sodium eye drops with 2% sodium cromoglycate and placebo eye drops in the treatment of seasonal allergic conjunctivitivitis. *Clin. Exp. Allergy*, **22**, 929–932

Limberg and Bugge (1994) Tear concentrations of topically applied ciprofloxacin. *Cornea*, **13**, 496–499

Mahajan, V. M. (1983) Bacterial infections of the eye: their aetiology and treatment. *Br. J. Ophthalmol.*, **67**, 191–194

Malet, F. *et al.* (1995) Bacterial keratitis therapy in guinea pigs with lomefloxacin by initially high- followed by low-dosage regimen. *Ophthalmic Res.*, **27**, 322–329

Martindale, W. (1977) *Extra Pharmacopoeia*, p. 517. London: The Pharmaceutical Press

McGill, J., Tormey, P. and Walker, C. B. (1981) Comparative trial of acyclovir and adenine arabinoside in the treatment of herpes simplex corneal ulcers. *Br. J. Ophthalmol.*, **65**, 610–613

McGhee, C. N. J. (1996) Widespread ocular use of topical chloramphenicol: is there justifiable concern regarding idiosyncratic aplastic anaemia? *Br. J. Ophthalmol.*, **80**, 182–184

McKinnon, J. P., McGill, J. I. and Jones, B. R. (1975) A coded clinical evaluation of adenine arabinoside and trifluorothymidine in the treatment of ulcerative herpetic keratitis. In *Adenin Arabinoside: An Antiviral Agent*. (D. Pavan-Langston, R. A. Buchanan and C. Alford, eds.). New York: Raven Press

McNeil, J. I. and Kaufman, H. E. (1979) Local antivirals in herpes simplex stromal keratitis model. *Arch. Ophthalmol.*, **97**, 727–729

Melamed, J. *et al.* (1994) Evaluation of nedocromil sodium 2% ophthalmic solution for the treatment of seasonal allergic conjunctivitis. *Ann. Allergy*, **73**, 57–66

Michelson, J. B. and Nozik, R. A. (1979) Experimental endophthalmitis treated with an implantable osmotic minipump. *Arch. Ophthalmol.*, **97**, 1345–1348

Miglior B. *et al.* (1993) Nedocromil sodium and astemizole, alone or combined, in the treatment of seasonal allergic conjunctivitis. *Acta Ophthalmol.*, **11**, 73–78

O'Brien, T. P. *et al.* (1988) Topical ciprofloxacin treatment of *Pseudomonas* keratitis in rabbits. *Arch. Ophthalmol.*, **106**, 1444–1446

O'Day, D. M. *et al.* (1991) Differences in response *in vivo* to amphotericin B among *Candida albicans*. *Invest. Ophthalmol. Vis. Sci.*, **32**, 1569–1572

Pang, R., Ten, L. B., Rajan, V. S. and Sng, E. H. (1979) Gonococcal ophthalmia neonatorum caused by β-lactamase producing *Neisseria gonorrhorue*. *Br. Med. J.*, 10th February, 380

Pavan-Langston, D. and Foster, C. S. (1977) Trifluorothymidine and idoxuridine therapy of ocular herpes. *Am. J. Ophthalmol.*, **84**, 818–825

Pavan-Langston, D., Lass. J. H. and Campbell, R. (1979) Antiviral drugs: competitive therapy of experimental herpes simplex keratouveitis. *Arch Ophthalmol.*, **97**, 1132–1135

Pavan-Langston, D. and Nelson, D. J. (1979) Intraocular penetration of trifluorothymidine. *Am. J. Ophthalmol.*, **87**, 814–818

Pierce, J. M., Ward, M. E. and Seal, D. V. (1982) Ophthalmia neonatorum in the 1980s: incidence, aetiology and treatment. *Br. J. Ophthalmol.*, **66**, 728–731

Power, W. J. *et al.* (1993) Evaluation of efficacy and safety of ciprofloxacin ophthalmic solution versus chloramphenicol. *Eur. J. Ophthalmol.*, **3**, 77–82

Power, W. J. *et al.* (1991) Bromovinyldeoxyuridine (BVDU) and trifluorothymidine (TFT) in dendritic corneal ulceration: A double blind controlled study. *Curr. Eye Res.*, **10** (Suppl.)., 183–187

Ramsell, T. G., Bartholomew, R. S. and Walker, S. R. (1980) Clinical evaluation of clobetasone butyrate; a comparative study of its effects in postoperative inflammation and on intraocular pressure. *Brit. J. Ophthalmol.*, **4**, 43–45

Raucher, H. S. and Newton, M. J. (1983) New issues in the prevention and treatment of ophthalmia neonatorum. *Ann. Ophthalmol.*, **15**, 1004–1009

Reidy, *et al.* (1991) The efficacy of topical ciprofloxacin and norfloxacin in the treatment of experimental *Pseudomonas* keratitis. *Cornea*, **10**, 25–28

Ronen, S. *et al.* (1985) Treatment of ocular inflammation with diclofenac sodium: Double blind trial following cataract surgery. *Ann. Ophthalmol.*, **17**, 577–581

Sand, B. B. and Krogh, E. (1991) Topical indomethacin, a prostaglandin inhibitor, in acute anterior uveitis. A controlled clinical trial of nonsteroid versus steroid anti-inflammatory treatment. *Acta Ophthalmol.*, **69**,145–148

Seal, D. V., Barrett, S. P. and McGill, J. T. (1982) Aetiology and treatment of acute bacterial infection of the external eye. *Br. J. Ophthalmol.*, **66**, 357–360

Sher, N. A. *et al.* (1992). Excimer laser photorefractive keratetcomy in high myopia. *Arch. Ophthalmol.*, **194**, 935–943

Sher, N. A. *et al.* (1993) Topical diclofenac in the treatment of ocular pain after excimer photorefractive keratectomy. *Refractive and Corneal Surgery*, **9**, 425–436

Sinclair, N. M. and Leigh, D. A. (1988) A comparison of fusidic acid viscous eye drops and chloramphenicol eye ointment in acute conjunctivitis. *Curr. Ther. Res. Clin. Exp.*, **44**, 468–474

Stern, G. A. and Buttross, M. (1991) Use of corticosteroids in combination with antimicrobial drugs in the treatment of infectious corneal disease. *Ophthalmology*, **98**, 847–853

Stern, G. A., Okumoto, M. and Smolin, G. (1979) Combined amphotericin B and rifampicin treatment of experimental *Candida albicans* keratitis. *Arch. Ophthalmol.*, **97**, 721–722

Struck, H. G. *et al.* (1994) Influence of diclofenac and flurbiprofen eye drops on the inflammation after cataract extraction. *Ophthalmology*, **31**, 482–485

Tadokoro, Y. *et al.* (1995) Topical vancomycin for ocular infection by methicillin resistant *Staphylococcus aureus*. *Jpn. J. Clin. Ophthalmol.*, **49**, 521–525

Tilden, M. E. *et al.* (1990) The effects of topical S(+)-ibuprofen on interleukin-1 induced ocular inflammation on a rabbit model. *J. Ocul. Pharmacol.*, **6**, 131–135

Titcomb, L. (1997) Ophthalmic vhloramphenicol and blood – A review. *Pharm. J.*, **258**, 28–35

Trope, G. E., Lawrence, J. R., Hind, V. M. D. and Bunney, J (1979) Systemic absorption of topically applied chloramphenicol eyedrops. *Br. J. Ophthalmol.*, **63**, 690–691

Trousdale, M. D., Newburn, A. B. and Miller. C. A. (1981) Assessment of acyclovir on acute ocular infections induced by drug-resistant strains of HSV-I. *Invest. Ophthalmol. Vis. Sci.*, **20**, 230–235

Vajpayee, R. B., Gupta, S. K., Beraja, U. and Mohan, M. (1989) Evaluation of acyclovir in the management of various types of herpetic corneal lesions: A prospective controlled clinical trial in 34 patients. *Med. Sci. Res.*, **17**, 93–94

van Bjisterveld and Post, H. (1980) Trifluorothymidine versus adenine arabinoside in the treatment of herpes simplex keratitis. *Br. J. Ophthalmol.*, **64**, 33–36

Van Bijsterveld *et al.* (1994) Nedocromil sodium treats symptoms of perennial allergic conjunctivitis not fully controlled by sodium cromoglycate. *Ocular Immunology and Inflammation*, **2**, 177–186

Van Gogh, E. R. and Smit, P. (1994) Topical antibiotics in ophthalmology. A review. *Pharm. Weekly*, **129**, 156–163

Vickers, F. F. *et al.* (1991) The effect of diclofenac sodium ophthalmic solution on the treatment of postoperative inflammation. *Invest. Ophthalmol.*, **32**, 793

Ward, J. B., Siojo, L. G. and Waller, S. G. (1993) A prospective, masked clinical trial of trifluridine, dexamethasone, and artificial tears in the treatment of epidemic keratoconjunctivitis. *Cornea*, **12/03**, 216–221

Wellings, P. C., Awdry, P. N., Bors, F. H., Jones, B. R., Brown, D. C. and Kaufman, H. E. (1972) Clinical evaluation of trifluorothymidine in the treatment of herpes simplex corneal ulcers. *Am. J. Ophthalmol.*, **73**, 932–942

Wright, M. M. *et al.* (1985) Acanthamoeba keratitis successfully treated medically. *Br. J. Ophthalmol.*, **9**, 778–782

Zhang, W., Wu, Y. and Zhao, J. (1995) Rapid diagnosis and treatment of chlamydial conjunctivitis. *Chi. Med. J.*, **108**, 138–141

Zuber, P. and Pecaud, A. (1988) Effect of levocabastine, a new H1 antagonist, in a conjunctival provocation test with allergens. *J. Allerg. Clin. Immun.*, **82**, 590–594

12

Drugs for the treatment of glaucoma

All glaucoma treatments are aimed at reducing intraocular pressure (IOP), even though it is generally agreed that there is no proven relationship between IOP reduction and visual field preservation. As the level of intraocular pressure is determined by both the rate of production and the rate of outflow, IOP can be lowered by reducing secretion or increasing outflow. Most glaucomas are considered to be due to a reduced outflow facility, but it is thought acceptable to approach the problem by modifying the inflow of aqueous humour. The effect of a reduced throughput of aqueous humour has not received a great deal of attention.

Of the primary glaucomas, only open angle glaucoma is amenable to chronic medical treatment. Although acute closed angle glaucoma can be relieved by a combined attack with both topical and systemic treatment, its long term relief will be from surgery. Surgical treatment of open angle glaucoma is also an option, especially when medical treatments appear to be losing their effect.

Whatever its form, an antiglaucoma treatment should satisfy certain criteria.

1. *Reduction of intraocular pressure.* The amount by which intraocular pressure must be reduced in order that the glaucoma can be deemed to be 'controlled' varies between different studies. IOPs of below 20 mm Hg are often taken to indicate control, but it is known that different individuals tolerate different tensions so a level of 20 mm Hg may not be control for a patient with normal tension glaucoma. It is probably more important that the pressure should remain stable and not vary greatly during the day.
2. *Duration of effect.* There is little doubt that if the treatment is to be effective then the reduction should last for some hours. As stated above, it is important that the pressure remains stable rather than oscillating. It is assumed, but not proven, that there is an inverse relationship between the number of doses per day and patient compliance. In other words, twice a day therapy is better than four times a day therapy but not as good as once a day.
3. *Preservation of visual field.* With modern diagnostic techniques, most glaucomas today are diagnosed before serious impairment of vision has occurred and the obvious aim of treatment is that no further loss will occur. Since visual field change is a slow insidious effect, it is important that it is monitored.

4. *No loss of effect with time*. Once a patient has been stabilized on a treatment, it is unfortunate if his therapy has to be modified because the original drug is no longer sufficiently effective.

5. *Compatibility with other treatments*. Because drugs can lose their effect with time and because some patients require more vigorous therapy, it is often necessary for more than one drug to be administered. As the possibility exists of modifying pressure by reducing secretion or by increasing outflow, drugs with antagonistic pharmacological actions may have synergistic therapeutic effects.

6. *Lack of topical adverse effects*. Often, due to the diligence of the optometrist, glaucoma is detected before the patient is aware of symptoms. The patient does not know that he has a problem which will require a lifetime course of continuing therapy. Having persuaded the patient that it is necessary to apply the drops every day, it is counterproductive if these drops cause problems to him which could lead to lack of patient compliance. Initial stinging is one of the problems that can occur with many eye drops. Some drops can cause a local anaesthetic effect (e.g. beta blockers) and this can lead to corneal problems. Eye drops contain other ingredients as well as the drug and water and these adjuvants may interfere with the anterior surface of the eye. For example, some of the preservatives used to maintain sterility can adversely affect the tear film and can thus exacerbate dry eye problems.

7. *Lack of systemic effects*. All topical antiglaucoma drugs used at the moment produce their action by modifying the effects of the autonomic nervous system. The ANS also innervates many other structures in the body, e.g. the cardiovascular system, the respiratory system and the gastrointestinal system, and serious systemic effects can result from the topical use of autonomic drugs.

8. *Patient compliance*. Treatments must be easy and pleasant to use and this requires attention not only to the active ingredient and its formulation but also to the container in which it is supplied.

Glaucoma treatments can be administered either systemically or topically.

Systemic treatments

Drugs administered in this manner are given by mouth for chronic treatment or by injection for acute use. Beta blockers will reduce intraocular pressure when given systemically and have been tested for use in this manner (Tutton and Smith, 1982). Williamson *et al.* (1985) compared topical treatment with timolol and systemic treatment with nadolol. They found that once a day systemic treatment was as efficacious as twice a day topical treatment, and suggested that systemic treatment would be useful for patients who had difficulty in administering drops. These findings were not confirmed in a later trial by Dowd *et al.* (1991). Of 30 newly diagnosed patients suffering from chronic open angle glaucoma, only one was controlled throughout the three month study and the authors rightly concluded that the drug was ineffective in controlling IOP in the patients undergoing the trial. The only drugs that have been used routinely as systemic treatments are the carbonic anhydrase inhibitors, acetazolamide and dichlorphenamide. Carbonic anhydrase is present in the ciliary epithelium and is necessary for the secretion of bicarbonate ions. If their secretion is reduced there is a concomitant reduction in the secretion of the accompanying sodium ions. In order to maintain the proper osmotic pressure, the volume of aqueous secreted is less than normal and intraocular pressure falls.

The carbonic anhydrase inhibitors have some unfortunate side effects. These include:

lack of appetite
paresthesia
gut disturbances
fatigue
kidney stones
aplastic anaemia.

Local treatments

Topical treatments, with one exception (the Ocusert device), consist of the application of drops to the anterior surface of the eye. There are a number of agents available for use in the treatment of glaucoma.

Miotics

These are the same drugs which can be used to reverse the action of mydriatics. Whereas for the reversal of mydriasis pupillary constriction is the desired effect, in the treatment of open angle glaucoma it is an unwanted side effect. It is the contraction of the ciliary muscle, putting tension on the trabecular meshwork, that is responsible for the increased outflow and reduced intraocular pressure. In addition, direct effects on the trabecular meshwork have been postulated by Barany (1962). Of course, if the filtration angle is narrow the miosis is an important component of the drug's action, but for the majority of patients it is the cyclospasm which produces the fall in IOP.

By far the most commonly used miotic is pilocarpine, which has been used in ophthalmology for well over 100 years. The concentration employed varies from 0.5% to 8% but the higher strengths are probably 'overkill' as a maximum effect has been reported at 4% (Harris and Galin, 1970). It produces a biphasic small rise followed by a persistent fall (Korczyn et al., 1982) which lasts for about six hours, requiring the drug to be administered four times a day. Its effect is on outflow rather than secretion and thus the drug restores the aqueous flow to a more physiological status.

The miosis and spasm of accommodation are fundamental to the mode of action of these drugs, and there is little that can be done to separate the beneficial effects from the adverse effects. Not only does the spasm of accommodation caused by miotics lead to pseudomyopia, but it also increases the risk of retinal detachment. Kraushar and Steinberg (1991) recommended peripheral retinal examination prior to prescribing miotics. Research into miotics has been aimed at the other disadvantages of pilocarpine, namely:

1. It is a natural product which means that:
   (a) it tends to be expensive
   (b) its supplies can be erratic
   (c) there is a greater possibility of allergic reaction.
2. Its effects only last for six hours and therefore:
   (a) patient compliance is reduced
   (b) the intraocular pressure goes up and down four times a day.

To avoid these problems, developments have been in two directions, viz. new presentations of pilocarpine and new miotics.

New presentations of pilocarpine

These developments have been aimed at increasing the contact time of the drug with the eye, leading to a greater and more prolonged effect. They include:

1. *Viscolized solutions.* Viscolizers such as hydroxyethylcellulose or polyvinyl alcohol have been added to make the drop more viscous and thus stay in the eye for longer (Davies *et al.*, 1977). Although a greater and more prolonged fall has been reported following the use of viscolized drops, the duration of effect does not seem to justify a reduction in the number of doses per day.
2. *Gels.* Polymers have been developed into which the pilocarpine can be incorporated and from which it is slowly released (Ticho *et al.*, 1979). *Pilogel* is the latest formulation to be introduced into which pilocarpine has been incorporated (pilocarpine 4%). It only requires a once a day treatment and is usually used at bedtime. It can be combined with other treatments such as beta blockers and carbonic anhydrase inhibitors.

   During early studies with pilocarpine-containing gels it was found that the amount of IOP reduction and the duration of effect were dose dependent up to 4% (Stewart *et al.*, 1984). With aqueous solutions the maximum is reached at a lower concentration in some patients, especially those with light irides.

   Although pilocarpine gels produce a reduction for 24 hours, the effect is greater at 12 hours than 24 hours (March *et al.*, 1982) and it may be necessary to carry out phasing studies to determine whether the effect is maintained sufficiently towards the end of the interdose period. Johnson *et al.* (1984) similarly found higher values in the afternoon than in the morning, but did nor consider the difference significant.

   Of course, apart from patient compliance, the principal advantage of a once a day therapy should be a reduction in the inconvenience of pseudomyopia induced four times a day. With the gel applied at bedtime, the worst of the myopia should occur at night time. Mandel *et al.* (1988) found that patients suffered less visual problems with the gel than with aqueous solutions. Aldrete *et al.* (1983) compared pilocarpine gel with 0.5% timolol and found the gel as effective as the beta blocker. Although the pupil diameter was reduced in the morning by the pilocarpine preparation, visual acuity was unaffected. Pilocarpine lacks some of the side effects linked with beta blockers, i.e. cardiovascular problems and corneal sensitivity effects, and taking into consideration that the gel only has to be used once daily, it must represent a useful development in the treatment of glaucoma.

3. *Oily solutions*. Not only are oils more viscous than water, but the actual alkaloid can be incorporated and thus be better absorbed by the corneal epithelium. Unfortunately oily drops are not as pleasant to use as the aqueous ones.

4. *Soft contact lenses*. Hydrogel lenses can be soaked in pilocarpine solutions and the lens applied to the eye (Marmion *et al.*, 1977), a method of application which does not seem to have been widely accepted.

5. *Ocusert*. This consists of a viscous solution surrounded by a membrane which allows a slow but constant delivery of pilocarpine into the conjunctival sac (Heilman and Sinz, 1975). The duration of treatment lasts for up to nine days and because the level of pilocarpine is constant, the side effects are smaller than from drop application. One of the problems that has been encountered is that sometimes the unit becomes lost and the patient is untreated until the loss is discovered.

Other miotics

Many other miotics have been tried in the treatment of glaucoma. These include the following.

1. Other parasympathomimetics:
   (a) *Aceclidine*. This synthetic drug has similar efficacy and duration of action to pilocarpine but does not seem to confer any particular advantage other than the fact that it can be tolerated when pilocarpine is not (Romano, 1970).
   (b) *Metachol*. A synthetic analogue of acetylcholine.
   (c) *Carbachol*. This drug is similar to metachol but is not broken down by cholinesterase. It is poorly absorbed across the cornea. Reichert *et al.* (1988) reviewed patients who had been switched from pilocarpine (four times a day) to carbachol (three times a day) when the former drug failed to produce adequate control. They found little improvement in control and an increased chance of side effects.

2. Short acting (reversible) anticholinesterases:
   (a) *Physostigmine*. This produces a marked miosis and a reduction in intraocular pressure which lasts for 12 hours. It is sometimes combined with pilocarpine.
   (b) *Neostigmine*. This is a weaker, synthetic analogue of physostigmine which does seem to have found favour in the treatment of glaucoma.

3. Long acting (irreversible) anticholinesterases:
   (a) *Dyflos*. DFP was the first organophosphorus compound but this is unstable in water and is administered in arachis oil.
   (b) *Ecothiopate*. This is similarly susceptible to hydrolysis and is supplied dry, being dissolved in a diluent just before use. Reichert and Shields (1991) replaced pilocarpine or carbachol with ecothiopate and found an improvement in intraocular pressure in 60% of

patients. Predictably, patients reported decreased vision and ocular irritation and one patient suffered retinal detachment.

(c) *Demecarium*. This is one of the shorter acting irreversible agents.

Sympathomimetics

The ability of adrenaline to reduce intraocular pressure has been known for a long time, but its application to the treatment of glaucoma was only possible following the development of the gonioscope lens. Because of the ability of adrenaline to cause a dilation of the pupil, it is vital that open angle glaucoma is differentiated from closed angle glaucoma. Sympathomimetics will reduce pressure in the former and increase it in the latter. They produce a triphasic response with a fall followed by a rise and then a more persistent fall. The effect lasts for at least 12 hours and thus the drops require administration twice a day. The time course of the ocular hypotensive effect is different from the mydriatic effect (Langham *et al.*, 1979). Many different sympathomimetics have been tried but only adrenaline and its derivatives are used routinely.

Adrenaline produces its pharmacological effects by stimulating both alpha and beta receptors and by a variety of biochemical effects, e.g. enhanced liver glycogenolysis leading to a higher blood sugar level and enhanced production of prostaglandins. Its best known biochemical effect is the enhanced production of cyclic adenosine monophosphate from adenosine triphosphate.

Adrenaline produces a beta mediated increase in secretion by stimulating chloride transport through cAMP production. This increase is however more than cancelled out by an alpha stimulated reduction. It also causes an increase in the facility of outflow by acting beta receptors. Phenylephrine, a predominantly alpha agonist, shares with timolol and betaxolol the ability to cause a vasoconstriction in the ciliary epithelium in rabbits during short term treatment (Van Buskirk *et al.*, 1990). However, tolerance develops to phenylephrine and betaxolol after several weeks treatment (but not to timolol!).

An interesting finding is that pretreatment with steroids can increase the ocular hypotensive effect of adrenaline (Bealka and Schwartz, 1991). Steroids on their own can cause a rise in IOP in some patients.

Adrenaline is not without its adverse effects, producing a red eye in some patients probably as a result of reactive hyperaemia. It will also cause black deposits in the cornea (Madge *et al.*, 1971), especially if old solutions are used (Krejci and Harrison, 1969). Maculopathy has been reported, especially in aphakic patients (Kolker and Becker, 1968; Mackool *et al.*, 1977).

In order to improve its efficacy adrenaline has in the past been combined with guanethidine, an adrenergic neurone blocker. It initially causes a release of noradrenaline from the nerve terminals and thus acts as an indirectly acting sympathomimetic. Mydriasis and a fall in intraocular pressure are the result. Since the noradrenaline is not replaced, a chemical denervation syndrome eventually exists. The intraocular pressure returns to normal and the pupil is constricted. The eye is now supersensitive to sympathomimetics and it will respond to a concentration of these agents which would normally have no effect. Crombie

(1974) used the combination of guanethidine and adrenaline to control patients who were previously difficult to control. Eltz *et al.* (1978) used a combination of 5% guanethidine and 1% adrenaline and found that the mixture was synergistic.

A recent development has been the production of prodrugs which are modifications of the drug with enhanced lipid solubility. An example is dipivefrin, which is inactive; when it enters the eye, it must be converted to active adrenaline by enzymes before it can produce its hypotensive effect. Kass *et al.* (1979) reported smaller falls with 0.1% dipivefrin than with 2% adrenaline. It was found to be less effective than timolol (Frumar and McGuinness, 1982). In terms of side effects, the results are disappointing. Reactive hyperemia (Azuma and Hirano, 1981), endothelial damage (Sasamoto *et al.*, 1981) and follicular conjunctivitis (Theodore and Leibowitz, 1979; Coleiro *et al.*, 1988) have been reported.

Beta blockers

Beta blockers were originally developed for the treatment of cardiovascular disorders and this is still the major use for this type of agent. Since it was found that propranolol reduced intraocular pressure, many other beta blockers have been tried for the treatment of glaucoma. These include atenolol, betaxolol, bupranolol, carteolol, labetalol, levobunolol, metipranolol, metoprolol, nadolol, pindolol, sotalol and timolol.

Beta blockers reduce intraocular pressure by reducing secretion (Liu *et al.*, 1980). This reduction is probably due to the blocking of the beta receptors, the stimulation of which causes an increased secretion of chloride ions. Beta blockers have no effect on outflow resistance (Reiss and Brubaker, 1983). The reduction in intraocular pressure is maintained in the absence of circulating adrenaline (Maus *et al.*, 1994), ruling out the importance of the natural hormone in the normal circadian rhythm.

Beta blockers are normally prescribed as a twice a day therapy, being applied morning and night. However there is some evidence to suggest that a once a day therapy would produce a satisfactory IOP reduction. Rakofsky *et al.* (1989) compared the use of levobunolol once a day and twice a day in patients with open angle glaucoma and found no significant difference between regimens in the reduction in IOP.

Of course, the reduction of intraocular pressure is not the only parameter which may have a bearing on the course of the condition. Retinal blood flow and its modification by drugs must also be important. Harris *et al.* (1995) studied perimacular blood flow in normal subjects after treatment with betaxolol, carteolol and levobunolol and found no significant alteration.

Not all beta blockers are the same and they vary in several ways.

1. *Selectivity*
Beta receptors can be divided into two groups – beta$_1$ and beta$_2$. Beta$_1$ receptors are found in the heart and kidneys while the bronchi contain beta$_2$. Most beta blockers are nonselective and have similar potency on both types of beta receptors.

However some have a greater affinity for beta receptors and are called cardioselective agents. One of the troublesome side effects of the use of beta blockers in the treatment of glaucoma is the blocking of the effect of beta$_2$ stimulants used to dilate bronchi during asthma attacks, leading to aggravation of such attacks (Fraunfelder and Barker, 1984). The use of beta blockers with reduced activity on beta receptors will have less effect on the bronchi and therefore have advantages in patients with obstructive airway disease (Berry *et al.*, 1984). However they are not completely safe and all beta blockers must be used with care on asthmatic patients. Harris *et al.* (1986) reported respiratory difficulties in patients receiving topical betaxolol.

2. *Intrinsic sympathomimetic activity (ISA)*
These drugs are partial agonists and can stimulate the receptor before blocking it. Many advantages have been claimed for drugs having this property, e.g. less bradycardia, less bronchoconstriction, but none would appear to have been substantiated by clinical trials. For example, carteolol (a beta blocker with ISA) causes an inhibition of exercise induced tachycardia (Brazier and Smith, 1987).

3. *Membrane stabilizing action (MSA)*
The membrane referred to here is the membrane of nerve fibres. Membrane stabilizing action is another name for local anaesthetic effect. Propranolol, the first medically used beta blocker, has marked local anaesthetic effects and because of this all beta blockers are suspect until proven innocent. Many beta blockers have small amounts of MSA but for most the effects are not clinically significant. As well as the embarrassment of respiratory problems, beta blockers may have effects on other systems, including the cardiovascular system. The effects on the heart are especially noted when increased demands are placed on the system. The heart at rest is often not significantly affected by beta blockers (Ros and Dake, 1979), but when exercise is taken the heart has difficulty in speeding up to cope with it. Fraunfelder and Meyer (1987) have reviewed the systemic side effects of topical timolol, and reported effects on the CNS, the skin and the gut as well as the cardiovascular and respiratory systems.

Because it was originally considered possible to separate the ocular hypotensive effects from the systemic effects of beta blockers by making use of different stereoisomers, Richards and Tattersfield (1987) compared timolol to its D isomer. The isomer is four times less potent in reducing IOP and is four times less potent in causing bronchoconstriction. It does not therefore offer any particular advantage for use in asthmatic patients.

Timolol

Timolol was the first beta blocker to be introduced as a topical solution in the early 1980s. Ophthalmic solutions of timolol are well tolerated by the eye, causing less irritation than betaxolol or artificial tears (Kendall *et al.*, 1987). When applied topically it produces an effect not only in the treated eye but also in the untreated contralateral eye. Woodward *et al.* (1987) demonstrated bilateral beta blockade in rabbits' eyes from unilateral application and concluded that this effect must be due to systemic absorption. In many trials the contralateral eye has been used as a control; these results would seem to call this practice into doubt.

Like all topical beta blockers timolol has a twice a day dose regimen. However, a long acting form Timoptol LA has been introduced which only requires application once a day. The drop is formulated with a polysaccharide to produce a viscous gel which retards drainage from the conjunctival sac.

Another interesting development of timolol is the study of the relative potencies of the two isomers of timolol, L-timolol and D-timolol. L-timolol is the normal isomer which has been used up to now and has by far the most affinity for the beta receptor. If the fall in IOP produced by timolol is due entirely due to blockade of the beta receptor, then the D form should be inactive. Chiou et al. (1990) found the two isomers to be equi-effective on topical instillation in lowering IOP. Furthermore, D-timolol had a beneficial effect on retinal and choroidal blood flows while the L isomer had the opposite effect. This finding confirms that of Martin and Rabineau (1989) who found that timolol had a vasoconstrictor effect on retinal arteries. Chiou (1990) concludes that D-timolol could be a better agent for the treatment of glaucoma than L-timolol.

Because timolol has been on the market for such a long time, long term studies are available which allow the real beneficial effects of treatment to be monitored, i.e. protection against disc cupping and visual field loss. This is especially true in the treatment of ocular hypotensive patients. Epstein et al. (1989) examined patients for over four years and found that timolol had a beneficial effect on visual fields and the optic disc compared with untreated patients. Similar findings were reported by Kass et al. (1989) who treated one eye of ocular hypotensive patients and found that medical treatment reduced the incidence of ocular change.

Other beta blockers

After the advent of timolol came a series of new topical beta blockers for the treatment of open angle glaucoma. There are many systemically used beta blockers, but only a few showed topical activity. Those which reached the market are, in alphabetical order, betaxolol, carteolol, levobunolol and metipranolol. The first three remain on the market in multidose form while metipranolol is only available in single dose units. Krieglstein et al. (1987) reported a higher incidence of stinging with metipranolol when compared with levobunolol although both were equally effective as ocular hypotensive agents.

Although there are minor differences between the individual beta blockers, they all produce their effect in the same manner, i.e. by reducing aqueous humour production and aqueous flow. Yablonski et al. (1987) found that levobunolol produced its effect in the same way as did timolol. Freyler et al. (1988) compared levobunolol and timolol and found little difference in efficacy. A similar result was reported by Savelsbergh-Filette and Demailly (1988). Duff and Newcombe (1988) however found that the hypotensive effect of carteolol was not as well maintained with twice a day therapy as it was with timolol.

Topical carbonic anhydrase inhibitors

Carbonic anhydrase inhibitors are useful drugs for lowering intraocular pressure, which in the past have had to be administered systemically.

Unfortunately when given by this route they produce some undesirable systemic side effects (see above), which can lead to a large proportion of patients discontinuing therapy. The traditional agents such as acetazolamide and dichlorphenamide were found not to be active when applied topically. Acetazolamide has poor lipid solubility and corneal penetration. In the early 1980s the development of trifluoromethazolamide produced some interest as it provided good lipid solubility as well as water solubility and potency. Unfortunately it was unstable and did not reach clinical use. However, this encouraged further research into newer compounds such as MK-927 which showed marked activity in lowering IOP in animals (Sugrue et al., 1990) and patients (Lippa et al., 1991). In both studies the effects were proportional to the concentration up to a maximum of 2% and were maintained for 12 hours after application. A 12 hour duration of action allows for a twice a day therapy and good patient compliance. Although this compound showed promise further chemical modifications were made which led to the development of dorzolamide. Maren (1995) has reviewed the development of the various intermediate carbonic anhydrase inhibitor compounds which showed gradual improvement over the earlier compounds. Dorzolamide is now marketed under the trade name of *Trusopt*. This preparation has good acceptability and can be used on its own (three times a day) or more commonly as adjunctive therapy (twice daily).

Apraclonidine

Apraclonidine is a derivative of clonidine, a central alpha$_2$ adrenergic agonist which reduces blood pressure and heart rate by reducing sympathetic tone. It is used systemically in the treatment of hypertension and, in lower doses, for the prophylaxis of migraine.

Apraclonidine has been found to produce a significant fall in IOP in patients following cataract surgery (Prata et al., 1992; Wiles et al., 1991). When applied topically to normal healthy volunteers it had no cardiovascular effects, unlike timolol (Coleman, 1990). It has also been trialled as adjunctive therapy with timolol and was found to be superior to dipivefrin in producing an additive effect (Morrison and Robin, 1989). However when used together with timolol in patients previously no additive effect was seen (Koskela and Brubaker, 1991). This suggests that apraclonidine shares in part the mode of action in reducing aqueous humour production. It is well tolerated in the eye with conjunctival hyperemia or conjunctival blanching, lid retraction and mydriasis being noted in a small percentage of patients.

Apraclonidine is marketed under the trade name *Iopidine* (apraclonidine 1%). It is available as single use units for the treatment or prevention of the postsurgical rise in intraocular pressure following anterior segment laser surgery. In multidose form it can be used as an adjunct therapy for primary open angle glaucoma where a single treatment produces inadequate control.

Table 12.1 Glaucoma treatments

Official name	Trade name	Mode of action	Dosage forms	Concentrations employed	Adverse reactions	Notes
Pilocarpine	Isoptocarpine Sno-pilo Minims	Miotic	drops	0.5%–4.0%	Spasm of accommodation, pinpoint pupils	Most often used as combination treatment
	Piloplex Ocusert	Miotic Miotic	viscous gel constant delivery	4% 20–40 mcg/hr		
Adrenaline	Epppy Simplene	Sympathomimetic	drops	0.5%–1%	Red eye, pupil dilation	Little used today
Dipivefrin	Propine	Prodrug sympathomimetic	drops	0.1%	Reactive hyperemia, follicular conjunctivitis	
Guanethidine and adrenaline	Ganda	Sympathomimetic + potentiator	drops	1% + 0.2% 3% + 0.5%	Red eye	
Brimonidine	Alphagen	Sympathomimetic				
Betaxolol	Betoptic	Beta blocker	drops	0.5%	Bronchoconstriction	
Carteolol	Teoptic	Beta blocker	drops	1%, 2%	Bronchoconstriction	
Levobunolol	Betagen	Beta blocker	drops (+ single units)	0.5%	Bronchoconstriction	
Metipranolol	Minims	Beta blocker	single units	0.1%, 0.3%	Bronchoconstriction uveitis	Limited indications
Timolol	Timoptol Glaucol Timoptol LA	Beta blocker	drops (+ single units) gel	0.25%, 0.5% 0.25%, 0.5%	Bronchoconstriction	
Dorzolamide	Trusopt	Carbonic anhydrase inhibitor	drops	2%		Most often used as adjunctive therapy
Latanoprost	Xalantan	Prostaglandin analogue				

Mixtures of agents

Because of their different modes of action, it is possible to mix drugs from different groups in order to achieve an enhanced effect. This is necessary where control is not achieved with a single medication or the effect of the original therapy wears off with time. It is possible to combine a drug from one group with another from one of the other two groups, e.g.

beta blockers and miotics
beta blockers and sympathomimetics
miotics and sympathomimetics.

The most common combination is pilocarpine and timolol. One matter of interest is the dose regimen if the drugs are administered in the same drop. Timolol is normally a twice daily therapy while pilocarpine requires administration four times a day. Airaksinen *et al.* (1987) compared timolol and pilocarpine with pilocarpine alone. Not only was a greater effect found with the combination, but the duration of effect was sufficient to allow twice daily administration. Leroy and Collignon-Brach (1990) found that a combination of timolol 0.5% and pilocarpine 2% was more effective in lowering IOP than timolol alone. Maclure *et al.* (1989) found similar results in patients who could not be controlled on timolol alone. Patients reported systemic effects consistent with those of beta blockers while the local ocular side effects were due to the miotic.

Studies of beta blockers with adrenaline (Allen and Epstein, 1986) and with dipivefrin (Ober and Scharrer, 1980; Parrow *et al.*, 1989) have also been undertaken and demonstrated advantages of these combinations. Drance *et al.* (1991) found that a mixture of timolol and epinephrine was more effective than either agent on its own.

Combining two compounds from the same group, e.g. two miotics or two beta blockers, is less successful.

It is possible to combine all four forms of medical treatment, i.e. beta blockers, miotics, sympathomimetics and carbonic anhydrase inhibitors, but usually surgery is employed before this stage is reached.

Treatments of the future?

Although great strides have been made in the medical treatment of open angle glaucoma, the present range of treatments is far from perfect, either from the point of view of efficacy or of side effects. Because of the complex nature of aqueous humour dynamics, a whole range of new compounds has been tested for ocular hypotensive effects.

Bromocriptine is a dopaminergic receptor stimulant which has been found to be effective in reducing the intraocular pressure in rabbits. It is a derivative of ergot and is used principally for the treatment of Parkinsonism. Given by mouth, it produces many side effects such as nausea, vomiting, dizziness, orthostatic hypertension and syncope. It has also been reported to cause blurred vision. The incidence of side effects is dose related and it may be possible for topical treatment to be given without inconveniencing the patient.

Brovincamine, a calcium channel blocker used in the treatment of cardiovascular problems, has been shown to prevent visual field defect in patients with normotensive glaucoma (Sawada *et al.*, 1996). Since this type of glaucoma is normally difficult to treat, such a result is very encouraging.

Cannabis, best known as a drug of abuse, contains tetrahydrocannabinol which lowers IOP, but until its effects on the CNS can be separated from the ocular hypotensive effect, there is little future for its clinical use.

Forskolin is a natural product which like adrenaline stimulates adenylate cyclase, causing an increase in the intracellular levels of cAMP, but does not involve the reaction with a receptor. It reduces IOP when injected or applied topically (Caprioli, 1985).

Bunazosin is an alpha blocker similar to prazosin, and has been tested in healthy subjects for ocular hypotensive effects (Trew et al., 1991). It produced significant falls in IOP without affecting blood flow, and the expected ocular effects of miosis, ptosis and conjunctival hyperemia.

A class of compounds which is now receiving attention is the eicosanoids, which are in the main endogenous derivatives of a fatty acid (arachidonic acid) with marked activity on many cell types and tissues. The group includes the leucotrienes and prostaglandins and it is the prostaglandins that have been tested for ocular hypotensive effect. Bito et al. (1990) found that certain derivatives of prostaglandin A2 (PGA2) were effective in lowering the pressure in cats' eyes. Camras et al. (1987) tested prostaglandin F2 alpha (PGF2alpha) in monkeys and found that it produced a significant reduction in IOP without tolerance or tachyphylaxis developing. This prostaglandin is a free fatty acid and thus will suffer absorption problems across the intact cornea. Bito and Baroody (1987) experimented with prostaglandin esters in rabbit eyes and found that the penetration of the ester was superior to that of the free acid. Siebold et al. (1989) tested prostaglandin F2 alpha isopropyl ester (PGF(2alpha)-IE) in patients with ocular hypertension or open angle glaucoma and found it to be a potent ocular hypotensive and a potential agent for treatment. Prostaglandins are also thought to be involved in the ocular hypotensive effect of other drugs. The ACE inhibitor (angiotensin converting enzyme inhibitor) enalapril produced a fall in IOP in monkeys (Lotti and Pawlowski, 1990). This effect was inhibited by pretreatment with indomethacin indicating the involvement of prostaglandins.

Another candidate for inclusion in the armamentarium of antiglaucoma drugs is acepromazine, which lowered the intraocular pressure in monkeys in which it had been artificially raised (Hayreh et al., 1991). It is a phenothiazine anxiolytic drug related to chlorpromazine. It is not on the market in the UK but has been used by veterinarians in conjunction with other drugs to immobilize large animals.

References

Aldrete, J., Mcdonald, T. O. and De Sousa, B. (1983) Comparative evaluation of pilocarpine gel and timolol in patients with glaucoma. *Glaucoma*, 236–241

Airaksinen, P. J. et al. (1987) A double masked study of timolol and pilocarpine. *Am. J. Ophthalmol.*, **104**, 587–590

Allen, R. C. and Epstein, D. L. (1986) Additive effect of betaxolol and epinephrine in primary open glaucoma. *Arch. Ophthalmol.*, **104**, 1178–1184

Azuma, I. and Hirumo, T. (1981) Long term topical use of DPE solution in open angle glaucoma. *Acta Soc. Ophthalmol., Jap.*, **85**, 1157–1164

Barany, E. H. (1962) The mode of action of pilocarpine on outflow resistance in the eye of a primate (*Cercopithecus ethiops*) *Invest. Ophthamol.*, **1**, 712–727

Bealka, N. and Schwartz, B. (1991) Enhanced ocular hypotensive response to epinephrine with prior dexamethasone treatment. *Arch. Ophthalmol.*, **109**, 346–348

Berry, D. P., van Bushkirk, M. and Shields, M. B. (1984) Betaxolol and timolol. *Arch. Ophthalmol.*, **102**, 42–45

Bito, L. Z. and Baroody, R. A. (1987) The ocular pharmacokinetics of eicosanoids and their derivatives. *Exp. Eye Res.*, **44**, 217–226

Bito, L. Z. *et al.* (1990) Eicosanoids as a new class of ocular hypotensive agents. 3. Prostaglandin A-1-isopropyl ester is the most potent reported hypotensive agent on feline eyes. *Exp. Eye Res.*, **50**, 419–428

Brazier, D. J. and Smith, S. E. (1987) Ocular and cardiovascular response to topical carteolol 2% and timolol 0.5% in healthy volunteers. *Br. J. Ophthalmol.*, **72**, 101–103

Camras, C. B. *et al.* (1987) Multiple dosing of prostaglandin F(2alpha) or epinephrine on cynomolgus monkeys. 1. Aqueous humour dynamics. *Invest. Ophthalmol.*, **28**, 463–469

Caprioli, J. (1985) The pathogenesis and medical management of glaucoma. *Drug Dev. Res.*, **6**, 193–215

Chiou, G. C. Y. (1990) Development of D-timolol for the treatment of glaucoma and ocular hypertension. *J. Ocul. Pharmacol.*, **6**, 67–74

Chiou, G. C. Y. *et al.* (1990) Effect of D-timolol and L-timolol on ocular blood flow and intraocular pressure. *J. Ocul. Pharmacol.*, **6**, 23–30

Coleiro, J. A., Sigurdsson, H. and Lockyer, J. A. (1988) Follicular conjunctivitis on dipivefrin therapy for glaucoma. *Eye*, **2**, 440–442

Coleman, A. L. *et al.* (1990) Cardiovascular and intraocular pressure effects and plasma concentrations of apraclonidine. *Arch. Ophthalmol.*, **108**, 1264–1267

Crombie, A. L. (1974) Adrenergic hypersensitisation as a therapeutic tool in glaucoma. *Trans. Ophthalmol. Soc. UK*, **94**, 570–572

Davies, D. J. G., Jones, D. E. P., Meakin. B. J. and Norton, D. A. (1977) The effect of polyvinyl alcohol on the degree of miosis and intraocular pressure induced by pilocarpine. *Ophthalmol. Dig.*, **39**, 13–26

Dowd, T. C., Harding, S. and Rennie, I. (1991) A prospective study of oral nadolol inn the management of patients with newly diagnosed chronic simple glaucoma. *J. Ocul. Pharmacol.*, **7**, 21–26

Drance, S. M. *et al.* (1991) Adrenergic and adrenolytic effects on intraocular pressure. *Exp. Ophthalmol.*, **229**, 50–51

Duff, G. R. and Newcombe, R. G. (1988) The 12 hour control of intraocular pressure on carteolol 2% twice daily. *Brit. J. Ophthalmol.*, **72**, 890–891

Eltz, H., Aeschlimann, J. and Gloor, B. (1978) Double blind trial of a guanethidine/ adrenaline combination, compared with the two separate components in glaucoma. *Acta Ophthalmol.*, (Kbh)., **56**, 191–200

Epstein, D. L. *et al.* (1989). A long term clinical trial of timolol therapy versus no treatment in the management of glaucoma suspects. *Ophthalmology*, **96**, 1460–1467

Fraunfelder, F. T. and Barber, A. F. (1984) Respiratory effects of timolol. *New Engl. J. Med.*, **311**, 1441

Fraunfelder, F. T. and Meyer, S. M. (1987) Systemic side effects from ophthalmic timolol and their prevention. *J. Ocul. Pharmacol.*, **3**, 177–184

Freyler, H. *et al.* (1988) Comparison of ocular hypotensive efficacy and safety of levobunolol and timolol. *Klin. Monatsbl. Augenheilk*, **193**, 257–260

Frumar, K. D. and McGuiness, R. (1982) A study of the intraocular pressure lowering effect of timolol and dipivalylepinephrine. *Aust. J. Ophthalmol.*, **10**, 121–123

Harris, L. S. and Galin, M. A. (1970) Dose response analysis of pilocarpine induced ocular hypotension. *Arch. Ophthalmol.*, **84**, 605–608

Harris, L. S., Greenstein, S. H. and Bloom, A. F. (1986) Respiratory difficulties with betaxolol. *Am. J. Ophthalmol.*, **102**, 274

Harris, A. *et al.* (1995) Acute effect of topical beta adrenergic antagonists on normal perimacular hemodynamics. *J. Glaucoma*, **4**, 36–40

Hayreh, S. S. *et al.* (1991) Acepromazine. Effects on intraocular pressure. *Arch. Ophthalmol.*, **109**, 119–124

Heilman, K. and Sinz, V. (1975) Ocusert – a new drug carrier for the treatment of glaucoma. *Klin. Monatsbl. Augenheilk.*, **166**, 289–292

Johnson, D. H. *et al.* (1984) A one-year multicenter clinical trial of pilocarpine gel. *Am. J. Ophthalmol.*, **6**, 723–729

Kass, M. A., Mandell, A. I., Goldberg, I., Paine, J. M. and Becker, B. (1979) Dipivefrin and epinephrine treatment of elevated intraocular pressure. *Arch. Ophthalmol.*, **97**, 1865–1866

Kass, M. A. *et al.* (1989) Topical timolol administration reduces the incidence of glaucomatous damage in ocular hypertensive individuals. A randomized double masked long term clinical trial. *Arch. Ophthalmol.*, **107**, 1590–1598

Kendall, K. *et al.* (1987) Tolerability of timolol and betaxolol in patients with chronic open angle glaucoma. *Clin. Ther.*, **9**, 651–655

Kolker, A. E. and Becker, B. (1968) Epinephrine maculopathy. *Arch. Ophthalmol.*, **79**, 552–562

Korczyn, A. D., Nemet, P., Carel, R. S. and Eyal, A. (1982) Effect of pilocarpine on intraocular pressure in normal humans. *Ophthal. Res.*, **14**, 182–187

Koskela, T. and Brubaker, R. F. (1991) Apraclonidine and timolol. Combined effects in previously untreated normal subjects. *Arch. Ophthalmol.*, **109**, 804–806

Kraushar, M. F. and Steinberg, J. A. (1991) Miotics and retinal detachment: Upgrading the community standard. *Surv. Ophthalmol.*, **35**, 311–316

Krejci, L. and Harrison, R. (1969) Corneal pigment deposits from topically administered epinephrine. *Arch. Ophthalmol.*, **82**, 836–839

Krieglstein, G. K. *et al.* (1987) Levobunolol and metipranolol. Comparative ocular hypotensive effects. *Br. J. Ophthalmol.*, **71**, 250–253

Langham, M. E., Simjee. A. and Joseph, S. (1979) The alpha and beta adrenergic responses to epinephrine in the rabbit. *Exp. Eye Res.*, **15**, 75–84

Leroy, C. and Collignon-Brach, J. (1990) Comparison between the effect of timolol pilocarpine combination vs. timolol alone on the intraocular pressure of open angle glaucoma patients. *J. Fr. Ophthalmol.*, **13**, 29–32

Lippa, E. A. (1991) Multiple dose, dose response relationship for the topical carbonic anhydrase inhibitor MK-927. *Arch. Ophthalmol.*, **109**, 46–49

Liu, H. K., Chiou, G. C. Y. and Garg, L. C. (1980) Ocular hypotensive effects of timolol in cats' eyes. *Arch. Ophthalmol.*, **98**, 1467–1469

Lotti, V. J. and Pawlowski, N. (1990) Prostaglandin mediates the ocular hypotensive effect of the angiotensin converting enzyme inhibitor MK-422 enalaprilat in African green monkeys. *J. Ocul. Pharmacol.*, **6**, 1–7

Mackool, R. J., Muldoon, T., Fortier, A. and Nelson, D. (1977) Epinephrine induced cystoid macular oedema in aphakic eyes. *Arch. Ophthalmol.*, **95**, 791–793

Maclure, G. M. *et al.* (1989) Effect on the 24-hour diurnal curve of intraocular pressure of a fixed combination of timolol 0.5% and pilocarpine 2% in patients with COAG not controlled on timolol 0.5% *Br. J. Ophthalmol.*, **73**, 827–831

Madge, G. E., Geeraets, W. J. and Guerry, D. (1971) Black cornea secondary to topical epinephrine. *Am. J. Ophthalmol.*, **71**, 402–405

Mandel, A. I. *et al.* (1988) Reduced cyclic myopia with pilocarpine gel. *Ann. Ophthalmol.*, **20**, 133–135

March, W. F. *et al.* (1982) Duration of effect of pilocarpine gel. *Arch. Ophthalmol.*, **9**, 1270–1271

Maren, T. H. (1995) The development of topical carbonic anhydrase inhibitors. *J. Glaucoma*, **4**, 49–62

Marmion, V. J. and Yurdakul, S. (1977) Pilocarpine administration by contact lens. *Trans. Ophthalmol. Soc.*, **97**, 162–163

Martin, X. D. and Rabineau, P. A. (1989) Vasoconstrictive effect of topical timolol on human retinal arteries. *Graefes Arch. Clin. Exp. Ophthalmol.*, **227**, 526–530

Maus, T. L. *et al.* (1994) Aqueous flow in humans after adrenalectomy. *Invest. Ophthalmol.*, **35**, 3325–3331

Morrison, J. C. and Robin, A. L. (1989) Adjunctive glaucoma therapy. A comparison of apraclonidine to dipivefrin when added to timolol maleate. *Ophthalmology*, **96**, 3–7

Ober, M. and Scharrer, A. (1980) The effect of timolol and dipivalyl-epinephrine in the treatment of the elevated intraocular pressure. *Graefes Arch. Ophthalmol.*, **213**, 273–281

Parrow, K. A. *et al.* (1989) Is it worthwhile to add dipivefrin 0.1% to topical beta$_1$, beta$_2$ blocker therapy. *Ophthalmology*, **96**, 1338–1342

Prata, J. A. *et al.* (1992) Apraclonidine and early postoperative intraocular hypertension after cataract extraction. *Acta Ophthalmol.*, **70**, 434–439

Rakofsky, S. I. (1989) A comparison of the ocular hypotensive efficacy of once daily and twice daily levobunolol treatment. *Ophthalmology*, **96**, 8–11

Reichert, R. W. and Shields, M. B. (1991) Intraocular pressure response to the replacement of pilocarpine or carbachol with echothiophate. *Graefes Arch. Clin. Exp. Ophthalmol.*, **229**, 252–253

Reichert, R. W., Shields, M. B. and Stewart, W. C. (1988) Intraocular pressure response to replacing pilocarpine with carbachol. *Am. J. Ophthalmol.*, **106**, 747–748

Reiss, G. R. and Brubaker, R. F. (1983) The mechanism of betaxolol, a new ocular hypotensive agent. *Ophthalmology*, **90**, 1369–1372

Richards, R. and Tattersfield, A. E. (1987) Comparison of the airway response to eye drops of timolol and its isomer L-714,465 in asthmatic subjects. *Br. J. Clin. Pharmacol.*, **24**, 485–491

Romano, J. H. (1970) Double blind crossover comparison of aceclidine and pilocarpine in open angle glaucoma. *Br. J. Ophthalmol.*, **54**, 510–521

Ros, F. E. and Dake, C. L. (1979) Timolol eye drops: bradycardia or tachycardia. *Documenta Ophthalmologica*, **48**, 283–289

Sasamoto, K., Akagi, Y. and Itoi, M. (1981) Effects of epinephrine and dipivalyl epinephrine on rabbit corneal endothelium. *Folio Ophthalmol., Jap.*, **32**, 1292–1297

Savelsbergh-Fillette, M. P. and Demailly, P. (1988) Levobunolol compared with Timolol for control of elevated intraocular pressure. *J. Fr. Ophthalmol.*, **11**, 587–590

Sawada, A. *et al.* (1996) Prevention of visual field defect progression with brovincamine in eyes with normal tension glaucoma. *Ophthalmology*, **103**, 283–288

Siebold, E. C. *et al.* (1989) Maintained reduction of intraocular pressure by prostaglandin f(2)-1 isopropyl ester applied in multiple doses in ocular hypertensive and glaucoma patients. *Ophthalmology*, **96**, 1329–1337

Stewart, R. H. *et al.* (1984) Long acting pilocarpine gel: a dose-response in ocular hypertensive subjects. *Glaucoma*, **6**, 182–185

Sugrue, M. F. *et al.* (1990) MK-927. A topically active ocular hypotensive carbonic anhydrase inhibitor. *J. Ocul. Pharmacol.*, **6**, 9–22

Theodore, J. and Leibowitz, H. M. (1979) External ocular toxicity of dipivalyl epinephrine. *Am. J. Ophthalmol.*, **88**, 1013–1016

Ticho, U. *et al.* (1979) A clinical trial with piloplex – a new long acting pilocarpine compound preliminary report. *Ann. Ophthalmol.*, **11**, 535–561

Trew, D. R., Wright, L. A. and Smith, S. E. (1991) Ocular responses in healthy subjects to topical bunazosin 0.3% – an alpha-adrenoceptor antagonist. *Br. J. Ophthalmol.*, **75**, 411–413

Tutton, M. K. and Smith, R. J. H. (1982) Comparison of ocular hypotensive effects of three dosages of oral atenolol. *Br. J. Ophthalmol.*, **67**, 664–667

Van Buskirk, E. M., Bacon, D. R. and Fahrenbach, W. H. (1990) Ciliary vasoconstriction after topical adrenergic drugs. *Am. J. Ophthalmol.*, **109**, 511–517

Wiles, S. B., Mackenzie, D. and Ide, C. H. (1991) Control of intraocular pressure with apraclonidine hydrochloride after cataract extraction. *Am. J. Ophthalmol.*, **111**, 184–188

Williamson, J., Young, J. D. H., Muir, G. and Kadom, A. (1985) Comparative efficacy of orally and topically administered beta blockers for chronic simple glaucoma. *Br. J. Ophthalmol.*, **69**, 41–45

Woodward, D. F. *et al.* (1987) Topical timolol at conventional unilateral doses causes bilateral ocular beta blockade in rabbits. *Exp. Eye Res.*, **44**, 319–329

Yablonski, M. E. *et al.* (1987) The effect of levobunolol on aqueous humour dynamics. *Exp. Eye Res.*, **44**, 49–54

13

Artificial tears

Reduced tear flow may go unnoticed by the patient or cause a variety of symptoms and signs, varying from the clinically trivial to the potentially sight threatening. It may be the result of the normal ageing process in which other exocrine glands function less well in addition to the tear glands, e.g. the salivary glands. However, it can be the sign of more fundamental problems such as trauma to the lacrimal gland, scarring of the conjunctiva or a congenital lack of lacrimal tissue.

Sjögren's syndrome is characterized by dry eye, dry mouth and rheumatoid arthritis. Dry eye is usually the first symptom to be noticed and there is a familial tendency (Bjerrum and Prause, 1990). When tear insufficiency is marked enough to lead to symptoms of inflammation then the term keratoconjunctivitis sicca (KCS) is used. The numerous causes of dry eye include the side effects of such drugs as some antihistamines, beta blockers, phenothiazines and oral contraceptives.

Diagnosis of dry eye used to be based on three tests

1. Schirmer's I test in which a strip of filter paper is placed in the conjunctival sac and the amount of wetting noted after five minutes. Some practitioners question the validity of this apparently crude test, being of the opinion that it really just confirms what is known already. It shows the quantity of tears without any assessment of their quality.
2. Tear break up time can be carried out with or without the aid of fluorescein stain. It is a measure of tear film stability which will be dependent to a large extent on mucin concentration.
3. Rose bengal staining (see Chapter 10) shows the extent of dead cells caused by the lack of tears. It is usually most marked in the exposed interpalpebral area of the cornea and conjunctiva.

As techniques have developed, more sophisticated tests have been used. Van Bijsterveld (1988) used lysozyme and lactoferrin assays in assessing patients with KCS. Heiligenhaus et al. (1994, 1995) performed a battery of tests on patients with dry eyes who were not stabilized with artificial tears. Few had aqueous deficiencies, while the majority lacked lipid. Such differentiation will lead to more sophisticated, targeted treatments of KCS.

Also indicative of dry eye is a predisposition to infection and the patients' complaints of 'gritty feelings' in the eye, especially in adverse environments such as smoky rooms. Environmental conditions may precipitate the problem for normally unaffected patients, such as visual display operators who usually work in dry atmospheric conditions. Rapinese et al. (1994) and Ferrari (1993) found that such workers benefited from artificial tear treatment.

Treatment

Where the dry eye is secondary to some primary cause then the latter must receive attention, as well as symptomatic relief. In severe cases, efforts are made to retain those tears which are present, e.g. by cauterizing the nasolacrimal duct openings or inserting collagen or silicone plugs into the puncta (Barnard 1996). Cauterization is a major step and is not undertaken lightly, as a return to normal secretion levels will cause the patient to suffer epiphora. A particularly novel treatment was the use of salivary secretion by transplanting the parotid duct into the conjunctival sac.

The most common treatment however is the use of tear supplements, normally in the form of aqueous eye drops, although modern developments have been towards the application of gels and ointments.

Formulation of tear supplements

Marquardt (1986) sets down four requirements for artificial tears:

1. They must not irritate the eye.
2. They must have a good lubricating effect.
3. They must have a long retention time.
4. They must not disturb the optics of the eye.

These ideals only relate to the short term benefits to the patient. Obviously the ultimate aim is to prevent damage to the cornea as well as giving the patient symptomatic relief. Much attention has been given to the measure of corneal permeability as an assessment of the degree of corneal epithelial damage. The normal intact healthy cornea provides a barrier to the passage of drugs and other solutes into the corneal stroma. If the epithelium is damaged then this barrier is disrupted and permeability is increased. Gobbels and Spitznas (1989) found that patients with dry eye had corneal permeabilities 2.8 times greater than normal patients. This was the parameter chosen by Gobbels and Spitznas (1991) in their comparison of different formulations.

Viscolizers

Many dry eye sufferers have a mucin deficiency and respond by producing copious aqueous tears. Ideally, tear supplements should contain a viscolizer in order to compensate for this deficiency. Mucin has several actions in tears, acting as a surface active agent making the hydrophobic surface of the corneal epithelium more hydrophilic in the same way that a wetting solution acts on a hard contact lens, and as a lubricant between the lids and the cornea. Additionally, it slows the rate of drainage of tears down the nasolacrimal duct and keeps them in contact with the corneal epithelium for longer. There have been many attempts to produce the 'perfect' viscolizer which would replace the mucin in dry eye patients. The original cellulose derivatives such as methylcellulose, carboxymethylcellulose, hydroxyethylcellulose and hydroxypropylmethylcellulose (hypromellose) are still widely used, while polyvinyl alcohol is said to have the advantage of being a surfactant as well as a viscolizer. Polyvinylpyrrolidine has also been used as a viscolizer.

The viscosity of some artificial tears has been increased to such an extent that they are no longer aqueous drops but gels. Hyaluronic acid, used extensively as a protective agent during intraocular surgery, has been used as artificial tears. Snibson *et al.* (1992) found solutions of 0.2% sodium hyaluronate had much greater retention times than solutions of hydroxypropylmethylcellulose and polyvinyl alcohol. Limberg *et al.* (1987), however, in comparing hyaluronic acid and chrondroitin sulphate formulations with polyvinyl alcohol, found that none of them were superior to the others in reducing the signs and symptoms, although they all provided improvements. Carbomer 940 (polyacrylic acid) is the viscolizer used in *Viscotears* and *Gel-tears*. The gel has good water binding properties which helps it to form a stable tear film. It shows thixotropic properties, i.e. the gel is reversible. During blinking, liquefaction of the gel occurs followed by a reformation of the gel to reduce elimination from the tear film. These more viscous presentations have two principal advantages; first, they provide relief for longer and thus require fewer doses. Marquadt (1986) found that liquid gels had a retention time seven times greater than polyvinyl alcohol and that patients could reduce dosing from 20 times a day to four times a day. Secondly, they provide protection during sleep when few natural tears are produced. This is particularly important for patients undergoing operations and in intensive care units who exist in dry atmospheres, and may be exposed to gases which cause drying. Ointments such as simple eye ointment have been used in the past, but it was found that gel artificial tears provided sufficient protection and were pleasant for the patient to use (Marquadt *et al.*, 1987). The gel film also made eye examination easier.

Solid insert viscolizers were developed which could be inserted into the conjunctival sac and dissolved over several hours. These products did not find much acceptance. Lindahl *et al.* (1988) found that while there was a relief of symptoms and a reduction in keratoconjunctival staining, Schirmer test results and tear break up were unaltered. Two thirds of their patients withdrew because of adverse effects. Hill (1989), however, found that the majority of patients experienced an improvement in their symptoms compared with the use of artificial tears.

The use of collagen shields for drug delivery has led to their possible use in dry eye products. Kaufmann *et al.* (1994) used small pieces of collagen with the inclusion of lipid suspended in a methylcellulose solution for the treatment of moderately severe KCS. A majority of patients preferred the formulation to the vehicle alone.

Tonicity

Most artificial tears have the same tonicity as natural tears and blood plasma, i.e. equivalent to a sodium chloride (NaCl) concentration of 0.9%, but one product, *Hypotears*, has a sodium chloride equivalent of 0.6%. Fassihi and Naidoo (1989) found a range of NaCl equivalents of 0.5% to 1.5%. Of course it not just the osmotic pressure that is important, as the individual electrolytes that contribute to the pressure play a part. Sodium is of course essential, but the findings of Green *et al.* (1992) suggest that potassium should also be incorporated into tear solutions.

pH

A pH just on the alkaline side of neutral, e.g. pH 7.4, is normally selected for the pH of artificial tears, but some products are made more alkaline. Fassihi and Naidoo (1989) found a pH range of 4–9 in commercial preparations. Ubels *et al.* (1995) found that bicarbonate vastly improved the recovery of damaged corneae when included in preservative free artificial tears.

Preservatives

There is an increasing trend towards the use of preservative free preparations either in the form of single use containers such as Minims, or in extemporaneously prepared eyedrops which are kept in the refrigerator after opening to reduce bacterial growth and discarded after one week.

However, normal multidose containers require the addition of an antibacterial preservative to prevent microbial contamination during use. Unfortunately, the one normally chosen is 0.01% benzalkonium chloride, which will at this concentration destabilize the tear film and shorten the tear break up time (Holly, 1978; Hollis and Lemp, 1977). In some formulations the concentration is reduced to 0.004% which does not interfere with tear film stability.

The toxic effects of preservatives have been studied. Bernal and Ubels (1991) found that 0.01% benzalkonium chloride markedly reduced the corneal epithelial barrier to the uptake of a fluorescein derivative, indicating corneal surface damage. They recommend that KCS patients should avoid benzalkonium chloride preserved solutions and that unpreserved solutions are preferable. This opinion is confirmed by Palmer and Kaufman (1995), who suggest that the disadvantages of benzalkonium chloride outweigh any beneficial effects from the tear preparations. Gobbels and Spitznas (1991, 1992) also came to the same conclusion after comparing 2% polyvinylpyrrolidone preserved with benzalkonium with the same viscolizer in an unpreserved solution.

Viscotears uses 0.01% w/w cetrimide as the preservative. Chlorbutanol has also been used in the preservation of artificial tears but this has been shown to cause irritation (Fassihi and Naidoo, 1989).

Other treatments

More active treatments have been suggested in order to repair the damage caused by the drying of the cornea. Leibowitz *et al.* (1993) carried out a pilot study on cyclosporin ophthalmic ointment and found a beneficial effect.

Cyclosporin is an immunosuppressant drug used to prevent the rejection of transplants.

Mucolytic agents

Overproduction of mucus can cause an excess of debris in the tear film and result in the presence of strands or filaments on the cornea (filamentary keratitis). Mucus molecules can be broken down by an agent such as acetylcysteine.

Table 13.1 Artificial tears

Official name	Trade name	Dosage form	Concentration
Acetylcysteine	Ilube	drops	5% (with 0.3% hypromellose)
Carbomers	Geltears Viscotears	gel	0.2%
Hydroxylethyl-cellulose	Minims Artificial Tears	drops (single use)	0.44%
Hypromellose	Isopto Alkaline Moisture Eyes Tears Naturale	drops (unpreserved drops often used)	Conc. varies between 0.3 and 1.0%
Liquid paraffin	Lacrilube	ointment	
Paraffin Yellow soft	Simple Eye Ointment	ointment	
Polyvinyl alcohol	Liquifilm Tears Sno Tears	drops	1.4%

References

Barnard, N. A. S. (1996) Punctal and intracanalicular occlusion – a guide for the practitioner. *Ophthal. Physiol. Opt.*, **16**, S15–S22

Bernal, D. L. and Ubels, J. L. (1991) Quantitative evaluation of the corneal epithelial barrier: Effect of artificial tears and preservatives. *Curr. Eye Res.*, **10**, 645–656

Bjerrum, K. and Prause, J. U. (1990) Primary Sjögren's syndrome: A subjective description of the disease. *Clin. Exp. Rheumatol.*, **8**, 283–288

Fassihi, A. R. and Naidoo, N. T. (1989) Irritation associated with tear replacement ophthalmic drops. A pharmaceutical and subjective investigation. *S. Afr. Med. J.*, **75**, 233–235

Ferrari, M. (1993) Artificial tears and antocianosides therapy in video display operators with one year follow-up. *Clin. Ocul. Pathol. Ocul.*, **14**, 295–299

Gobbels, M. and Spitznas, M. (1989) Influence of artificial tears on corneal epithelium in dry eye syndrome. *Graefes Arch. Exp. Ophthalmol.*, **227**, 139–141

Gobbels, M. and Spitznas, M. (1991) Effects of artificial tears on corneal epithelial permeability in dry eyes. *Graefes Arch. Clin. Exp. Ophthalmol.*, **229**, 345–349

Gobbels, M. and Spitznas, M. (1992) Corneal epithelial permeability of dry eyes before and after treatment with artificial tears. *Ophthalmology*, **99**, 873–878

Green, K. *et al.* (1992) Tear potassium contributes to maintenance of corneal thickness. *Ophthalmic Res.*, **24**, 99–102

Heiligenhaus, A. *et al.* (1994) Therapy in tear film deficiencies. *Klin. Monatsbl. Augenheilk.*, **204**, 162–168

Heiligenhaus, A. *et al.* (1995) Diagnosis and differentiation in tear film deficiencies. *Ophthalmologie*, **92**, 6–11

Hollis, F. J. and Lemp, M. A. (1977) Tear physiology and dry eyes. *Survey of Ophthalmology*, **22**, 69–87

Holly, F. J. (1978) The preocular tear film. *Contact Lens J.*, 52–55

Hill, J. C. (1989) Slow release artficial tear inserts in the treatment of dry eyes in patients with rheumatoid arthritis. *Br. J. Ophthalmol.*, **73**, 151–154

Kaufman, H. E. *et al.* (1994) Collagen based drug delivery and artificial tears. *J. Ocul. Pharmacol.*, **10**, 17–27

Leibowitz, R. A. (1993) Pilot trial of cyclosporine 1% ophthalmic ointment in the treatment of keratoconjunctivitis sicca. *Cornea*, **12**, 315–323

Limberg, M. B. *et al.* (1987) Topical application of hyaluronic acid and chrondroitin sulphate in the treatment of dry eyes. *Am. J. Ophthalmol.*, **103**, 194–197

Lindahl, G., Calissendorff, B. and Carle, B. (1988) Clinical trial of sustained release artificial tears in keratoconjunctivitis sicca and Sjögren's syndrome. *Acta Ophthalmol.*, **66**, 9–14

Marquadt, R., Christ, T. and Bonfils, P. (1987) Gel-like tear substitute products and nonspecific eye ointments in intensive care units and in perioperative usage. *Anaesth. Intensivther. Notfallmed.*, **5**, 236–251

Marquadt, R. (1986) The treatment of dry eye with a new liquid gel. *Klinische Monatsbl. Augenheilk.*, **189**, 51–54

Palmer, R. M. and Kaufman, H. E. (1995) Tear film, pharmacology of eye drops and toxicity. *Curr. Opin. Ophthalmol.*, **6**, 11–16

Rapinese, M. *et al.* (1994) Effects of artificial tears on lacrimal film in VDU workers. *Ann. Ophthalmol. Clin. Ocul.*, **120**, 109–112

Snibson, G. R. *et al.* (1992) Ocular surface residence times of artificial tear solutions. *Cornea*, **11**, 288–293

Ubels, J. L. *et al.* (1995) Effects of preservative free artificial tear solutions on corneal epithelial structure and function. *Arch. Ophthalmol.*, **113**, 371–378

Van Bijsterveld (1988) Action of carbopolymer gel therapy (*Vidisc*) on the lacrimal function parameters in keratoconjunctivitis sicca. *Z. Prakt. Augen.*, **9**, 151–154

14

Contact lens solutions

Contact lens solutions are as old as contact lenses. The first description of a contact lens was given by Fick in 1888 who experimented with different solutions to fill the space between the cornea and the back surface of the glass scleral shell. He found that a 2% solution of 'grape sugar' (i.e. dextrose) was suitable for this purpose. In 1892, Dor reported that having first tried a glucose solution and then an artificial serum, 'physiological saline' was satisfactory and it formed the basis of contact lens solutions for many years thereafter.

It was the advent of rigid corneal lenses manufactured from the oxygen-impermeable material polymethylmethacyrlate (PMMA), in the late 1940s which encouraged the popular use of contact lenses as an alternative to spectacles. Commercially produced contact lens solutions date from this period. Initially two types of solution were introduced, one for 'wetting' which was intended to promote tear flow over the PMMA surfaces and another for 'soaking' with which the storage case was filled in order to achieve disinfection of the contact lenses. A later development was the introduction of daily surfactant cleaners and subsequently dual-, triple- and multipurpose solutions were introduced in an endeavour to simplify the lens care regimen and to enhance compliance with its proper use. Gas permeable rigid materials, which evolved rapidly from the 1970s, tend to be more susceptible to deposits than PMMA but less so than hydrogels.

Hydrogel, or soft, contact lenses were introduced in the 1960s and became widely available a decade later. Their arrival necessitated the development of new systems of lens care. For example, benzalkonium chloride, an effective preservative which had been used extensively in rigid contact lens solutions, was found to bind to the hydrogel polymer. Soft lenses have a greater affinity for surface deposits than rigid lenses and this problem has been addressed by means of the following, alternative strategies:

1. The introduction of enzymatic cleaners intended for use about once a week.
2. The development of various 'deposit resistant' hydrogels.
3. Limitation of the 'lifetime' of the lenses. This option ranges from the 'planned replacement' of lenses after an interval of, for example, six months, to 'disposable lenses' which are discarded after one month of use or after one day's use.

The functions of the care products required by a contact lens patient will, therefore, vary according to the type of lens worn and its 'lifetime', and are illustrated in Table 14.1. The reasons for the use of contact lens solutions are as follows:

Table 14.1 The functions which need to be provided by care products in relation to the type of contact lens worn

Lens type	Daily cleaning	Disinfection	Enzymatic cleaning	'Comfort'
Rigid				
scleral	Essential	Essential	Optional	Optional
corneal	Essential	Essential	Optional	Optional
Soft				
planned or unscheduled replacement	Essential	Essential	Essential	Optional
monthly disposable	Essential	Essential	Not required	Optional
daily disposable	Not required	Not required	Not required	Optional

1. To facilitate contact lens wear (e.g. wetting solution for rigid lenses).
2. To maintain the optical and physical properties of the contact lens (e.g. storage solutions for hydrogel lenses).
3. To reduce the risk of infection (e.g. overnight storage of lenses in a solution which disinfects them).

Contact lens solutions should have the following ideal properties:

1. They should be sterile.
2. They should not discolour the lens (Wardlow and Sarver, 1986), or change its properties or parameters.
3. They should not be toxic or irritative to the eye.
4. Their mode of use should encourage patient compliance.

The daily routine for contact lens care

The hands are washed thoroughly and dried with a clean towel.

The contact lenses are removed from the storage case (or blister pack in the case of daily disposable soft lenses).

In the case of rigid lenses only, wetting solution (or one which performs this function) is applied to the lenses.

The lenses are inserted.

At the end of the wearing period, the hands are washed and dried thoroughly.

A surfactant cleaner (or a multipurpose one which performs this function) is applied and the lens is rubbed between the fingers to remove all debris. This step is not required with daily disposable lenses.

The lenses are rinsed with sterile saline and inspected. If they do not appear to be clean and clear, the previous step is repeated The lenses are placed in a storage case filled with a disinfecting solution (or one which performs this function) or simply discarded if they are of the daily disposable type.

All planned or unscheduled replacement soft lenses and some rigid gas permeable lenses will require the use of enzymatic cleaners, usually on a weekly basis.

Contact lens care solutions are now considered in a sequence which reflects this routine. While the various solutions required for contact lens care are described for convenience as dedicated purpose products, the reader should bear in mind the fact that an increasing number of solutions claim to fulfil more than one function. The use of multipurpose solutions has become popular since they are perceived to be a means of ensuring patient compliance with lens care.

Wetting solutions

Wetting solutions (or solutions which incorporate this function) are only required for rigid contact lenses. Such solutions contain a surface active agent which reduces the contact angle of tears on the contact lens surface. They provide the lens with a viscous 'coating' which encourages the lens to adhere to the finger during insertion. The solution also acts as a lubricant between the contact lens and cornea, thereby enhancing comfort.

Prior to the advent of wetting solutions, patients were sometimes encouraged to use saliva for this purpose. While being available at no cost and having good wetting and viscoelastic properties, its use involves an unacceptable microbiological hazard. It remains necessary to warn patients not to lick a lens in order to remove foreign matter on its surfaces.

Wetting solutions contain a wetting agent, a viscosity increasing agent and a preservative. The usual wetting agent used in wetting solutions is polyvinyl alcohol (PVA). This agent has been employed extensively in artificial tear formulations and also in eye drops to prolong the contact time in the conjunctival sac, achieving increased penetration. Thus, as well as acting as the wetting constituent, PVA also acts as the viscosity increasing agent. In some solutions, other agents such as cellulose derivatives are incorporated. There has been little agreement as to the proper level of viscosity that is required for wetting solutions.

Wetting solutions are applied to the lens following its removal from the storage case (i.e. to a disinfected lens). The function of the antimicrobial agent in a wetting solution is not therefore to disinfect the lens, but only to maintain the initial sterility of the solution in the bottle. The solution in the bottle is expected to be sterile, while that on the lens is not. It is important that the level of preservative is kept as low as possible while remaining effective in its function.

Benzalkonium chloride is an effective preservative which can be made more efficient by the addition of the chelating agent ethylene diamine tetra acetic acid (EDTA), but will interfere with tear film integrity if its concentration is too high. A concentration of 0.004% w/v benzalkonium chloride combined with EDTA will give both effectiveness and minimal adverse effect on the tear film.

Other preservatives may also be incorporated into rigid lens wetting solutions. Irrespective of any effect on the tear film, it is imperative that the concentration is kept to a minimum in order to reduce any toxic or allergic effects. Wetting solutions, by their very method of use, will be in contact with the eye for a prolonged period. Furthermore, they are used on a daily basis and the total exposure time to the eye is quite high.

Daily surfactant cleaner

With the exception of daily disposable soft lenses, the use of a daily cleaner is essential prior to disinfection of all contact lenses. These surfactant cleaners have a detergent action which enables them to emulsify lipids and some organic deposits.

Contact lenses attract a variety of contaminants, including fats and proteins from tears. Other contaminants will occur depending on the patient's lifestyle, e.g. nicotine (Broich *et al.*, 1980). Deposits occur both on rigid lenses (Fowler *et al.*, 1984) and on soft lenses of either low or high water content (Hosaka *et al.*, 1983). The level of deposit formation appears to be proportional to the water content of soft lenses (Fowler *et al.*, 1985), and is also influenced by the surface charge of the hydrogel. Ionic, high water content lenses have a greater affinity for protein deposits than nonionic lenses, and nonionic low water content lenses attract the least protein (Minarik and Rapp, 1989).

Daily cleaning of contact lenses:

1. Improves the clarity of the lens by removing mucus, lipids and other contaminants. These can become bound to the surface of the lens by the subsequent process of disinfection.
2. Prolongs the successful wearing time (Hesse *et al.*, 1982).
3. Reduces the level of microbiological contamination by physically removing contaminated debris. The preservatives in the solution are, of course, capable of achieving some disinfection. Indeed, Vogt *et al.* (1986) demonstrated the efficacy of cleaners on both rigid and soft lenses which had been contaminated with the AIDS virus (identified at that time as HTLV-III). A cleaner containing 20% isopropyl alcohol has been shown to be effective against the cyst of *Acanthamoeba culbertsoni* (Connor *et al.*, 1991). Although the AIDS virus, HIV, has been recovered from soft contact lenses and from tears, no case has yet been reported in which they were identified as the means of transmission of the disease (Slonim, 1995). The same alcohol based cleaner has been found to kill both trophozoites and cysts of *Acanthamoeba polyphaga* and *Acanthamoeba castellanii* (Penley *et al.*, 1989). It has been suggested (Donzis *et al.*, 1989) that bacterial and fungal contamination within the contact lens care system may be an important factor in the survival and growth of acanthamoebae. Such an assertion underlines the importance of rigorous daily cleaning.
4. Improves the efficacy of subsequent disinfection by exposing clean surfaces to this process.
5. Removes possible nutrients on which organisms can grow.
6. May reduce toxic effects from disinfection solutions since contaminants to which preservatives might bind have been removed.
7. Reduces the adherence of organisms to the lens. It has been shown that tear components absorbed onto the lens surface enhance the adherence of micro-organisms to lenses (Butrus and Klotz, 1986), but some may adhere even to clean lenses (Duran *et al.*, 1987).

These considerations demonstrate that daily cleaning is not just a prelude to the disinfection process but is an integral part of it. Failure to remove protein prior to disinfection with heat or hydrogen peroxide allows it to become denatured and act as an antigen.

Daily cleaners contain a surface active agent or detergent which reduces the surface tension of fats and other lipophilic substances. The surfactants may be nonionic, anionic or amphoteric. Nonionic surfactants are usually used with soft lenses in order to minimize interaction with the hydrogel material. As multi use solutions, they will also contain a preservative similar to those found in disinfecting solutions.

The formulations commonly include a chelating agent such as EDTA, phosphate or borate buffers, and sodium or potassium chloride which determines the tonicity of the solution.

There is no concern about toxicity of cleaning solutions since they should be rinsed thoroughly from the lens surface before it is disinfected. This step avoids the possibility of contaminating the soaking solution.

The mode of use of daily cleaners requires that after their application to the contact lens, its surface is rubbed between the fingers for some moments. An efficient rubbing action plays a role in decreasing contamination by micro-organisms such as *Acanthamoeba polyphaga* (Liedel and Begley, 1996). The rubbing with cleaner is followed by rinsing with a suitable solution such as sterile saline.

A study which compared the use of a dedicated cleaner as part of a care system with a multipurpose product showed that use of the former resulted in more comfortable and cleaner lenses (Lebow and Christenson, 1996).

Disinfecting solutions

With the exception of daily disposable soft lenses, all contact lenses need to be disinfected following their removal and cleaning. These solutions have also been described as soaking solutions since they act as a storage medium when the contact lenses are not being worn. If rigid lenses were stored dry, any organic contaminants on them would support the growth of micro-organisms. The surface wetting properties of some rigid gas permeable materials would be impaired by dry storage.

Wet storage of soft lenses is essential in order to maintain their hydration since they have a water content which can range from 38 to 80%.

There are three types of solution used to achieve disinfection of contact lenses:

1. A stable solution containing a preservative which has been formulated for use either with rigid contact lenses or with soft lenses.
2. A transient solution containing an antimicrobial agent which is inherently unstable and which is broken down by a neutralizer until none of the active ingredient remains. Such solutions were originally introduced for use with soft lenses but may also be used with rigid lenses.
3. A saline solution in which the lens is heated to at least 100°C. This thermal disinfection procedure can only be used with soft lenses.

Any system of disinfection should be effective not only on commonly used challenge bacteria such as *Staph. aureus, Pseud. aeruginosa* and *Escherichia coli*, but also on bacteria such as *Serratia marcescens* (Ahearn *et al.*, 1986; Parment *et al.*, 1986), *Haemophilus influenzae* (Armstrong *et al.*, 1984) and other organisms such as fungi (Churner and Cunningham, 1983; Brooks *et al.*, 1984) and acanthamoebae. Fungi in particular are a problem, as organisms can actually penetrate soft lenses (Bernstein, 1973; Filppi *et al.*, 1973).

Stable disinfecting solutions

These solutions contain one or more preservatives. Lenses may need several hours exposure to the solution in order to ensure adequate disinfection, whereas oxidative methods and thermal disinfection are much quicker (Kreis, 1972). The efficacy of this type of solution will be affected by several factors: the level of microbial contamination, the volume of solution in the storage case and the temperature.

As mentioned earlier, the use of a daily cleaner will do much to reduce the bacterial contamination before the lens is immersed in the disinfection solution. Attention has previously been drawn to the importance of good personal hygiene such as thorough hand washing before the lens is handled. This precaution can reduce the burden placed upon the disinfecting solution.

Storage solutions must be changed regularly. Although it may look the same as when it was poured from the bottle, it steadily loses its effectiveness. In over half of the 217 cases (reported by Barry and Ruben, 1978) who exhibited contact lens related problems, bacteria were isolated from the storage cases. Some of the preservatives will have been taken up by contamination and dead bacteria. Contaminants will also provide protection for bacteria from the antimicrobial agent. Reports of eye infections in contact lens wearers are often the result of the use of contaminated storage cases. The storage case must be compatible with both the solution and the lens, which must be completely immersed to ensure its disinfection.

Disinfecting solutions formulated for rigid lenses contain a variety of preservatives, including chlorhexidine, benzalkonium chloride, thiomersal and chlorbutol. EDTA is often present as a synergistic agent.

Norton *et al.* (1974) tested the antimicrobial efficacies of contact lens solutions containing a variety of preservatives, including those mentioned above. They found a range of activity ranging from adequate to very inadequate. Studies on solutions of preservatives alone have shown benzalkonium chloride to be the most effective against *Staph. aureus* and *Pseud. aeruginosa*.

The original disinfecting solutions for soft lenses contained the same preservatives, with the exception of benzalkonium chloride which binds to hydrogel materials. It has been claimed by Rosenthal *et al.* (1986) that benzalkonium chloride also binds to rigid gas permeable materials in a manner different to that of chlorhexidine. Chlorhexidine binding is limited to a monomolecular layer, but benzalkonium chloride builds a self propagating multilayer which reduces surface wettability. In a study of *in vivo* and *in vitro* absorption of benzalkonium chloride, Wong *et al.* (1986) demonstrated that rigid gas permeable lenses did not accumulate significant levels of the preservative. A study by Chapman *et al.* (1990) showed that the level of benzalkonium chloride which can be released from either soft or rigid lenses is of sufficient concentration to be at, or near, the upper limit of safety.

It is of course important that preservatives do not react with any container in which they are placed. Richardson *et al.* (1977) found that some preservatives, particularly thiomersal, reacted markedly with the plastic bottle, with the result that the concentration fell below the labelled value.

Disinfecting solutions have been implicated in the development of toxic or allergic reactions, especially solutions intended for use with soft lenses. Wilson *et al.* (1981) examined 38 patients with ocular signs and symptoms related to soft lens wear. All the solutions used by the patients contained thiomersal, and 27 of the patients responded positively to thiomersal patch testing.

Wright and Mackie (1982) examined patients with conjunctival irritation and reduced lens tolerance. They found that organic mercurials such as thiomersal were heavily implicated as the cause of the symptoms. Similar results were reported by Mondino and Groden (1980), who reported conjunctival hyperemia and anterior stromal infiltrates in three soft lens wearers who had used solutions containing thiomersal.

Soaking solutions have traditionally been rendered isotonic by the addition of sodium chloride or other electrolytes, but a non-electrolyte tonicity agent has been used for this purpose. It had been assumed that a sodium chloride equivalent of 0.9% would provide the best solution but Kempster (1984) studied the effect of soaking lenses in solutions of different tonicities and found that those between 1.0 and 1.1% w/v produced minimal changes in corneal thickness. A randomized double masked study by Fletcher and Brennan (1993) demonstrated that both hypotonic and hypertonic solutions can produce ocular discomfort. Discomfort was minimal with a saline solution having a 1.3% (w/v) concentration.

Multipurpose solutions which are intended to both clean and disinfect soft contact lenses commonly use polyquaternium (polyquad) or polyaminopropyl biguanide (polyhexanide/*Dymed*) as the preservative in concentrations of 0.0011% and 0.0001%, respectively. These polyquats are related to chlorhexidine but have a larger molecular size which does not allow them to penetrate the matrix of hydrogels. While a relatively high concentration (0.0005%) of polyhexanide is effective against acanthamoebae, its use appears to be associated with significantly higher levels of corneal staining, especially with nonionic high water content lenses (Jones *et al.*, 1997). High molecular weight surfactants such as poloxamine/poloxamer are included in multipurpose solutions. Parment *et al.* (1996) found that lenses treated with polyquaternium preserved solutions can still harbour bacteria such as *Pseudomonas aeruginosa* and *Serratia marcescens*.

Multipurpose solutions for use with rigid lenses have similarly adopted preservatives such as polyhexanide and also polixetonium chloride.

Transient disinfecting solutions

Oxidizing agents such as iodine, hydrogen peroxide and chlorine have antimicrobial effects especially against anaerobes. Various iodine based products have been introduced from time to time, but all have fallen into disuse. The brown coloured iodine solution was reduced by a neutralizing agent to the inactive colourless iodide, the reaction producing a mixture of electrolytes, none of which were foreign to the eyes.

Solutions of hydrogen peroxide continue to be used extensively. Hydrogen peroxide has been used for many years as a surface disinfectant and for its bleaching effect. Its strength can be described in terms of volumes (i.e. 10 volume, 20 volume, etc.). A 10 volume solution possesses 10 times its volume of oxygen when it breaks down. In terms of percentage, a 10 volume solution is about 3% w/v. Tragakis et al. (1973) found that hydrogen peroxide was very effective against all the organisms used in their tests and similar results were obtained by Penley et al. (1985). A further advantage of hydrogen peroxide is that it employs no preservatives, which can always pose the threat of a toxic or allergic reaction.

When used to disinfect contact lenses, it is necessary to neutralize the peroxide after an interval of time and various methods have been used to achieve its breakdown. Originally, having soaked the lenses in peroxide for five minutes, they were then exposed to sodium bicarbonate (0.5% w/v) to accomplish neutralization (Isen, 1972). Following two changes of saline, the lenses were stored overnight in fresh saline. The time consuming nature of this multistep process prevented the popular use of hydrogen peroxide until simpler means of neutralization were developed.

One system (AOSept) uses a platinum disc in the storage case as a catalyst to break down the peroxide into oxygen and water. Having filled the case with 3% (w/v) peroxide, there is an initial rapid phase of neutralization resulting in a concentration of 0.9% (w/v) after two minutes which is followed by a slow phase to approximately 15 parts per million (ppm) after six hours. Such a level is below the threshold of subjective sensitivity (50–300 ppm) and that at which adverse effects on the mitotic activity and movement of epithelial cells occur (30 ppm) (Tripathi and Tripathi, 1989). In order to maintain efficacy of neutralization, the disc is replaced every time further supplies of peroxide are purchased. Since the patient is required to undertake only one procedure, this is described as a 'one step' system.

Another 'one step' system uses a coated tablet containing catalase which is slowly released with reactive neutralization to a final peroxide level of 1 ppm after about two hours.

Sodium pyruvate (0.5% w/v) is also used as an agent to reactively neutralize hydrogen peroxide in a 'two step' system. Pyruvic acid is an intermediate in the breakdown of glucose in the glycolytic cycle and is a normal constituent of cells. Another 'two step' system utilizes sodium thiosulphate to neutralize the hydrogen peroxide.

It is important that neutralization of the peroxide does not take place too rapidly, since Holden (1990) has warned that a short exposure of 10 to 15 mins is inadequate to ensure disinfection of fungi and acanthamoebae, and he recommended a period of at least two hours.

The pH of hydrogen peroxide is in the range of 3.5 to 4.5 (McKenney, 1990), and the patient who omits to neutralize it before inserting a lens into the eye will make this mistake only once due to the resultant degree of discomfort! After neutralization, the final pH is between 6.15 to 7.64 and the level of residual peroxide is 0 to 70 ppm (Harris, 1990). Any discomfort experienced by patients using hydrogen peroxide is therefore likely to be due to pH rather than the residual concentration. It would appear to be a wise precaution to advise patients to rinse their lenses liberally with sterile saline prior to insertion.

Although a two step hydrogen peroxide system is compatible with non-ionic high water content soft lenses, ionic high water content lenses undergo marked hydration changes. Lowe et al. (1993) concluded that the latter lens type should not be used with this peroxide method.

Microbiological contamination of the contact lens storage case regularly receives attention as a possible source of infection in wearers. Wilson et al. (1990) found that cases disinfected with peroxide systems showed a lower level of microbial contamination than those in which other methods of disinfection had been used. Frequent replacement of the storage case remains the best means of avoiding the risk of its contamination (Devonshire et al., 1993) .

Chlorine, which like other halogens acts a disinfectant and mild cleaning agent, is liberated by two products one of which contains dichloro-sulphamoyl benzoic acid (halozone) and another containing sodium dichloro-isocyanurate. Both products liberate their active agents from tablets which are dissolved in unpreserved saline. According to Copley (1989) and Ferreira et al. (1991), chlorine provides effective disinfection of clean soft lenses, but one such system tested by Lowe et al. (1992) failed to meet the United States Food and Drug Administration recommendations for bacterial challenge.

Although all transient disinfecting solutions were developed for use with soft lenses, they may also be used with rigid lenses.

Saline solutions

Mention has already been made of the important role played by sterile saline solutions in 'rinsing' contact lenses.

Saline is also used as a medium for various enzymatic cleaners which are mentioned later. Another use of saline is to fill the storage case of soft lenses when they are subjected to thermal disinfection. This method of disinfection requires that the lenses in their storage case are placed in either an electrical heater or in a small vacuum flask which is filled with boiling water.

In a study of nine different heating units, the maximum temperature of the contents of the case were found to be between 78°C and 92°C (Liubinas et al., 1987). These temperatures were considered to be too high and these authors recommended one between 70°C and 80°C over a period of five minutes. Similarly, Stone et al. (1984) recommended that the lenses should be subjected to temperatures over 50°C for a minimum time and 80°C for 10 minutes has been recommended by other authors (Busschaert et al., 1978). Even higher temperatures were recorded in a study by Garner (1982). The temperatures attained are sufficient to kill all vegetative organisms and most spores, providing the biological burden is not too great. Thermal disinfection is an effective method against

Acanthamoeba culbertsoni but some cysts can survive this procedure (Connor *et al.*, 1989).

Although heat disinfection of soft contact lenses offers the advantages of efficacy, low cost and absence of preservatives, it is now seldom used. The fact that heating tended to shorten the lifetime of lenses is no longer a disadvantage in view of the common use of disposable or planned replacement types.

Saline solutions should have a pH between 6.8 and 8 and an osmolarity between 280 and 320 milliosmoles per litre in order to ensure comfort and compatibility with hydrogels. Saline has been made available in various forms.

Salt tablets

In the early 1970s, salt tablets were supplied so that they could be dissolved in the correct amount of purified water in order to produce normal saline for use with heat disinfection. However, purified water is water that has been purified chemically and not microbiologically; it can thus be heavily contaminated (Jenkins and Phillips, 1986). Indeed, this method of producing saline was implicated in the outbreak of *Acanthamoeba* keratitis in contact lens wearers. Three such cases were reported by Moore *et al.* (1986) in which patients were initially diagnosed as suffering from Herpes simplex keratitis or 'overwear syndrome', whereas cultures from the solution bottles revealed the presence of acanthamoebae. The authors concluded that the use of patient prepared saline should be discouraged. Salt tablets for such use are no longer sold in the United Kingdom.

Preserved saline

Preserved saline has been used to enhance the efficacy of heat disinfection but is generally used today to rinse contact lenses. The function of preservatives in saline solutions is to maintain solution sterility and not to provide a means of contact lens disinfection. Preservatives can pose the risk of allergic and toxic reactions. Shaw (1980) demonstrated the relationship between preservatives and the incidence of solution allergy. In a double masked randomized crossover study, six subjects used an unpreserved saline solution and a preserved saline solution (0.001% thiomersal and 0.1% EDTA). These subjects had a probable history of sensitivity to preserved solutions which was confirmed in this investigation.

Preserved saline solutions containing EDTA as part of the preservative system have a useful deposit resistant effect compared with an unpreserved saline solution (Moore *et al.*, 1980).

Purite, a form of stabilized chlorite, has been adopted as the preservative in a saline solution. The chlorite acts as an oxidizing agent and is combined with chlorate and a trace amount of chlorine dioxide. Chlorine dioxide free radicals which are effective against bacteria, viruses, yeasts and fungi are generated in the presence of microbial contamination.

Hydrogen peroxide (0.006%) is present in one saline being derived from the buffer system following the conversion of sodium perborate to boric acid. When the solution is in contact with the eye, the hydrogen peroxide is rapidly reduced to water and oxygen by catalase and other enzymes present in the conjunctival sac. This saline might impair the action of chlorine based disinfection systems.

Single use sachets   Available both preserved and unpreserved, sachets have the major advantage of remaining sterile until opened. Their disadvantage is the greater cost.

Pressurized containers   Both buffered and unbuffered forms of sterile saline are available in aerosol type containers. This mode of presentation of saline requires no preservatives.

Enzymatic cleaners   Tablets containing an enzyme are dissolved in either saline or distilled water in order to remove protein deposits from the surfaces of contact lenses. They were originally introduced for use about once a week with hydrogel lenses, but may if necessary also be used with rigid contact lenses. Fluorine is present in rigid gas permeable lenses in order to provide good oxygen permeability and has relatively low surface energy, which reduces the adhesion of deposits.

A film of protein, mainly lysozyme (Hosaka *et al.*, 1983) but with amounts of albumin and globulin from the tears, can build up on lenses and be difficult to remove with the surfactants in the daily cleaning solutions. Treatment with proteolytic enzymes is necessary to remove this form of contamination. Proteins are macromolecules composed of chains of amino acids which are linked by peptide bonds. Proteolytic enzymes hydrolyse these bonds either at the end of the molecule, stripping off units of amino acids each time, or by breaking the protein into smaller and smaller multi amino acid segments. The former are called exopeptidases and the latter endopeptidases. Like all enzymes, the proteolytic enzymes have optimum working conditions, i.e. temperature and pH. Tonicity does not seem to be so important, as some tablets can be used in saline while others can be used in purified water. Another property which enzymes share with all proteins is the possibility of producing allergic reactions. Bernstein *et al.* (1984) reported a case of local anaphylaxis resulting from the use of papain and a similar case was reported by Santucci *et al.* (1985).

Papain, one of the enzymes used in protein remover tablets, is a thermostable endopeptidase found in the pawpaw fruit. Other enzymatic cleaners utilize pronase, pancreatin or subtilisin. Pronase is comprised of a bacterial protease, a lipase and a pronase and pancreatin is composed of protease, a lipase and an amylase. Subtilisin is derived from the bacterium *Bacillus lichenformis*. In a comparison of the efficacy of papain and subtilisin, the former proved to be better with medium and heavy deposits and the latter was better with light deposits (Larcabal *et al.*, 1989).

Although hydrogen peroxide cannot be used as a solvent for papain since it is rendered ineffective, it can be used with pronase and subtilisin resulting in enhanced disinfectant action.

It has been suggested that enzymatic cleaners are unnecessary when hydrogen peroxide is used for disinfection because this agent causes swelling which is followed by shrinkage upon neutralization and these changes might be thought to dislodge surface contamination. However, when chemical disinfection and enzymatic cleaning was compared with oxidative disinfection alone (Lasswell *et al.*, 1986), the lenses treated by the former method were significantly cleaner than those treated by the latter.

The use of protein removing tablets is not an alternative to daily cleaners since the two agents are complementary. Lenses treated with either type of cleaner were contaminated more than those treated with both (Fowler and Allansmith, 1981).

Comfort drops

These drops, which are also referred to as conditioning or cushioning drops, may be instilled into the eyes of contact lens wearers in order to enhance comfort.

The eye can tolerate adverse atmospheric conditions, and while it can also tolerate the wearing of contact lenses, it sometimes has difficulty in coping with both. In particular, dry smoky environments can produce changes in the lens-tears system which turns an acceptable situation into an intolerable one. Certain drugs such as antihistamines, which have an antimuscarinic effect, can reduce contact lens tolerance. Hormonal changes in women can also modify the quantity or quality of tears. In such situations an in use comfort drop may be used. They are in reality artificial tears with one extra property, i.e. lens compatibility. They contain a viscosity increasing substance and, if intended for use with rigid lenses, a wetting agent. If they are in a multidose presentation, the drops will contain a suitable preservative.

As comfort drops are for 'in use', that is to be applied to the eye while the lens is being worn, the requirement for preservative concentration is the same as for wetting solutions, i.e. the concentration must be kept as low as possible. For rigid lenses, there are formulations containing polyvinyl alcohol and benzalkonium chloride. The concentration of the latter should not exceed 0.004% w/v for reasons considered in the section on wetting solutions. In the case of soft lenses, the problem of preservative binding to the hydrogel reduces the available options. For this reason, single dose unpreserved saline can be used as comfort drops.

Sibley and Lauck (1974) reviewed the usefulness of comfort drops and concluded that their use reduced patient problems and increased comfort. However, Efron *et al.* (1990) found that any enhancement of the pre-lens tear film is only transient and that the level of hydration of soft lenses is unchanged.

Alternative methods of soft contact lens disinfection

Electrical systems employing ultraviolet light and/or ultrasound have been shown to be only partially effective when subjected to a microbiological challenge (Phillips *et al.*, 1989; Palmer *et al.*, 1991; Scanlon, 1991).

However, Dolman and Dobrogowski (1989) found that a 253.7 nm ultraviolet light with an intensity of 1100 $\mu W/cm^2$ achieved satisfactory disinfection with short exposure times. A suspension of 104/ml *Acanthamoeba polyphaga* was sterilized in less than three minutes. Harris *et al.* (1993) similarly concluded that ultraviolet radiation of this wavelength is an effective and rapid method of disinfecting contact lenses.

According to Harris *et al.* (1989), a standard 600 W microwave oven can provide effective and rapid (90 secs) disinfection of soft lenses and up to 40 lenses can be disinfected at the same time.

Hygienic care of trial lenses

The simplest method of care of rigid trial lenses is to make thorough use of a surfactant cleaner before and after their use, to dry them thoroughly and store them dry. Disinfection can be provided by 10 mins immersion in hydrogen peroxide. Peroxide disinfection of rigid corneal lenses can cause a clinically insignificant flattening of the back optic zone radius (Boltz *et al.*, 1993). Certain rigid gas permeable materials may require constant immersion in a liquid in order to maintain optimal surface wetting. When trial lenses are stored in a preserved soaking solution, it must be changed regularly in order to maintain active disinfection.

The use of disposable soft lenses allows the practitioner to undertake fitting and wearing trials with freshly opened, sterile lenses. After assessment or a period of wear the lenses are discarded. Nondisposable soft trial lenses should be thoroughly cleaned after use and autoclaved. An autoclave sterilizes soft lenses by heating them to a temperature of about 121°C which is maintained for 15 to 20 minutes.

In a comparison of heat disinfection, hydrogen peroxide and a multipurpose solution for the disinfection of soft trial lenses, heat was shown to produce the lowest rate of bacterial contamination. It was concluded by Simmons *et al.* (1996) that practitioners using a hydrogen peroxide or multipurpose system should disinfect trial lenses at least once a month.

Patient education

It is the practitioner's responsibility to train patients in order to ensure that contact lens care products are used correctly and safely. It is important to mention the risks associated with contact lens wear and to review signs and symptoms of ocular infection. At each aftercare appointment it is essential to review the procedures actually being followed by the patient in an endeavour to maintain compliance with advice previously given. When contact lens wear is terminated for a period of more than 24 hours, the patient must be advised of the need to disinfect them before further wear. All solutions and the contact lens storage case should be replaced frequently. It is inadvisable to use simultaneously lens care products from different manufacturers due to possible incompatibility of preservatives, pH, etc. Patients should be warned not to use solutions which have passed their expiry date.

References

Ahearn, D. G., Penley, C. A. and Wilson, L. A. (1986) Growth and survival of *Serratia marcescens* in hard contact lens wetting solutions. *CLAO J.*, **10**, 172–174

Armstrong, J. R., Cohen, K. C. and McCarthy, L. R. (1984) *Haemophilus influenzae* corneal ulcer in a therapeutic contact lens wearer. *Br. J. Ophthalmol.*, **68**, 188–191

Barry, D. J. and Ruben, M. (1978) Contact lens injuries. An analysis of 217 consecutive patients presenting to Moorfields casualty department. *Contact Lens J.*, **9**, 6–10

Bernstein, D. I., Gallagher, J. S., Grad, M. and Bernstein, I. L. (1984) Local ocular anaphylaxis to papain enzyme contained in a contact lens cleaning solution. *J. Allerg Clin. Immunol.*, **74**, 258–260

Bernstein, H. N. (1973) Fungal growth into a bionite hydrophilic contact lens. *Ann. Ophthalmol.*, March, 317–322

Boltz, R. L., Leach, N. E., Piccolo, M. G. and Peltzer, B. (1993) The effect of repeated disinfection of rigid gas permeable lens materials using 3% hydrogen peroxide. *Internat. Contact Lens Clinic*, **20**, 215–221

Broich, J. R., Weiss, L., and Rapp, J. (1980) Isolation and identification of biologically active contaminants from soft contact lenses. *Invest. Ophthalmol. Vis. Sci.*, **19**, 1328–1335

Brooks, A. M. V., Lazarus, M. G. and Weiner, J. M. (1984) Soft contact lens contamination by *Alternaria alternaria*. *Med. J. Aust.*, **2**, 490–491

Busschaert, S. C., Good, R. C. and Szabocsik, A. (1978) Evaluation of thermal disinfection procedures for hydrophilic contact lenses. *Appl. Environ. Microbiol.*, **35**, 618–621

Butrus, S. I. and Klotz, S. A. (1986) Blocking *Candida* adherence to contact lenses. *Curr. Eye Res.*, **5**, 745–750

Chapman, J. M., Cheeks, L. and Green, K. (1990) Interactions of benzalkonium chloride with soft and hard contact lenses. *Arch. Ophthalmol.*, **108**, 244–246

Churner. R. and Cunningharn. R. D (1983) Fungal contaminated soft contact lenses. *Ann. Ophthalmol.*, **15**, 724–727

Connor, C. G., Blocker, Y. and Pitts, D. G. (1989) *Acanthamoeba culbertsoni* and contact lens disinfection systems. *Optom. Vis. Sci.*, **66**, 690–693

Connor, C. G., Hopkins, S. L. and Salisbury, R .D. (1991) Effectivity of contact lens disinfection systems against *Acanthamoeba culbertsoni*. *Optom. Vis. Sci.*, **68**, 138–141

Copley, C. A. (1989) Chlorine disinfection of soft contact lenses. *Clin. Exp. Optom.*, **72**, 3–7

Devonshire, P., Munro, F. A., Abernethy, C. and Clark, B. J. (1993) Microbial contamination of contact lens cases in the west of Scotland. *Br. J. Ophthalmol.*, **77**, 41–45

Dolman, P. J. and Dobrogowski, M. J. (1989) Contact lens disinfection by ultraviolet light. *Am. J. Ophthalmol.*, **108**, 665–669

Donzis, P. B., Mondino, B. J., Weissman, B. A. and Bruckner, D. A. (1989) Microbial analysis of contact lens care systems contaminated with acanthamoeba. *Am. J. Ophthalmol.*, **108**, 53–56

Dor, H. (1892) Sur les verres du contact. *Rév. Gen. d'Ophthalmol.*, **11**, 493–497

Duran, J. A., Refojo, M. F., Gipson, I. K. and Kenyon, K. R. (1987) *Pseudomonas* attachment to new hydrogel contact lenses. *Arch. Ophthalmol.*, **105**, 106–108

Efron, N., Golding, T. R. and Brennan, N. A. (1990) Do in–eye lubricants for contact lens wearers really work? *Transactions BCLA Conference*, 14–19

Ferreira, J. T., Kriel, F., van der Merwe, D. and Pheiffer, G. (1991) Efficacy of chlorine disinfection of soft contact lenses. *Optom. Vis. Sci.*, **68**, 718–720

Fick, A. E. (1888) Eine Contactbrille. *Arch. Augenheilk.*, **18**, 279–289

Filippi, J. A., Pfister, R. M. and Hill, R. M. (1973) Penetration of hydrophilic contact lenses by *Aspergillus fumagatus*. *Am. J. Optom.*, **50**, 553–557

Fletcher, E. L. and Brennan, N. A. (1993) The effect of solution tonicity on the eye. *Clin. Exp. Optom.*, **76**, 17–21

Fowler, S. A. and Allansmith, M. R. (1981) The effect of cleaning soft contact lenses. *Arch. Ophthalmol.*, **99**, 1382–1386

Fowler, S. A., Korb, D. R., Finnemore, D. R. and Allansmith, M. R. (1984) Surface deposits on worn hard contact lenses. *Arch. Ophthalmol.*, **102**, 757–759

Fowler, S. A., Korb, D. R., Finnemore, V. M. and Allansmith, M. R. (1985) Deposits on soft contact lenses of various water contents. *CLAO J.*, **11**, 124–127

Garner, L. F. (1982) A comparison of some heat disinfection methods for soft contact lenses. *Aust. J. Optom.*, **65**, 32–34

Harris, M. G., Kirby, J. E., Tornatore, C. W. and Wrightnour, J. A. (1989) Microwave disinfection of soft contact lenses. *Optom. Vis. Sci.*, **66**, 82–86

Harris, M. G. (1990) Practical considerations in the use of hydrogen peroxide disinfection systems. *CLAO J.*, **16**, S53–S60

Harris, M. G., Fluss, L., Lem, A. and Leong, H. (1993) Ultraviolet disinfection of contact lenses. *Optom. Vis. Sci.*, **70**, 839–842

Hesse, R. J., Kneisser, G., Fukushima, A. and Yamaguchi, T. (1982) Soft contact lens cleaning. A scanning electron microscope study. *Contact and Intraocular Lens Medical Journal*, **8**, 23–28

Holden, B. (1990) A report on hydrogen peroxide for contact lens disinfection. *CLAO. J.*, **16**, S61–S64

Hosaka, S. *et al.* (1983) Analysis of deposits on high water content contact lenses. *J. Biomed. Mat. Res.*, **17**, 261–274

Isen, M. G. (1972) The Griifin lens. *J. Am. Optom. Assoc.*, **43**, 275–286

Jenkins, C. and Phillips, A. J. (1986) How sterile is preserved saline? *Clin. Exp. Optom.*, **69**, 131

Jones, L., Jones, D. and Houlford, M. (1997) Clinical comparison of three polyhexanide preserved multipurpose contact lens solutions. *Contact Lens Anterior Eye*, **20**, 23–30

Kempster, A. J. (1984) The effect of soft contact lens soaking solutions on corneal thickness. *J. Contact Lens Assoc.*, **7**, 137–142

Kreis, F. (1972) La stérilisation des lentilles souples hydrophiles. *Arch. Ophthalmol. Paris*, **32**, 825–829

Larcabal, J. E., Hinrichs, C. A., Edrington, T. B. and Kurishige, L. T. (1989) A comparison study of enzymatic cleaners: papain versus subtilisin A. *Int. Contact Lens Clinic*, **16**, 318–321

Laswell, L. A., Tarantino, N., Kono, D. L., Frank, J. and Nelson, N. E. (1986) Chemical vs. oxidative disinfection of high water content extended wear lenses. *Int. Eyecare*, **2**, 615–618

Lebow, K. and Christenson, B. (1996) Cleaning efficacy and patient comfort: a clinical comparison of two contact lens care systems. *Int. Contact Lens Clinic*, **23**, 87–92

Liedel, K. K. and Begley, C. G. (1996) The effectiveness of soft contact lens disinfection systems against acanthamoeba on the lens surface. *J. Am. Optom. Assoc.*, **67**, 135–142

Liubinas, J., Swenson, G. and Carney, L. G. (1987) Thermal disinfection of contact lenses. *Clin. Exp. Optom.*, **70**, 8–14

Lowe, R., Vallas, V. and Brennan, N. A. (1992) Comparative efficacy of contact lens disinfection solutions. *CLAO J.*, **18**, 34–40

Lowe, R., Harris, M. G., Lindsay, R. and Brennan, N. A. (1993) Hydration of high water content nonionic soft lenses during hydrogen peroxide disinfection. *Int. Contact Lens Clinic*, **20**, 145–148

McKenney, C. (1990) The effect of pH on hydrogel lens parameters and fitting characteristics after hydrogen peroxide disinfection. *Transactions BCLA Conference*, 46–51

Minarik, L. and Rapp, J. (1989) Protein deposits in individual hydrophilic contact lenses: effects of water and ionicity. *CLAO J.*, **15**, 185–188

Mondino, B. J. and Groden, L. R. (1980) Conjunctival hyperemia and corneal infiltration with chemically disinfected soft contact lenses. *Arch. Ophthalmol.*, **98**, 1767–1770

Moore, M., McCulley, J., Kaufman, H and Robin, J. (1980) Radial keratoneuritis as a presenting sign in *Ancanthamoeba* keratitis. *Ophthalmologica*, **93**, 1310

Moore, R. A., Satterberg, L. B., Weiss, S. and Shivery, C. D. (1986) Novel temperature dependent model for examining soilant deposition deterrant action. I. Preserved thermal disinfecting solutions. *Contacto*, **30**, 23–30

Norton, D. A., Davies, D. J. S., Richard. N. E., Meakin, B. J. and Keall, A. (1974) The antimicrobial efficiencies of contact lens solutions. *J. Pharm. Pharmacol.*, **26**, 841–846

Palmer, W., Scanlon, P. and McNulty, C. (1991) Efficacy of an ultraviolet light contact lens disinfection unit against microbial pathogenic organisms. *J. Br. Contact Lens Assoc.*, **14**, 13–16

Parment, P. A., Colucci, B. and Nystrom, B. (1996) The efficacy of soft contact lens disinfection solutions against *Serratia marcescens*. *Acta Ophthalmol.*, **74**, 235–237

Parment, P., Ronnerstam, R. and Walder, M. (1986) Persistance of *Serratia marcescens* and *E. coli* in solutions for contact lenses. *Acta Ophthalmol.*, **64**, 456–462

Penley, C. A., Llabres, C., Wilson, L. A. and Ahearn, D. G. (1985) Efficacy of hydrogen peroxide disinfection system for soft contact lenses contaminated with fungi. *CLAO J.*, **11**, 65–68

Penley, C. A., Willis, S. W. and Sickler, S. G. (1989) Comparative antimicrobial efficacy of soft and rigid gas permeable contact lens solutions against acanthamoeba. *CLAO J.*, **15**, 257–260

Phillips, A. J., Badenoch, P. and Copley, C. (1989) Ultrasound cleaning and disinfection of contact lenses: a preliminary report. *Trans. BCLA Conference*, 20–23

Richardson, N. E., Davies, D. J. G., Meakin, B. J. and Norton, D. A. (1977) Loss of antibacterial preservatives from contact lens solutions during storage. *J. Pharm. Pharmacol.*, **29**, 717–722

Rosenthal, P., Chou, M. H., Salamore, J. C. and Israel, S. C. (1986) Quantitative analysis of chlorhexidine gluconate and benzalkonium chloride adsorption on silicone/acrylate polymers. *CLAO J.*, **12**, 43–50

Santucci, B., Cristando, J. and Piccardo, A. (1985) Contact urticaria from papain in a soft lens solution. *Contact Dermatitis*, **12**, 233–237

Scanlon, P. (1991) Microbiological aspects of combined ultrasonic contact lens disinfection units. *J. Br. Contact Lens Ass.*, **14**, 55–59

Shaw, E. I. (1980) Allergies induced by contact lens solutions. *CLAO J.*, **6**, 273–277

Sibley, M. J. and Lauck, D. E. (1974) Contact lens conditioners. New solutions for old problems. *Contact Lens J.*, **8**, 10–12

Simmons, P. A., Edrington, T. B., Lao, K. F. and Le Concepcion, L. (1996) The efficacy of disinfection systems for in office storage of hydrogel contact lenses. *Int. Contact Lens Clinic*, **23**, 94–97

Slonim, C. B. (1995) AIDS and the contact lens practice. *CLAO J.*, **21**, 233–235

Stone, R. P., Braun, A., Kreutzer, P. and Smith, L. (1984) A new concept in heat disinfection. *Contact Lens J.*, **12**, 5–9

Tragakis, M. P., Brown, S. I. and Pearce, D. B. (1973) Bacteriologic studies of contamination associated with soft contact lenses. *Am. J. Ophthalmol.*, **75**, 496–499

Tripathi, B. J. and Tripathi, R. C. (1989) Hydrogen peroxide damage to human corneal epithelial cells *in vitro*. *Arch. Ophthalmol.*, **107**, 1516–1519

Vogt, M. W., Ho, D. D., Bakar, S. R. *et al.* (1986) Safe disinfection of contact lenses after contamination with HTLV–III. *Ophthalmology*, **93**, 771–774

Wardlow, J. C. and Sarver, M. D. (1986) Discolouration of hydrogel contact lenses under standard care regimens. *Am. J. Optom. Physiol. Opt.*, **63**, 403–408

Wilson, L. A., McNatt, J. and Reitschel, R. (1981) Delayed hypersensitivity to thiomersal in soft contact lens wearers. *Trans. Ophthalmol. Soc. UK*, **102**, 3–6

Wilson, L. A., Sawant, A. D., Simmons, R. B., and Ahearn, D. G. (1990) Microbial contamination of contact lens storage cases and solutions. *Am. J. Ophthalmol.*, **110**, 193–198

Wong, M. P., Dziabo, A. J. and Kirai, R. M. (1986) Adsorption of benzalkonium chloride by RGP lenses. *Contact Lens Forum*, **11** (5), 25–32

Wright, P. and Mackie, I. (1982) Preservative related problems in soft contact lens wearers. *Trans. Ophthalmol. Soc. UK*, **102**, 3–6

15

UK law

The use of drugs by optometrists in the United Kingdom is subject to control and regulation by Acts of Parliament in the same manner as the use of drugs by other health professionals or by patients. Much of the sale and supply of drugs is covered by the Medicines Act 1968, which is set out in eight parts and deals not only with sale and supply but also with the licensing of medicinal products, their manufacture or import and other matters such as advertising.

Part I   – Administration of the Act and setting up of Medicines
             Commission
Part II   – Licensing
             Manufacture
             Product licenses
             Import and export
             Clinical trial
Part III   – Sale and supply (see below)
Part IV   – Pharmacies
Part V   – Containers, labelling
Part VI   – Promotion and advertising
Part VII   – Publications, e.g. *British Pharmacopoeia*
Part VIII – Miscellaneous provisions

A medicinal product is a product intended for one or more of the following purposes:

treating medical conditions
preventing medical conditions
diagnosing medical conditions
contraception
otherwise modifying the physiological state of the body.

In addition, orders may be made to include products and devices not falling into one of the groups above. For example, an order made in 1976 brought contact lenses and contact lens solutions under some of the provisions of the Medicines Act.

Sale and supply of medicinal products is covered by Part III of the Act which categorizes products into three groups:

General Sale List
Pharmacy Medicines
Prescription Only Medicines.

General Sale List (GSL) – section 51

The medicines which are considered to be sufficiently safe that they can be supplied to the general public without supervision of a pharmacist are incorporated into a list of medicines called the General Sale List (SI 1980/1922). This list is very detailed and can for instance limit the quantity supplied in a container. For example 25 aspirin tablets are a General Sale List medicine, but a bottle of 100 such tablets is excluded from the list and becomes a pharmacy medicine. The list is constantly being updated and amended. Any retailer may sell a GSL medicine providing that he has lockable permanent premises. An optometric practice will certainly satisfy this criterion.

Eye drops and eye ointments are specifically excluded from the General Sale List, whether for human or animal use, irrespective of the drug they contain.

Pharmacy Medicines (P) – section 52

Pharmacy medicines are only available to the general public from a person lawfully conducting the business of a retail pharmacy, and the sale must be under the supervision of a registered pharmacist. Whereas there are legal lists of GSL and POM medicines, there is no legal list of Pharmacy medicines. Optometrists may supply any pharmacy medicine providing that the supply is (a) in line with his professional practice and is (b) in an emergency. This ability to supply P drugs is due to an amendment order made in 1978 (SI 1978/988).

Prescription Only Medicines (POM) – section 58

As its name suggests, these products are only available to the public on the prescription of a doctor, dentist or veterinary surgeon. The Prescription Only Medicine List (SI 1983/1212) is very detailed. For many agents there are exemptions from the requirements for a prescription if a maximum dose is specified or if the drug is presented in a particular form. A number of products are exempted, becoming pharmacy medicines if they are intended for external use, providing the external use is not ophthalmic. Eye drops and eye ointments of such compounds remain POM products.

Many of the mydriatics/cycloplegics, miotics, local anaesthetics and antimicrobial agents which the optometrist may wish to use are POM drugs. In order that he may have access to these drugs, specific exemptions are made for registered optometrists. One exemption allows the optometrist to supply the patient (directly or via a signed order to the pharmacist) with certain medicinal products, e.g. atropine or pilocarpine. The direct sale or supply must satisfy the same restrictions as for pharmacy medicines, namely that it must be in the course of the optometrist's professional practice and be in an emergency.

There is another group of drugs which the optometrist may obtain for use in his practice but may not supply to his patients under any circumstances, for example local anaesthetics.

The following is a list of drugs which the optometrist may supply (under the conditions stated above) to his patient as well as using them in practice.

Atropine sulphate
Bethanecol chloride
Chloramphenicol
Carbachol
Cyclopentolate hydrochloride
Homatropine hydrobromide
Hyoscine hydrobromide
Naphazoline hydrochloride or nitrate
Neostigmine methylsulphate
Physostigmine sulphate or salicylate
Pilocarpine nitrate or hydrochloride
Sulphacetamide sodium
Tropicamide
Any P medicine
Any GSL medicine.

The list of drugs covered by this regulation was initially much longer and included such drugs as ecothiopate, but it was amended in 1978 (SI 1978/987) and is currently incorporated in SI 1983/1212.

The following may only be used by the optometrist in his practice:

Amethocaine hydrochloride
Benoxinate hydrochloride (oxybuprocaine hydrochloride)
Framycetin sulphate
Lignocaine hydrochloride
Proxymetacaine hydrochloride
Thymoxamine hydrochloride.

This particular list of drugs is not included in the Prescription Only Medicines list, but is the subject of a miscellaneous order provision originally made in 1977 (SI 1977/2132) and subsequently modified in 1978 (SI 1978/989), and currently incorporated in SI 1980/1923. The modifications removed some obscure local anaesthetics and added framycetin.

Diagnostic drug formulary

Tables 15.1 and 15.2 list common drugs and preparations that are available for use as diagnostic and prophylactic agents. The normal volume of a container for eye drops is 10 ml and the weight of a tube of eye ointment is 4 g. Unit dose preparations are usually packed in boxes of 20. When the volumes of branded preparations vary from the above they will be stated. Products that are only available by special manufacture are excluded.

Acts of Parliament and statutory instruments

Medicines Act 1968, chapter 67.
The Medicines (General Sale List) Order 1984/769.
1980/1924. The Medicines (Pharmacy and General Sale–Exemptions) Amendment Order.
1983/1212. The Medicines (Products Other than Veterinary Drugs) (Prescription Only Order) The Medicines (Sale or Supply) (Miscellaneous Provisions) Amendment Regulations 1978/989.

Table 15.1 Mydriatics/cycloplegics, miotics and local anaesthetics

Category	Drug	Availability	Branded preparations	Unit dose	Legal category	See page
Mydriatics/ cycloplegics	Atropine sulphate	0.5% w/v drops 1.0% w/w ointment	Isopto atropine 1.0% w/v 5 ml (contains a viscolizer)	Minims 1.0% w/v	POM	84
	Cyclopentolate hydrochloride		Mydrilate 0.5% w/v 5 ml Mydrilate 1.0% w/v 5 ml	Minims 0.5% w/v Minims 1.0% w/v	POM	86/103
	Homatropine hydrobromide	1.0% w/v drops		Minims 2.0% w/v	POM	91/103
	Phenylephrine hydrochloride	2.0% w/v drops 10.0% w/v drops		Minims 2.5% w/v Minims 10.0% w/v	P	90/103
	Tropicamide		Mydriacil 0.5% w/v 5 ml Mydriacil 1.0% w/v 5 ml	Minims 0.5% w/v Minims 1.0% w/v	POM	90/102
Miotics	Carbachol		Isopto carbachol 3.0% w/v (contains a viscolizer)		POM	115
	Pilocarpine Hydrochloride (or nitrate)	0.5% w/v drops 1.0% w/v drops 2.0% w/v drops 3.0% w/v drops 4.0% w/v drops	Isopto carpine 0.5% w/v Isopto carpine 1.0% w/v Isopto carpine 2.0% w/v Isopto carpine 3.0% w/v Isopto carpine 4.0% w/v (all viscolized preparations) Sno pilo 1.0% w/v Sno pilo 2.0% w/v Sno pilo 4.0% w/v (all viscolized preparations)	Minims 1.0% w/v Minims 2.0% w/v Minims 4.0% w/v	POM	113
Local anaesthetics	Amethocaine hydrochloride	0.5% w/v drops 1.0% w/v drops		Minims 0.5% w/v Minims 1.0% w/v	POM	128
	Benoxinate hydrochloride			Minims 0.4%	POM	127
	Lignocaine hydrochloride			Minims 4.0% with fluorescein sodium 0.25%	POM	128
	Proxymetcaine hydrochloride	0.5% w/v drops	Ophthaine 0.5% w/v 15 ml	Minims 0.5% w/v	POM	126

Table 15.2 Stains, antimicrobials, artificial tears and saline

Category	Drug	Availability	Branded preparations	Unit dose	Legal category	See page
Stains	Fluorescein sodium			Flurets (paper strips containing 1 mg) Minims 1.0% w/v Minims 2.0% w/v	P	133
	Rose bengal			Minims 1.0% w/v	P	136
Antimicrobials	Framycetin sulphate		Soframycin 0.5% w/v drops 8 ml Soframycin 0.5% w/w ointment 5 g		P	142
	Propamidine isethionate		Brolene 0.1% w/v drops		P	140
Artificial tears	Hypromellose	0.3 w/v drops 1.0% w/v drops	Isopto Alkaline 1.0% w/v drops Isopto Plain 0.5% w/v drops Tears Naturale 0.3% w/v drops (with dextran)		P	185
	Liquid paraffin		Lacrilube ointment 3.5 g		P	188
	Polyvinyl alcohol		Hypotears 1.0% w/v drops (with macrogol) Liquifilm Tears 1.4% w/v drops 15 ml Sno tears 1.4% w/v drops		P	186
	Carbomers		Gel Tears Viscotears		P	186
	Hydroxethyl-cellulose			Minims Artificial Tears	P	185
Saline	Sodium chloride			Minims 0.9% w/v		198
Miscellaneous	Antalozoline sulphate		Otrivine-Antistine 0.5% w/v drops (with xylometazoline 0.05% w/v)		P	157

16

Ocular first aid

As a professional involved in health care who is easily accessible to the public, the optometrist will from time to time be confronted by a variety of emergency situations, both ocular and general. The term 'First Aid' is very apt and it is important that procedures should be kept simple and to a minimum.

It is worth stating the underlying principles of first aid, which should govern the optometrist's action in an emergency situation.

1. *Separate the patient from the cause of the trauma*. If there is an external cause this should whenever possible be removed from the patient (e.g. a foreign body), or the patient from it. The important words are 'whenever possible' as there are situations in which this aim cannot be achieved or to do so would exacerbate the patient's condition. For example, intraocular and deeply embedded foreign bodies should be left for ophthalmological removal. On the other hand, superficial foreign bodies should be removed if possible and the elimination of chemical splashes on the eye must not be delayed, as in both cases damage will continue to develop while they are in contact with the eye.
2. *Relieve the patient's distress and make him as comfortable as possible*. This can be achieved to a great extent by reassurance from the optometrist. In many simple emergency cases, the patient will believe that he is more badly injured than he really is, so a confident approach will do much to dispel these fears. The commendable desire to relieve the patient's symptoms should not, however, lead to indiscriminate use of local anaesthetics.
3. *Seek medical assistance as soon as possible*. The implementation of first aid procedures should not delay the patient's referral for medical assistance.

The optometrist will of course be confronted by general emergencies as well as ocular ones. His patients are not immune from such conditions such as epistaxis (nosebleed), syncope (fainting) and heart attacks. It would thus be useful for the optometrist to periodically attend a short course in first aid techniques. In this chapter only ocular emergencies will be covered.

Whatever the emergency, traumatic or medical, serious or trivial, proper records must be kept of each case encountered and should include the following details.

1. Name and address of patient requesting attention.
2. Date of treatment.
3. Brief history and nature of injury, including the time it occurred.

4. Unaided vision and visual acuity with spectacles, if worn, of affected eye, at earliest suitable opportunity (usually after treatment, before bandaging).
5. The treatment administered, including any drugs used and advice given.
6. In all except minor cases the patient must be referred with a brief note, covering the details listed above, to his own doctor or a hospital eye department as appropriate. If the latter, as when specialized ophthalmological treatment is necessitated (for example, in the case of a perforating foreign body or severe chemical burn), a further report must be sent the same day to the patient's own general medical practitioner, with full details of the case including the procedure followed.

Equipment

A well equipped optometric practice will as a matter of course contain most of the instruments and drugs to cope with first aid requirements.

In addition, the following will be useful:

glass rods for everting the upper lids
cotton wool buds
nylon loop
small forceps
sterile cotton wool balls.

Careful clinical judgement is necessary in deciding as to whether or not an injured eye should be bandaged. Alternatively, the sterile cotton wool/gauze eyepad may be kept in place with a two inch wide (5.1 cm) strip of zinc oxide adhesive plaster extending diagonally from inner forehead to cheek. As Havener (1978) emphasizes, 'patching of an eye promotes the growth of any micro-organisms that may happen to be in this conjunctival sac'. After instillation of an anti-infective preparation, only the more seriously injured or painful eyes should be patched and then only for the shortest period appropriate for that particular case. Sometimes an eyepad is necessitated for superficial corneal abrasions to prevent the pain elicited by movements of the lid across the denuded area. Three hourly instillation of antibacterial eyedrops must be continued until epithelial healing and accompanying absence of discomfort allow discontinuation of drugs and removal of the eyepad.

In addition to the above, certain pharmaceutical agents will be required:

1. Local anaesthetics, e.g. benoxinate, amethocaine.
2. Fluorescein in some form, e.g. single use eyedrops or paper strips.
3. Antibacterial agents, e.g. chloramphenicol, framycetin.
4. Emollient drops, e.g. castor oil, liquid paraffin.
5. Normal saline for irrigation.

In most cases where irrigation is required, running water is probably the best medium as it is unlikely that sufficient volume of normal saline will be stocked.

Specific antidotes to cope with chemical injuries to the eye are not worth keeping, as dilution by irrigation is probably the best method.

Common ocular emergencies

The common ocular emergencies are:

superficial foreign body
intraocular foreign body
blow with a blunt instrument
chemical burns
thermal burns
exposure keratitis
acute closed angle glaucoma.

Superficial foreign body

This is the most common ocular emergency that is likely to be encountered and the stages of dealing with it are as follows:

history
local anaesthetic (if necessary)
location
removal
staining
visual acuity assessment
prophylaxis
records
corneal sensitivity.

History

It is very important to ascertain the circumstances in which the foreign body came in contact with the eye because in every case of superficial foreign body there is always the possibility of an intraocular foreign body, and the latter must be positively discounted rather than assumed to be absent. Foreign bodies which result from any kind of explosion however mild, or those thrown up by moving machinery can sometimes penetrate the eye rather than remaining on the surface.

Local anaesthetic

Foreign bodies cause discomfort and this in turn leads to reflex tearing and blepharospasm. The optometrist is thus confronted by an eye which is closed and difficult to open. Under these circumstances a local anaesthetic can be used to facilitate examination and to alleviate the patient's discomfort. Any of the usual topical anaesthetics are suitable – amethocaine, benoxinate, proxymetacaine or lignocaine.

   The use of local anaesthetic is only justified prior to the removal of a foreign body. Problems arise when local anaesthetics are used to relieve the discomfort which may remain after the foreign body has been removed. Attention has been drawn to the dangers of the overuse of local anaesthetics in the chapter on these agents (Chapter 9).

Location

The foreign body should be located if possible. It is not unknown for the reflex tearing to dislodge the object and do the optometrist's job for him. If the foreign body is not immediately visible on inspection it is probably trapped under the upper lid, necessitating eversion of the lid or even double eversion in order to locate it.

Removal

Providing that it is not embedded, the object can be removed either by irrigation with eye lotion or with the end of a cotton bud or nylon loop. If the particle is embedded, the patient should be immediately referred to the hospital accident and emergency department for medical treatment.

Staining

After removal of the foreign body, staining with fluorescein should be carried out in order to assess the extent of any disturbance to the corneal epithelium. This information will enable the optometrist to decide whether to refer the patient to his general practitioner or whether to ask the patient to return on a subsequent visit for re-examination.

Visual acuity assessment

The patient's visual acuity, both distance and near, should be included in the records kept of the incident.

Prophylaxis

In order to supplement the natural antibacterial action of tears, an antimicrobial such as chloramphenicol or framycetin may be instilled. It is debatable how much protection one drop will give considering the turnover rate of the tear film when the eye is inflamed. It will do no harm, providing it does not lead the practitioner into a false sense of security.

Records

As stated above, full and accurate records are essential and the point is reinforced here because it may be thought that a trivial event such as a foreign body which is easily removed does not warrant the writing up of records. It is just this kind of case which could lead to problems subsequently if full details of the history, drugs used, procedures carried out and the results of visual acuity measurement and corneal examination cannot be recalled.

Corneal sensitivity

Finally, if a local anaesthetic has been used it is important to check that sensitivity has returned to the eye. It would be ironic to say the least if the patient, having had a foreign body removed, were sent out onto the street in a condition in which he would be unaware of the entry of another one.

Intraocular foreign body

Whereas a superficial foreign body may be considered as a relatively trivial problem, an intraocular foreign body is a very serious event which always requires medical attention. Admittedly the eye will tolerate pieces of glass and plastic (for example intraocular lenses) relatively well compared with metals such as copper or iron or organic materials (vegetable or animal), but there is always the threat of infection either from the foreign body itself or by opportunistic organisms gaining access through the entry wound.

There is little an optometrist can do for a patient with an intraocular foreign body other than refer the patient for medical treatment. His greatest service to the patient is the discovery of such an invasion in doubtful cases. The foreign body may be visible by ophthalmoscopic examination, or the entry wound may be visible as a rivulet of aqueous. The entry wound may however not be visible, and the only indication of an intraocular foreign body may be the history. Any suspect case must be referred.

Blow with a blunt instrument   Although the bony orbit provides good protection against damage, some-times objects, e.g. squash balls, may penetrate this protection and impact on the eye. Even larger objects can exert such a force to the surrounding tissue as to cause fractures and ocular damage.

The result of a blow can be alarming, with marked swelling and bruis-ing. These will normally resolve spontaneously but there are serious sequelae to blows, e.g.

detached retina
cataract or lens subluxation
commotio retinae
traumatic macular degeneration
blowout fracture
iris damage (iridodialysis)
haemorrhage.

It is important after such an injury that careful ophthalmoscopy is carried out followed by an examination of ocular motility and eye position. If a blowout fracture has occurred, one or more extraocular muscles may become trapped, impeding eye movements, and herniation of orbital con-tents may result in enophthalmos. It is essential that visual acuity is also measured and recorded.

If there is any doubt about the integrity of the eye or other orbital struc-tures, the patient must be referred.

Chemical burns   Both strong acids and strong alkalis can cause damage, but the latter are far more harmful to ocular tissues. Chemical splashes can occur in indus-try and so the provision of safety glasses is necessary to reduce their occurrence. Potentially harmful substances can also be found in the home and the use of ammonia in 'mugging' constitutes another source of chemical splashes in the eye.

Whether acid or alkali, dilution is the best method of neutralization, preferably using running water. Specific antidotes are necessary and are unlikely to be kept in sufficient quantities to be effective. Irrigation should be maintained for about 20 minutes before referring the patient for medical attention.

Thermal burns   Thermal burns usually involve the face as well as the eye and the patient will probably be in great discomfort. There is no specific treatment and the patient should be referred for medical care as soon as possible.

Exposure keratitis   If the cornea is exposed to short wavelength ultraviolet light for a certain time, it develops a form of keratitis which normally occurs as snow blind-ness or arc eye (welder's flash). The patient will complain of a dry, gritty feeling. Arc eye drops containing adrenaline (a vasoconstrictor) and zinc sulphate (an astringent) have been used in the past, but these are not necessary as the condition is self resolving.

Acute closed angle
glaucoma

This condition can arise spontaneously or as a result of the use of a mydriatic in an eye with a very shallow anterior chamber. Incidence from both causes is very rare but the optometrist must be aware of the signs and symptoms in order to recognize this medical emergency. The patient experiences intense pain which may be severe enough to induce vomiting. The conjunctival blood vessels are dilated, giving the appearance to the inexperienced observer of conjunctivitis. The cornea loses transparency slightly because the high intraocular pressure causes it to imbibe water and swell, which the patient may report as seeing haloes around lights. Through the hazy cornea the pupil can be seen, often mid-dilated (Chandler, 1952) and probably noncircular. The pupil will not constrict to light, accommodation or to the action of miotics. The intraocular pressure, whether measured with a tonometer or assessed digitally, is very high. The situation is an emergency one, but does not require panic measures. Providing the intraocular pressure is reduced over the ensuing few hours, there should be no long lasting damage.

Although the iris will not react to miotics because of ischaemia, one should still be administered. When the pressure is reduced by systemic methods it will be present in the aqueous ready to exert its action. A drop of 2% pilocarpine eyedrops should be given to both eyes and repeated at 10 minute intervals (Norden, 1978). There are several first aid methods of trying to reduce the pressure systemically and the decision whether to use one of these or not will depend on the proximity and availability of expert medical help. The use of glycerol (glycerine) has been recommended as an osmotic agent which can be given orally in orange juice in order to reduce the intraocular pressure sufficiently to allow the miotic to act. About 250 ml of glycerol has been suggested as the amount required for a 70 kg adult (Norden, 1978), but this may not be acceptable to the patient and 100 ml may be more appropriate. If the patient is diabetic, it may be advisable to omit this part of the treatment. In any case, the patient should be referred to an ophthalmologist as an emergency.

References

Chandler, C. (1952) Narrow angle glaucoma. *Arch. Ophthalmol.*, **47**, 695–716
Havener, W.H. (1978) *Ocular Pharmacology*, 4th edn. St. Louis: Mosby
Norden, L. C. (1978) Adverse reactions to topical autonomic agents. *JAOA*, **48**, 75–80

Adverse ocular reactions to systemic drug treatment

For a long time it has been realized that some systemic conditions such as diabetes and systemic hypertension may have ophthalmic complications, and it has been essential for the optometrist to take a general medical history before examining the patient. With the realization that the drugs used to treat these systemic conditions can also have effects on the eye, it is now also necessary to find out which drugs the patient may be taking. It is important that patients should be questioned on drugs which they purchase for themselves (over the counter or o.t.c. drugs) as well as prescription medicines. Kofoed (1986) reported that 40% of patients over 60 use o.t.c. medicines every day. Because they are not considered drugs by patients, they are thought to be safe.

In taking history with regard to medicine, the three 'Ds' are important: namely Drug, Dosage and Duration.

Drug

Patients on long term therapy are very often most knowledgeable about the medicines they are taking, especially if they are being purchased over the counter instead of being prescribed. For any particular drug, the likelihood of a drug causing an undesirable ocular side effect depends on three factors: prevalence of the condition for which it is prescribed, prescribing habits, and therapeutic index.

Prevalence of the condition

Some pathological conditions are far more common than others, although this may depend on the particular geographical location. In the United Kingdom, patients are far more likely to be suffering from systemic hypertension, rheumatoid arthritis and upper respiratory tract infections than they are from leprosy and malaria.

Prescribing habits

Many drugs have a definite life cycle and go through phases of introduction and growth before becoming standard treatments. Afterwards they go into decline as newer agents are developed and may eventually be discontinued. The amount of drug prescribed during the different phases will vary greatly. Some drugs, however, endure for a long time, notable examples being pilocarpine, aspirin and penicillin.

Therapeutic index

This is a measure of the drug's safety and is the ratio of the lethal dose (LD50) to the effective dose (ED50). The higher the ratio, the safer the drug. Some agents such as the antibiotics have a very high therapeutic index, while drugs used in the treatment of neoplasms have a very low ratio and their use is only justified by the very serious nature of the condition for which they are given. Much pharmaceutical research is aimed at producing drugs with a better therapeutic ratio or formulating existing drugs to maximize the useful effects while reducing as far as possible the unwanted ones.

Dosage

Some drugs have more than one indication and the dosage used for these indications varies greatly. For example, hydroxychloroquine can be used in three ways: to prevent malaria, to treat malaria and to relieve rheumatoid arthritis. The dose for malaria prophylaxis is much lower than for its treatment, with the antiarthritic dose being somewhere in the middle. A patient taking a low dose for a few weeks during and after a trip abroad is most unlikely to exhibit any retinal effects.

Duration

Patients can become tolerant to the side effects of drugs, especially if they are relatively mild, e.g. small pupil size changes and a loss of accommodation. Such effects are often noted when the treatment is first commenced but as it continues, they become less and less noticeable.

On the other hand, some side effects are cumulative and only make an appearance when the drug is taken for a long time. For example, steroid cataracts are only normally seen after a year's treatment.

Patient variability

Not all patients will exhibit adverse ocular effects. In fact, even when the patient is taking a drug with a well established causal relationship with a particular side effect, it is by no means certain that the patient will eventually develop that problem.

Factors which can influence the occurrence of adverse reactions are:

age
sex
weight
general state of health
ophthalmic state of health
concurrent medication
contact lenses.

Age

Children's metabolism is different to that of adults and they can be subject to certain adverse drug reactions that would not affect adults. For example, aspirin is contraindicated in children under 12 because it may cause a serious condition called Reye's syndrome, but is safe for patients over that age.

At the other end of the age spectrum, elderly people may not be able to metabolize and detoxify pharmaceutical agents as quickly as younger patients.

Sex

Some drugs interfere with tear production; this is more likely to embarrass middleaged women who have a greater tendency to become tear deficient than men. Of course, sex hormones may have bizarre effects on the opposite sex. There is another way in which the sexes differ and that is in the fat/water ratio of the body. For a given weight, women contain a slightly higher level of fat than men. Drugs which partition between fat and water will behave slightly differently in the two sexes. Sometimes drugs can be taken up by fat stores.

Weight

Weight can influence the incidence of adverse effects in two ways. Overweight people contain proportionally more fat than thin people and therefore variation in the fat/water ratios will occur. Secondly, the larger the body, the smaller will be the plasma levels resulting from the administration of a given dose of drug. This is especially important in the case of children, who will require proportionally less drug to produce the same effect.

General state of health

Liver and kidney problems will reduce the rate of clearance of drugs and lead to cumulative problems with some drugs.

Ophthalmic state of health

A dilated pupil may be annoying and if the patient has a narrow anterior chamber angle closure is a possibility, although this is not a common occurrence. Similarly, a slightly constricted pupil may only cause a minor problem in normal patients, but if an early central lens opacity is present then the miosis will be a greater problem.

Concurrent medication

Drug interaction is always a possibility when the patient is receiving more than one medicament, even if they are being given by two different routes.

Contact lenses

The successful wearing of contact lenses relies on a normal tear film. If this is reduced in quantity or quality (e.g. a lack of mucin) then the patient may experience problems which a non-wearer would not.

Adverse ocular effects of drugs

These can vary from the mildly irritating, transient effects to the serious, cumulative, toxic, sight threatening effects. Unfortunately, in much of the general literature on drugs, ocular adverse side effects are listed merely as 'visual disturbances', 'decreased vision' or 'blurred vision'. There are many underlying causes of such a report. The following are just some of them:

cyclospasm
cycloplegia
corneal oedema
media changes
optic neuritis
retinal changes.

Additionally, a patient may also complain of blurred vision if he fails to wear his proper refractive correction.

The causes vary from the trivial to the very serious and the optometrist is in an ideal situation to be able to differentiate between them.

The most common ocular effects are:

decreased tolerance to contact lenses
cataract
decreased accommodation and/or mydriasis
raised intraocular pressure
retinal pathologies
diplopia.

Sources of information

The number and range of products on the market is ever changing and it is difficult always to be aware of the changes in medicinal products. There are many sources of information which are produced mainly with the medical practitioner in mind but which will be a valuable aid to the optometrist if he gains access to them.

Data sheets are produced by the manufacturing company and must be supplied to a doctor if requested. A data sheet carries information such as trade mark, ingredients, indications, dosage and warnings, adverse effects, etc. They are constantly updated where necessary as new information becomes available.

Data Sheet Compendium is a collation of all the data sheets of the products produced by the member companies of the Association of British Pharmaceutical Industry.

MIMS (Monthly Index of Medical Specialities) is a list of all branded medicines (and some unbranded ones) currently on the United Kingdom market. It carries similar information to the data sheet but in a much more concise form. This reference source is published in a magazine format by Haymarket Publishing Services Ltd.

BNF (British National Formulary) covers all drugs, both branded and generic, and gives a comparison between agents having similar therapeutic effects. It is published every six months jointly by the British Medical Association and the Royal Pharmaceutical Society of Great Britain. The *BNF* carries a supply of yellow cards for the reporting of adverse effects to the Committee on the Safety of Medicines (CSM). If the drug is considered to be a new chemical entity (NCE) then an inverted black triangle will be displayed alongside the approved name of the compound in any product literature or publication. The CSM requires reporting of all adverse reactions to the drug, irrespective of the nature of severity.

For existing well established drugs, only serious side effects are reported. Well known trivial side effects do not need to be notified to the CSM.

Yellow cards have also been issued to optometrists for reporting unwanted side effects of contact lenses, contact lens solutions and other medicinal products used or sold by optometrists or dispensing opticians. This will of course include diagnostic drugs, although the emphasis of the optometrist reporting scheme appears to be on contact lens wear. The form requires the following information:

1. Name, sex and age of the patient.
2. Type of contact lens and reason for wearing it.

3. Contact lens fluid used.
4. Other ophthalmic medication.
5. Systemic medication.
6. Adverse reaction.
7. Comments.
8. Details of reporting practitioner.

The optometrist yellow card scheme only covers medicinal products which the optometrist uses himself. It does not cover drugs prescribed by the medical practitioner or over-the-counter drugs.

The College of Optometrists has a reporting scheme of ocular adverse effects of all drugs which has been in operation for some years.

Both *MIMS* and the *BNF* have a classification in which drugs are broken down into groups according to the anatomical system on which they act. A similar classification will be used in this text to describe some of the more important drugs and their possible ocular effects. The list is not exhaustive and the examples quoted merely give a guide to the more common drugs and their side effects. Under each heading, the following information will be included:

Indications and usage
Common examples and trade marks and
Common ocular adverse reactions.

Drugs acting on the alimentary tract

When drugs are administered orally, the alimentary tract is the first system with which they come in contact. Medicines such as antacids, ulcer healing drugs, laxatives and preparations for the relief of diarrhoea are administered for their action on the gut and often do not require absorption to produce their effect. For this reason they can be considered as topical agents. Modern drugs are designed or formulated to remain in the gut and to be poorly absorbed. Occasionally absorption does take place from the gut and adverse reactions are possible.

The gut is innervated by the autonomic nervous system and stimulation of the parasympathetic division causes increased motility and secretions. Antispasmodics are drugs which have antimuscarinic actions and are used to relieve gastrointestinal spasms, peptic ulceration and irritable bowel syndrome.

Examples

Dicyclomine (Merbentyl)
Hyoscine (Buscopan)
Propantheline (Probanthine)

Ocular adverse effects

As would be predicted, the ocular adverse effects are mydriasis and cyclo-plegia, which are mild and transitory. There is a theoretical contra-indication for glaucoma sufferers, but there have been few actual cases of closed angle glaucoma resulting from their use.

Drugs acting on the cardiovascular system

These drugs can influence the eye in two ways. First, they can have direct pharmacological effects on the ocular tissues, but they can also cause effects indirectly by producing fluctuations in blood pressure and blood flow. For example, systemic hypertension and glaucoma can coexist, with the former condition masking the other by maintaining the ocular perfusion. If the blood pressure is reduced by antihypertensives, then symptoms of glaucoma may become manifest.

Drugs in this class can be divided into the following groups:

cardiotonic drugs
diuretics
antiarrhythmic drugs
beta blockers
antihypertensives
anticoagulants.

Cardiotonic drugs

The best known drugs in this group are the cardiac glycosides which are found in digitalis, in particular digoxin.

Examples

Digoxin (Lanoxin)
Lanatoside C (Cedilanid)
Disopyramide (Rythmodan)

Ocular adverse effects

Digitalis produces toxic effects on the retina which are manifested by a disturbance in colour vision and a glare phenomenon in which objects appear to be surrounded by a white halo. Changes in the ERG and visual field may be recorded. Intraocular pressure is reduced, but digitalis produces insufficient effect to be considered as a glaucoma treatment. A case of mydriasis and cycloplegia equal to that of atropine eye drops was reported after using large doses of disopyramide (Frucht *et al.*, 1984).

Diuretics

Diuretics promote the flow of urine and are prescribed to reduce oedema in heart failure, essential hypertension, renal dysfunction and other conditions where the water/electrolyte balance of the body is disturbed. There are several different types of diuretic, varying from the very potent loop diuretics through the moderate diuretics such as the thiazides and carbonic anhydrase inhibitors to the mild potassium sparing agents.

Examples

Acetazolamide (carbonic anydrase inhibitor) (Diamox)
Bendrofluazide (thiazide) (Aprinox)
Bumetanide (loop diuretic) (Burinex)
Spironolactone (potassium sparing) (Aldactone)
Triamterene (potassium sparing) (Dytac)

Ocular adverse effects

Diuretics are used extensively in modern medicine but produce few ocular adverse reactions. A slight myopia is the most common effect but this usually regresses spontaneously.

Anti-arrhythmic drugs

There are several types of cardiac arrhythmia, e.g.

atrial fibrillation
atrial flutter

supraventricular tachycardia and
ventricular arrhythmias.

Different drugs are used for the different types.

Examples	Amiodarone (Cordarone X) Disopyramide (Rythmodan) Verapamil (Cordilox)
Ocular adverse effects	Disopyramide is used in ventricular arrhythmias and has a membrane stabilizing effect. It also has an anticholinergic action which can affect the eye, producing blurred vision and mydriasis. If the filtration angle is narrow then glaucoma is a possible problem. Amiodarone produces yellow brown deposits in the cornea. This is a fairly common occurrence, and is related to the total dose given. Vortex patterns of deposits are produced in 90% of patients who take the drug for more than a few weeks (Wright, 1978). The deposits will disappear slowly after discontinuation. There have been a few cases of blurred vision.

Beta blockers

These drugs will be well known to the optometrist for their use in the treatment of glaucoma. Their major use however is in the treatment of cardiovascular problems such as hypertension, angina and cardiac arrhythmias.

Examples	Atenolol (Tenormin) Labetalol (Trandate) Metoprolol (Betaloc) Oxprenolol (Trasicor) Propranolol (Inderal)
Ocular adverse reactions	Most beta blockers are relatively safe and the unwanted ocular side effects they produce are mild and transient. Practolol (which now has very restricted use) produced an oculomucocutaneous syndrome which was very severe in a number of patients, depending on the duration of treatment. The effect was reversible in the early stages, but if the treatment continued then blindness ensued.

Antihypertensives

Essential benign hypertension is one of the most commonly occurring conditions, for which there is a variety of methods of treatment including beta blockers, diuretics (mentioned above) and centrally acting drugs. Severe hypertension is treated with vasodilator drugs such as hydralazine.

Examples	Clonidine (Catapres) Methyldopa (Aldomet) Hydralazine (Apresoline)
Ocular adverse reactions	Retinal changes have been reported following the use of clonidine, leading to visual loss. Methyldopa on the other hand affects the anterior eye,

possibly being involved with cases of keratoconjunctivitis sicca. Both drugs reduce IOP.

Hydralazine produced a syndrome resembling systemic lupus erythematosus, with accompanying bilateral retinal vasculitis (Doherty *et al.*, 1985).

Drugs acting on the respiratory system

Respiratory tract infections and bronchospastic conditions figure highly amongst the general practitioner workload. For the latter condition, inhalers and insufflators are often the route of administration, and because this form of treatment is more local than systemic, side effects tend to be limited.

The following drugs are administered systemically for the treatment of respiratory disorders:

corticosteroids (see below)
antihistamines and
bronchodilators.

Antihistamines

Antihistamines are employed in the treatment of hay fever and are combined with vasoconstrictors for the topical relief of some upper respiratory tract conditions. Many antihistamines have antimuscarinic actions and it is this property which can lead to ocular adverse side effects.

Examples

Chlorpheniramine (Piriton)
Promethazine (Phenergan)
Terfenadine (Triludan)
Trimeprazine (Vallergan)

Ocular adverse effects

Many drugs in this group have antimuscarinic actions as well as antihistaminic and, as would be predicted, a slight mydriasis and cycloplegia are the most common adverse reactions. In addition the lacrimal gland may be affected, leading to depressed secretion of tears. Contact lens wearers may be particularly affected, but sometimes the tear flow is so reduced that the signs and symptoms of keratoconjunctivitis sicca appear.

Bronchodilators

Bronchoconstriction is brought about by the contraction of the smooth muscle which is innervated by the parasympathetic nervous system. This effect can be reversed by antimuscarinic drugs or by sympathomimetic amines. The tendency today is to use sympathomimetic agents because their effects are less. Sympathomimetics are also used in some common cold remedies which are purchased over the counter.

Examples

Ephedrine
Orciprenaline (Alupent)
Pseudoephedrine (Sudafed)
Salbutamol (Ventolin)
Terbutaline (Bricanyl)

Ocular adverse effects   A slight mydriasis is the principal adverse effect arising from the use of antihistamines. Large doses of ephedrine can lead to visual hallucinations (Chaplin, 1984).

Drugs acting on the central nervous system

There are many different types of central nervous system agents and together they represent a large proportion of the prescriptions issued in the United Kingdom. Many of the tissues in the eye, particularly the retina, have neural origins and it is therefore likely that these agents will have effects on the eye. They can also affect the centres in the brain which are responsible for controlling the eye, producing such effects as diplopia.

CNS drugs can be divided into the following groups:

Hypnotics and sedatives
Anti-Parkinsonism agents
Antipsychotic agents
Anxiolytic agents
Anticonvulsants
Antidepressants.

Hypnotics and sedatives

Hypnotics are drugs prescribed to treat insomnia. In the past, the barbiturates were the major group of drugs used for this purpose. However, because of their addictive properties they have fallen out of favour to a large extent and have been replaced by the benzodiazepines.

Examples

Amylobarbitone (Amytal)
Flurazepam (Dalmane)
Glutethimide (Doriden)
Nitrazepam (Mogadon)
Quinalbarbitone (Tuinal)
Temazepam (Normison)
Zolpidem (Stilnoct)
Zopiclone (Zimovane)

Ocular adverse effects

Hypnotics are designed to be used short term and when used in this manner will produce few unwanted side effects. Habitual users of barbiturates may experience problems of the extraocular musculature leading to decreased convergence or nystagmus.

Benzodiazepines have relatively few effects and if they do occur they are normally reversible. Patients sometimes complain of blurred vision caused by either loss of accommodation or abnormal extraocular movements.

Anti-Parkinsonism agents

Drugs used to treat Parkinson's disease can be divided into antimuscarinic drugs and dopaminergic drugs, which either increase the levels of dopamine in the brain or act directly with the dopamine receptors.

Examples

Amantadine (Symmetrel)
Benzhexol (Artane)

Levodopa (Larodopa) (levodopa is often combined with benserazide as
co-beneldopa or carbidopa as co-careldopa)
Orphenadrine (Disipal)

Ocular adverse effects   Amantadine produces few adverse effects apart from visual hallucinations. Antimuscarinic agents include benzhexol and orphenadrine, and
their effects include a loss of accommodation and a mydriasis which can
be sufficient to cause a closed angle glaucoma in patients whose angle
is narrow.

Levodopa produces variable effects. On the pupil, an initial mydriasis is
followed by a more persistent miosis. Effects on the lid include ptosis in
some patients and intense blepharospasm in others. Involuntary eye
movements have also been reported (Davidson and Rennie, 1986).

Antipsychotic agents

This group is sometimes called the major tranquillizers or neuroleptics.
The term tranquillizer is confusing as often this effect is secondary to
the principal antipsychotic action. They do not have a hypnotic effect
and are used to relieve conditions such as schizophrenia and severe
anxiety.

Examples   Chlorpromazine (Largactil)
Haloperidol (Serenace)
Promazine (Sparine)
Thioridazine (Melleril)
Trifluoroperazine (Stelazine)

Ocular adverse effects   Most of the drugs listed above (with the exception of haloperidol) belong
to the group known as the phenothiazines, of which the best known is
chlorpromazine. The use of these agents is relatively safe in the short
term, but with longer use the possibility of adverse effects increases.
Like many other classes of drugs, phenothiazines have varying degrees
of antimuscarinic effects and these can affect the iris and ciliary muscles,
producing mydriasis and cycloplegia.

Chlorpromazine, in chronic therapy, produces pigmentary deposits in
the eye which first appear on the lens surface, usually in the pupillary
area, then Descemet's membrane becomes affected. The deposits are
rarely found in the corneal epithelium. This effect may continue even
after the drug is discontinued. Skin pigmentation can also occur and
this affects up to 1% of patients who have received large doses for long
periods. Corneal deposits occur in 15% of such patients. As the total
dosage increases, so does the percentage of patients affected (Bernstein,
1977). The deposits do not appear to interfere with vision and the lens
deposits are unlikely to lead to development of cataract (Davidson,
1980). Phenothiazines can however cause a retinopathy which is dependent on the total dose administered, and results in visual problems
(Spiteri and Geraint James, 1983).

Haloperidol (a member of the butyrophenone group) may produce
mydriasis.

Anxiolytic agents

In contrast to the foregoing group, anxiolytics are sometimes known as the minor tranquillizers. By far the biggest group of drugs in this class is the benzodiazepines, which are some of the most widely prescribed drugs, and there is a tendency to prescribe them for any stress related condition. They are really intended for short term use but unfortunately become used chronically, with the development of dependence and withdrawal symptoms on discontinuation.

Examples

Clorazepate (Tranxene)
Diazepam (Valium)
Lorazepam (Ativan)

Ocular adverse effects

There are few ocular adverse reactions to these drugs and those which do occur are reversible. Decreased accommodation and a reduction in corneal reflex may be noted. Some patients can exhibit an allergy to these drugs which can manifest in the eye as allergic conjunctivitis and can cause particular problems to contact lens wearers.

Anticonvulsants

These are drugs used to treat epilepsy by suppressing fits. It is important that the dose of drug be titrated for each patient. The dosage and frequency should be the lowest possible in order to achieve control.

Examples

Carbamazepine (Tegretol)
Ethosuximide (Zarontin)
Lamotrigine (Lamictal)
Phenytoin (Epanutin)
Primidone (Mysoline)
Sodium Valproate (Epilim)
Vigabatrin (Sabril)

Ocular adverse effects

Nystagmus and diplopia are more commonly the result of overdose than normal side effects, and will often regress if the dosage is reduced. Phenytoin had a transient effect on the ERG when the drug was perfused through the retinae of rabbits (Honda *et al.*, 1973). A case of Stevens-Johnson syndrome following phenytoin therapy has been reported (Greenberg *et al.*, 1971). Blurred vision is a reported side effect to most drugs in this group.

Antidepressants

The more modern tricyclic antidepressants have to a large extent superseded the use of monoamine oxidase inhibitors (MAOI) because of the latter's potentially dangerous interactions with some drugs and particular foods (e.g. cheese). Antidepressants are used to treat depressive illnesses, and like the previous group of drugs it is vital that the dosage is carefully controlled. Some of these drugs have marked sedative properties (e.g. amitriptyline), while in others this effect is much less (e.g. imipramine).

These in turn have been replaced by the selective serotonin reuptake inhibitors such as fluoxetine (Prozac).

Examples	Amitriptyline (Tryptizol)
	Fluoxetine (Prozac)
	Imipramine (Tofranil)
	Nortriptyline (Aventyl)
	Paroxetine (Seroxat)
	Sertraline (Lustral)
	Tranylcypromine (Parnate)
	Trimipramine (Surmontil)
	Venlafaxine (Efexor)

Ocular adverse effects

All tricyclic antidepressants have anticholinergic effects to some extent and because they can produce mydriasis and cycloplegia, they are contra-indicated in glaucoma. The effects are reversible and will subside even with continuation of therapy. The lacrimal gland can become affected and the tear flow embarrassed, leading to problems for contact lens wearers.

Monoamine oxidase inhibitors potentiate the effects of sympatho-mimetics and anticholinergics and care should be taken with the use of mydriatics.

Drugs used in the treatment of infections

There are many different types of organism which can cause infections and a whole range of different compounds must be used to treat them. Although anti-infective drugs are widely prescribed, side effects are relatively rare. The course of treatment tends to be short and cumulative effects do not have time to develop. Also, anti-infective agents, because of their normally high specificity for the invading micro-organism, have a high therapeutic index.

However, some anti-infectives do require long term therapy and ocular adverse reactions can appear. The following groups will be considered:

antibiotics
urinary antiseptics
antitubercular drugs
anthelminthics
antimalarials.

Antibiotics

Agents in this class are used for the treatment of bacterial infections and are some of the most widely prescribed compounds in medicine. For most indications (e.g. upper respiratory tract infections) the treatment lasts for a few days, but in the treatment of acne, antibiotics are prescribed for months rather than days. Ideally the organism should be tested for sensitivity before an antibiotic is prescribed, but in practice therapy is started and modified if necessary.

Examples

These are groups rather than individual drugs:

Penicillins, e.g. penicillin, ampicillin, amoxycillin
Cephalosporins, e.g. cephaloridine, cephalexin, cefuroxime

Tetracyclines, e.g. chlortetracycline, tetracycline, oxytetracycline
Aminoglycosides, e.g. gentamicin, neomycin
Macrolides, e.g. erythromycin
4-quinolones e.g. ciprofloxacin
Metronidazole
Others, e.g. clindamycin
Sulphonamides

Ocular adverse effects

Of the above, only tetracyclines have been reported to cause ocular adverse reactions. As well as transient myopia and colour vision defects, ocular effects secondary to the penetration of the drug into the cerebro-spinal fluid (such as papilloedema and diplopia) have been reported. Tetracyclines can be secreted in tears and stain soft contact lenses (Aucamp, 1980).

Some antibiotics, e.g. penicillin, can produce allergic responses which may involve ocular tissues.

Sulphonamides have been reported to cause keratoconjunctivitis sicca in dogs (Slatter and Blogg, 1978).

Urinary antiseptics

As their name suggests, these agents are used in the treatment of urinary tract infections.

Examples

Nalidixic acid (Negram)
Nitrofurantoin (Furadantin)

Ocular adverse effects

Ocular irritation and profuse lacrimation leading to problems for contact lens wearers can result from the use of nitrofurantoin, but such problems will regress on drug discontinuation.

Nalidixic acid can affect colour vision and produce symptoms of glare, effects which are also reversible when the drug is stopped.

Antitubercular agents

The treatment of tuberculosis is a very long term problem because the causative organism, *Mycobacterium tuberculosum*, has a very slow meta-bolism and grows at a very slow rate. It takes a long time to eradicate the organism and resident strains can occur. Multitherapy is often applied to overcome the latter problem.

Examples

Ethambutol (Myambutol)
Rifampicin (Rifinah)
Isoniazid (used in combination with other drugs)
Streptomycin

Ocular adverse effects

Rifampicin produces a pink coloured byproduct which can be excreted in tears and will colour soft contact lenses (Ingram, 1986). It can also cause a conjunctivitis which varies in severity.

Ethambutol is well known for producing optic neuritis, which is slowly reversible in some patients but permanent in others. The optic neuritis takes two forms, an axial and a paraxial form. The axial form affects the central fibres of the optic nerve producing changes in colour vision. Loss of central visual acuity and macular degeneration are often the result. The paraxial form on the other hand produces visual field defects, with central acuity and colour vision remaining unaffected.

Toxic effects on the optic nerve can also develop from the use of isoniazid and streptomycin (Spiteri and Geraint James, 1983).

Antimalarials

Probably the main use of these compounds is for the prophylaxis of malaria by travellers to malaria endemic regions, rather than in the treatment of the condition. There are also other uses for some of the antimalarials, e.g. quinine can be used for the relief of night cramps and chloroquine and hydroxychloroquine can be used in the treatment of rheumatoid arthritis.

Examples

Chloroquine (Avlocor, Nivaquine)
Hydroxychloroquine (Plaquenil)
Mefloquine (Lariam)
Quinine

Ocular adverse effects

The adverse effects of these drugs are well known. Both retina and cornea can be affected, although the two effects are unrelated and can appear independently of one another. Effects on the cornea include deposits in the superficial cornea and subepithelial layers, which appear greyish white (Sinabulya, 1977), as well as an increased touch threshold and aggravation of existing keratoconjunctivitis sicca. The corneal deposits are often symptomatic (Bernstein, 1977) and do not indicate the discontinuation of therapy.

Pigmentary changes occur in the retina, giving rise to the well-known 'bulls eye maculopathy' (Sinabulya, 1977). Constricted visual fields and scotomata are accompanied by changes in the ERG. The condition is dose related and will continue to develop even if the drug is discontinued. One case of retinopathy, the onset of which was delayed for seven years after cessation of therapy, has been reported (Ehrenfeld et al., 1986). An early sign of chloroquine retinopathy is blurring of vision.

Quinine amblyopia due to a direct effect on the ganglion cells has been known for a long time and several cases of blindness due to overdosage were reported by Dyson et al. (1985). Blindness occurred within hours of ingestion and characteristically the patients had normal fundi when examined. Some of them had dilated unreactive pupils. One case exhibited cholinergic supersensitivity, like Adie's pupil in which the pupil miosed with 0.125% pilocarpine (Canning and Hague, 1988).

As patients recover, paradoxically the fundal appearance changes to show narrowing of the retinal arterioles and optic atrophy. Iris atrophy can occur (Bernstein, 1977).

Anthelminthics

These compounds are used in the treatment of worm infections which in the UK tend to be fairly minor, and are usually more embarrassing than medically dangerous.

Examples	Mebendazole (Vermox) Piperazine (Antepar, Pripsen)
Ocular adverse effects	With piperazine, cycloplegia and extraocular muscle paralysis can produce visual problems, but these effects are very rare and only occur in overdosage.

Drugs acting on the endocrine system

These are agents which replace or supplement the natural hormones produced by the endocrine system. Included in this section are:

drugs used to treat diabetes
corticosteroids
oral contraceptives.

Drugs used to treat diabetes

The best known agent for treating diabetes is of course insulin, but certain forms can be treated with drugs given by mouth rather than injected – the oral hypoglycaemic agents.

Examples

Glibenclamide (Daonil, Euglucon)
Chlorpropamide (Diabinese)
Tolbutamide (Rastinon)
Metformin (Glucophage)

Ocular adverse effects

Diabetes itself has well known ophthalmic complications and it is important to differentiate any ocular adverse effect of the drug from the problems caused by the condition. Chlorpropamide may produce toxic amblyopia (Davidson, 1971). Overdosage can produce hypoglycaemic attacks, with ocular effects of diplopia and loss of visual acuity.

Corticosteroids

Corticosteroids can be used either physiologically or pharmacologically. In the former manner they are employed for replacement therapy in Addison's disease or after adrenalectomy. For this use, both mineralocorticoid and glucocorticoid activity is required.

The suppression of disease processes such as inflammation is termed pharmacological use, and corticosteroids are used in this manner in the treatment of rheumatoid arthritis, systemic lupus erythematosus, ulcerative colitis, polyarteritis and chronic hepatitis.

Examples

Betamethasone (Betnelan)
Cortisone (Cortelan)
Dexamethasone (Decadron)
Prednisolone (Deltacortril)
Fludrocortisone (Florinef)
Triamcinolone (Ledercort)
Methylprednisolone (Medrone)

Ocular adverse effects

Corticosteroids are notorious for the adverse effects they produce. Systemic use of these agents can result in a cataract which is situated below the posterior capsule and normally occurs after a year's treatment.

It affects up to 30% of patients receiving these agents, especially children. Topical use rarely leads to cataract (David and Berkowitz, 1969).

Topical ophthalmic use of steroids can lead to a rise in intraocular pressure in a percentage of patients (steroid responders). This effect can also occur with systemic use, albeit less frequently and after a greater duration of treatment (David and Berkowitz, 1969; McDonnell and Kerr Muir, 1985). Patients who exhibit this reaction are not necessarily in early glaucoma, although like glaucoma there is a familial tendency for the reaction to occur. The increase is due to a reduction in outflow which itself is thought to be due to an accumulation of insoluble, polymerized, acid mucopolysaccharides (Francois, 1984). Newer corticosteroids have been developed which have less tendency to produce a rise in IOP (Morrison and Archer, 1984).

The list of other reported adverse reactions from steroids is long and they would appear to have the ability to produce any and every effect on the eye.

Oral contraceptives

The contraceptive pill has been in use in the UK for many years and it is now the most common method of birth control. There are a large number of pills available today but they can be divided into just two groups – the combined pills and the progestogen only pills. Many of the unwanted side effects reported following the use of combined pills are from the oestrogen component and the other type is often recommended for individuals who are most at risk from side effects.

Examples

Combined pills

Ethinyloestradiol/norethisterone (Brevinor, Gynovlar)
Ethinyloestradiol/levonorgestrel (Microgynon, Eugynon)

Progestogen only

Norethisterone (Micronor)
Levonorgestrel (Microval)

Ocular adverse effects

The contraceptive pill has been taken by millions of women for several years, and with all this patient experience it is surprising that better cause-effect relationships with ocular effects cannot be established. There have been many publications about the possible incompatibility between the pill and the wearing of contact lenses. Goldberg (1970) reviewed the problems of fitting contact lenses to patients taking the pill and suggested that sometimes there is a difficulty, but his findings are based on 'observation and conjecture'. Chizek and Franceschetti (1969) considered that the signs and symptoms which were reportedly due to the contraceptive pill could be due to overwear, humidity changes and infection. Peturrson et al. (1981) reviewed the evidence for the relationship between contact lens intolerance and oral contraceptives. A prospective study of 517 patients failed to show any difference in contact lens tolerance between patients taking the pill and those who were not. A similar study by Frankel and Ellis (1978) found no significant difference in tear production or tear break up time between women taking oral contraceptives and women who did not. There is some suggestion that the quality and quantity of tears may be adversely affected, especially during the early stages of their use. Davidson (1971) reviewed the reported ocular adverse effects of oral contraceptives. The Committee on Safety of Medicines recorded effects secondary to cerebral vascular and neurological events as well as localized vascular problems and visual disturbances. A very small number of patients reported contact lens intolerance. Faust and Tyler (1966) examined 212 patients taking various pills and considered that no pathology existed which would not normally exist in a healthy random sample. Connell and Kelman (1969), in carrying out a similar study, were surprised at the occurrence of abnormalities in the control group but also found no difference between therapy and control groups.

Anti-inflammatory drugs

These are agents which have been developed as alternatives to steroids for the treatment of conditions such as rheumatoid arthritis, to avoid the undesirable effects of steroids. They produce their effects in a slightly different manner to steroids and are not as potent. They are referred to as the nonsteroidal anti-inflammatory drugs (NSAIDs).

Examples

Diclofenac (Voltarol)
Ibuprofen (Brufen)
Indomethacin (Indocid)
Ketoprofen (Orudis)
Naproxen (Naprosyn)
Sulindac (Clinoril)

Ocular adverse effects

Reduced colour vision and visual acuity have been reported following the use of ibuprofen and indomethacin. Retinopathy (similar to that produced by chloroquine) has been reported following the use of indomethacin (Bernstein, 1977), involving visual field restrictions, depressed EOGs and a granular appearance of the fundus, effects which are transitory as is the diplopia which can also be recorded. Fraunfelder (1980) considered most of the ibuprofen related effects to be unimportant and consistent with 'blurred vision'. Cataract and optic neuritis are serious adverse reactions which have been linked with naproxen, but the actual causal relationship is yet to be established. Benaxaprofen (Opren) has had to be withdrawn because of very serious photoallergic reactions. Optic neuropathy has been reported following the use of this particular compound.

Drugs acting on the blood

Patients with some conditions require regular blood transfusions. As the donated corpuscles are broken down, the iron is stored and iron overload can develop. To remove this excess iron, a compound which will chelate the iron has to be given regularly. This compound is known as desferrioxamine, and when it reacts with iron it changes to ferrioxamine, which can be excreted in the bile and urine.

Examples   Desferrioxamine (Desferal)

Ocular adverse effects   Arden *et al.* (1984) reported minor alterations in the retinal function as
                              evidenced by alterations in the pattern ERG.

References
Arden, G. B., Wonke, B., Kennedy, C. and Huehns, E. R. (1984) Ocular changes in
    patients undergoing long term desferrioxamine treatment. *Br. J. Ophthalmol.*, **68**,
    873–877
Aucamp, A. (1980) Drug excretion in human tears and its meaning for contact lens
    wearers. *Die Suid Afrikaanse Oogkundige*, **39**, 128–136
Bernstein, H. N. (1977) Ocular side effects of drugs. In *Drugs and Ocular Tissues*.
    2nd Meeting of International Society for Eye Research, 1976
Canning, C. R. and Hague, S. (1988) Ocular quinine toxicity. *Br. J. Ophthalmol.*, **72**,
    23–26
Chaplin, S. (1984) Adverse reactions to sympathomimetics in cold remedies.
    Adverse Drug Reaction Bulletins, **No 107**, 369–399
Chizek, D. J. and Franceschetti, A. T. (1969) Oral contraceptives. Their side effects
    and ophthalmological manifestations. *Surv. Ophthalmol.*, **14**, 90–105
Connell, E. B. and Kelman, C. D. (1969) Eye examination in patients taking oral
    contraceptives. *Fertility and Sterility*, **20**, 67–74
David, D. S. and Berkowitz, J. S. (1969) Ocular effects of topical and systemic
    corticosteroids. *Lancet*, **2**, 149–151
Davidson, S. I. (1971) Reported adverse effects of oral contraceptives on the eye.
    Trans. Ophthalmol. Soc. UK, **91**, 561–574
Davidson, S. I. (1980) Drug induced disorders of the eye. *Br. J. Hospital Med.*, 24–28
Davidson, S. I. and Rennie, I. G. (1986) Ocular toxicity from systemic drug therapy.
    Medical Toxicology, **1**, 217–224
Doherty, M., Maddison, P. J. and Grey, R. H. B. (1985) Hydrazaline induced lupus
    syndrome with eye disease. *Br. Med. J.*, **290**, 675
Dyson. E. H., Proudfoot, A. T., Prescott, L. F. and Heyworth, R. (1985) Death and
    blindness due to overdose of quinine. *Br. Med. J.*, **291**, 31–33
Ehrenfeld, M., Nesher, R. and Merin, S. (1986) Delayed onset chloroquine
    retinopathy. *Br. J. Ophthalmol.*, **70**, 281–283
Faust, J. M. and Tyler, E. T. (1966) Ophthalmic findings in patients using oral
    contraceptives. *Fertility and Sterility*, **17**, 1–6
Francois, J. (1984) Corticosteroid glaucoma. *Ophthalmologica*, **188**, 76–81
Frankel, S. H. and Ellis, P. P. (1978) Effect of oral contraceptives on tear production.
    Ann. Ophthalmol., **10**, 1585–1588
Fraunfelder, F. T. (1980) Interim reports. National Registry of possible drug induced
    ocular side effects. *Ophthalmology*, **87**, 87–90
Frucht, J., Freimann, I., and Merin, S. (1984) Ocular side effects of disopyramide.
    Br. J. Ophthalmol., **68**, 890–891
Goldberg, J. B. (1970) A commentary on oral contraceptive therapy and contact lens
    wear. *J. Am. Optom. Assoc.*, **41**, 237–241
Greenberg, L. M., Mauriello, D. A., Cinattia, A. A. and Burton, J. N. (1971)
    Erythema multiforme exudativum (Stevens Johnson syndrome) following
    sodium diphenylhydantoin therapy. *Ann. Ophthalmol.*, **3**, 137–139
Honda, Y., Podos, S. M. and Becker, B. (1973) The effect of diphenylhydantoin on
    the electroretinogram of rabbits. *Invest. Ophthalmol.*, **12**, 567–572
Ingram, D. V. (1986) Spoiled soft contact lenses. *Br. Med. J.*, **292**, 1619
Kofoed, L. L. (1986) OTC drugs: a third of the elderly are at risk. *Ger. Med.*,
    February, 37–42
McDonnell, P. J. and Kerr Muir, M. G. (1985) Glaucoma associated with systemic
    corticosteroid therapy. *Lancet*, **2**, 386–387
Morrison, E. and Archer, D. B. (1984) Effect of fluorometholone (FML) on the
    intraocular pressure of corticosteroid responders. *Br. J. Ophthalmol.*, **168**, 581–584

Petursson, G. J., Fraunfelder, F. T. and Meyer, B. M. (1981) Oral contraceptives. *Ophthalmology*, **88**, 368–371

Sinabulya, P. M. (1977) Chloroquine retinopathy Case report. *E. African J. Ophthalmol.*, **2**, 29–30

Slatter, D. H. and Blogg, J. R. (1978) Keratoconjunctivitis sicca in dogs associated with sulphonamide administration. *Aust. Vet. J.*, **54**, 444–447

Spiteri, M. A. and Geraint James, D. (1983) Adverse ocular reactions to drugs. *Postgrad. Med. J.*, **59**, 343–349

Wright, P. (1978) Effect of drug toxicity on the cornea. *Trans. Ophthalmol. Soc. UK*, **98**, 377–378

Index